Autoimmune Blistering Diseases: Part II – Diagnosis and Management

Guest Editor

DÉDÉE F. MURRELL, MA, BMBCh, FAAD, MD, FACD

DERMATOLOGIC CLINICS

www.derm.theclinics.com

Consulting Editor
BRUCE H. THIERS, MD

October 2011 • Volume 29 • Number 4

SAUNDERS an imprint of ELSEVIER, Inc.

W.B. SAUNDERS COMPANY
A Division of Elsevier Inc.

1600 John F. Kennedy Boulevard ● Suite 1800 ● Philadelphia, PA 19103-2899

http://www.theclinics.com

DERMATOLOGIC CLINICS Volume 29, Number 4
October 2011 ISSN 0733-8635, ISBN-13: 978-1-4557-1034-8

Editor: Stephanie Donley
Developmental Editor: Teia Stone

Dermatologic Clinics (ISSN 0733-8635) is published quarterly by Elsevier Inc., 360 Park Avenue South, New York, NY 10010-1710. Months of publication are January, April, July, and October. Business and editorial offices: 1600 John F. Kennedy Blvd., Suite 1800, Philadelphia, PA 19103-2899. Customer service office: 11830 Westline Drive, St. Louis, MO 63146. Periodicals postage paid at New York, NY, and additional mailing offices. Subscription prices are USD 317.00 per year for US individuals, USD 474.00 per year for US institutions, USD 371.00 per year for Canadian individuals, USD 568.00 per year for Canadian institutions, USD 434.00 per year for international individuals, USD 568.00 per year for international institutions, USD 148.00 per year for US students/residents, and USD 214.00 per year for Canadian and international students/residents. International air speed delivery is included in all *Clinics* subscription prices. All prices are subject to change without notice. **POSTMASTER:** Send address changes to *Dermatologic Clinics*, Elsevier Health Sciences Division, Subscription Customer Service, 3251 Riverport Lane, Maryland Heights, MO 63043. **Customer Service: 1-800-654-2452 (U.S. and Canada); 314-447-8871 (outside U.S. and Canada). Fax: 314-447-8029. E-mail: journalscustomerservice-usa@elsevier.com (for print support); journalsonlinesupport-usa@elsevier.com (for online support).**

Reprints. For copies of 100 or more, of articles in this publication, please contact the Commercial Reprints Department, Elsevier Inc., 360 Park Avenue South, New York, New York 10010-1710. Tel.: (212) 633-3813; Fax: (212) 462-1935; Email: repritns@elsevier.com.

The *Dermatologic Clinics* is covered in *MEDLINE/PubMed (Index Medicus), Current Contents/Clinical Medicine, Excerpta Medica, Chemical Abstracts,* and *ISI/BIOMED.*

Printed and bound by CPI Group (UK) Ltd, Croydon, CR0 4YY

Transferred to Digital Print 2011

Contributors

CONSULTING EDITOR

BRUCE H. THIERS, MD
Professor and Chairman, Department of
Dermatology and Dermatologic Surgery,
Medical University of South Carolina,
Charleston, South Carolina

GUEST EDITOR

**DÉDÉE F. MURRELL, MA, BMBCh,
FAAD, MD, FACD**
Professor and Head, Department of
Dermatology, St George Hospital, University
of New South Wales, Kogarah, Sydney,
New South Wales, Australia

AUTHORS

V. AHLGRIMM-SIESS, MD
Department of Dermatology, Paracelsus
Medical University Salzburg, Salzburg, Austria

MASAYUKI AMAGAI, MD, PhD
Department of Dermatology, Keio University
School of Medicine, Tokyo, Japan

J.W. BAUER, MD
Department of Dermatology, Paracelsus
Medical University Salzburg, Salzburg, Austria

STEFAN BEISSERT, MD
Department of Dermatology, University of
Muenster, Muenster, Germany

LUCA BORRADORI, MD
Department of Dermatology, Inselspital and
University of Bern, Bern, Switzerland

MICHAEL J. CAMILLERI, MD
Assistant Professor, Department of
Dermatology, Mayo Clinic, Rochester,
Minnesota

ADELA RAMBI G. CARDONES, MD
Assistant Professor, Department of
Dermatology, Duke University Medical Center,
Durham, North Carolina

CHEYDA CHAMS-DAVATCHI, MD
Professor, Department of Dermatology,
Autoimmune Bullous Disease Research
Center, Razi Hospital, Tehran University for
Medical Sciences, Tehran, Iran

SHIEN-NING CHEE, MBBS (UNSW)
Department of Dermatology, St George
Hospital, Kogarah; Faculty of Medicine,
University of New South Wales, Kensington,
Sydney, New South Wales, Australia

TIFFANY CLAY, MD
Meharry Medical College, Nashville,
Tennessee

**BENJAMIN S. DANIEL, BA, BCom, MBBS,
MMed (Clin Epi)**
Dermatology Research Fellow, Department
of Dermatology, St George Hospital, Kogarah;
Conjoint Associate Lecturer, Faculty of
Medicine, University of New South Wales,
Sydney, New South Wales, Australia

MICHAEL DAVID, MD
Professor, Department of Dermatology, Rabin
Medical Center, Petah Tiqwa; Department of
Dermatology, Sackler Faculty of Medicine,
Tel Aviv University, Tel Aviv, Israel

ANDREW DERMAWAN
Medical Student, Faculty of Medicine, University of New South Wales; Department of Dermatology, St George Hospital, Kogarah, Sydney, New South Wales, Australia

MARINA ESKIN-SCHWARTZ, MD, PhD
Resident, Department of Dermatology, Rabin Medical Center, Petah Tiqwa; Department of Dermatology, Sackler Faculty of Medicine, Tel Aviv University, Tel Aviv, Israel

AGUSTÍN ESPAÑA, MD
Department of Dermatology, University Clinic of Navarra of School Medicine, University of Navarra, Pamplona, Spain

JOHN W. FREW, MBBS, MMed (Clin Epi)
Resident Medical Officer, St George Hospital, Kogarah; Faculty of Medicine, University of Sydney, Sydney, New South Wales, Australia

RUSSELL P. HALL III, MD
J. Lamar Callaway Professor and Chair, Department of Dermatology, Duke University Medical Center, Durham, North Carolina

JOSEP E. HERRERO-GONZÁLEZ, MD
Department of Dermatology, Hospital del Mar, Parc de Salut Mar, Institut Municipal d'Invetigació Mèdica Passeig Maritim, Barcelona, Spain

HELMUT HINTNER, MD
Department of Dermatology, Paracelsus Medical University Salzburg, Salzburg, Austria

LIZBETH R.A. INTONG, MD, DPDS
Dermatology Fellow, Department of Dermatology, St George Hospital, Kogarah; Associate Lecturer, Faculty of Medicine, University of New South Wales, Sydney, Australia

PILAR IRANZO, MD
Department of Dermatology, Hospital Clínic and Barcelona University Medical School, Barcelona, Spain

PASCAL JOLY, MD, PhD
Professor, Dermatology Department, INSERM U905, Rouen University Hospital, Rouen, France

INES LAKOS JUKIC, MD, MSc
Department of Dermatology and Venereology, University Hospital Centre Zagreb, School of Medicine, University of Zagreb, Zagreb, Croatia

AMER N. KALAAJI, MD
Assistant Professor, Department of Dermatology, Mayo Clinic, Rochester, Minnesota

A. SHADI KOUROSH, MD
Department of Dermatology, University of Texas Southwestern Medical Center in Dallas, Dallas, Texas

LUKAS KRAUS, MD
Department of Dermatology, Paracelsus Medical University Salzburg, Salzburg, Austria

MARTIN LAIMER, MD
Department of Dermatology, Paracelsus Medical University Salzburg, Salzburg, Austria

JULIA S. LEHMAN, MD
Assistant Professor, Department of Dermatology, Mayo Clinic, Rochester, Minnesota

JASNA LIPOZENCIC, MD, PhD
Department of Dermatology and Venereology, University Hospital Centre Zagreb, School of Medicine, University of Zagreb, Zagreb, Croatia

BRANKA MARINOVIC, MD, PhD
Department of Dermatology and Venereology, University Hospital Centre Zagreb, School of Medicine, University of Zagreb, Zagreb, Croatia

LINDA K. MARTIN, MBBS, MMed (Clin Epi)
Dermatology Registrar, St John's Institute of Dermatology, St Thomas' Hospital, London, England, United Kingdom

JOSÉ M. MASCARÓ Jr, MD
Department of Dermatology, Hospital Clínic and Barcelona University Medical School, Barcelona, Spain

TESS MCPHERSON, MD, MRCP
Clinical Lecturer of Dermatology, Department of Dermatology, Churchill Hospital, Oxford, United Kingdom

NICOLAS MEYER, MD
Dermatologist, UMR 1037-CRCT; Dermatology Department, Larrey Hospital, Toulouse, France

VOLKER MEYER, MD
Department of Dermatology, University of Muenster, Muenster, Germany

DANIEL MIMOUNI, MD
Professor, Department of Dermatology, Rabin
Medical Center, Petah Tiqwa; Department of
Dermatology, Sackler Faculty of Medicine,
Tel Aviv University, Tel Aviv, Israel

EMILY M. MINTZ, MD
Dermatology Resident, Department
of Dermatology, Columbia University,
New York, New York

KIMBERLY D. MOREL, MD, FAAD, FAAP
Associate Professor of Clinical Dermatology
and Clinical Pediatrics, Department of
Dermatology, Columbia University, New York,
New York

**DÉDÉE F. MURRELL, MA, BMBCh,
FAAD, MD, FACD**
Professor and Head, Department of
Dermatology, St George Hospital, University
of New South Wales, Kogarah, Sydney,
New South Wales, Australia

SUE YIN NG, MBBS, BSc, MRCP (UK)
Dermatology Registrar, Department of
Dermatology, Churchill Hospital, Oxford,
United Kingdom

ELKE NISCHLER, MD
Department of Dermatology, Paracelsus
Medical University Salzburg, Salzburg, Austria

AMIT G. PANDYA, MD
Professor, Department of Dermatology,
University of Texas Southwestern Medical
Center, Dallas, Texas

CARLE PAUL, MD, PhD
Professor, Paul Sabatier-Toulouse III
University; Dermatology Department, Larrey
Hospital, Toulouse, France

EVAN W. PIETTE, MD
Department of Dermatology, University of
Pennsylvania, Philadelphia, Pennsylvania

GABRIELA POHLA-GUBO, PhD
Department of Dermatology, Paracelsus
Medical University Salzburg, Salzburg, Austria

ENNO SCHMIDT, MD, PhD
Department of Dermatology; Comprehensive
Center for Inflammation Medicine, University of
Lübeck, Lübeck, Germany

DESHAN F. SEBARATNAM, MBBS (Hons)
Research Student, Department of
Dermatology, St George Hospital, Sydney,
New South Wales, Australia

JANET SEGALL, BA
International Pemphigus Pemphigoid
Foundation, Sacramento, California

DAVID SIROIS, MD, PhD
Department of Dentistry, New York University,
New York, New York

MOLLY STUART, JD
International Pemphigus Pemphigoid
Foundation, Sacramento, California

RICARDO SUÁREZ, MD
Department of Dermatology, Hospital
General Universitario Gregorio Marañón,
Madrid, Spain

AKIKO TANIKAWA, MD, PhD
Department of Dermatology, Keio University
School of Medicine, Tokyo, Japan

VANESSA V. VENNING, BMBCh, DM, FRCP
Consultant Dermatologist and
Honorary Senior Lecturer, Department
of Dermatology, Churchill Hospital,
Oxford, United Kingdom

VICTORIA P. WERTH, MD
Chief, Division of Dermatology,
Philadelphia Veterans Affairs Medical
Center; Professor, Department of
Dermatology, University of Pennsylvania,
Philadelphia, Pennsylvania

KIM B. YANCEY, MD
Department of Dermatology, University of
Texas Southwestern Medical Center in Dallas,
Dallas, Texas

DETLEF ZILLIKENS, MD
Department of Dermatology, University of
Lübeck, Lübeck, Germany

WILL ZRNCHIK, MBA
International Pemphigus Pemphigoid
Foundation, Sacramento, California

Contents

Corticosteroid Use in Autoimmune Blistering Diseases   535

John W. Frew and Dédée F. Murrell

Corticosteroids, while providing rapid remission and ongoing control of symptoms of autoimmune blistering diseases (AIBD), have numerous potentially serious acute and long-term side effects. Evidence-based medicine has reevaluated the various types of corticosteroids and forms of corticosteroid delivery in AIBD to ascertain whether any advantages of specific delivery systems or regimens exist. Careful monitoring of patients and simple preventive measures are effective in minimizing the adverse outcomes associated with their use. This article outlines the current level of evidence for corticosteroid use in AIBDs, and discusses appropriate investigations and interventions to minimize or prevent the associated adverse effects.

Azathioprine in the Treatment of Autoimmune Blistering Diseases   545

Volker Meyer and Stefan Beissert

Although there are no standard guidelines for the treatment of autoimmune blistering diseases, azathioprine has shown good efficacy in acquired autoimmune blistering diseases, and is well tolerated. Side effects of azathioprine normally occur in mild variants. Severe reactions are due to reduced thiopurine *S*-methyltransferase (TPMT) or inosine triphosphate pyrophosphohydrolase (ITPA) activity. Therefore, screening for TPMT activity should be conducted in white patients and Africans, whereas Japanese should be screened for ITPA activity before therapy with azathioprine is started. Azathioprine is clinically meaningful for the treatment of pemphigus.

Mycophenolate Mofetil for the Management of Autoimmune Bullous Diseases   555

Marina Eskin-Schwartz, Michael David, and Daniel Mimouni

Immunosuppressive agents such as azathioprine, cyclophosphamide, and mycophenolate mofetil (MMF) are now widely used in the treatment of autoimmune bullous diseases. This article reviews the use of MMF for the treatment of several bullous conditions, and assesses the evidence gathered from clinical trials and case series. According to numerous case series, MMF could be of value in treating refractory disease. The few randomized clinical trials conducted to date of patients with pemphigus and bullous pemphigoid report a similar efficacy for MMF to other immunosuppressants.

Dapsone in the Management of Autoimmune Bullous Diseases   561

Evan W. Piette and Victoria P. Werth

Dapsone is used in the treatment of autoimmune bullous diseases (AIBD), a group of disorders resulting from autoimmunity directed against basement membrane and/or intercellular adhesion molecules on cutaneous and mucosal surfaces. This review summarizes the limited published data evaluating dapsone as a therapy for AIBD.

Intravenous immunoglobulin (IVIG) has been shown to be effective in the treatment of autoimmune blistering diseases and may be an option if disease is refractory to conventional treatment. IVIG effectiveness appears to increase when administered concurrently with a cytotoxic drug and used in multiple treatment cycles (though a single cycle may give benefit). Tapering administration may improve the duration of remission and subcutaneous injections may be an option. This article provides an introduction to the make-up and use of IVIG, and reviews previous studies.

Rituximab is a chimeric, murine-human, monoclonal antibody against the CD20 antigen of B lymphocytes. It has been used off-label to treat and manage autoimmune and dermatologic diseases as an alternative or adjuvant therapy to systemic treatments. Due to cost, potential complications, and lack of data rituximab is used after standard systemic therapies have failed or the patient is absolutely contraindicated for corticosteroids. More research is required.

Autoimmune blistering diseases (AIBD) often require high-dose corticosteroids and immunosuppressive agents for adequate control. These diseases cause significant morbidity but treatment can also lead to side effects and complications. This article reviews the supportive management of AIBD and the management of corticosteroid-induced side effects. The prevention and management of secondary effects from some of the more commonly used steroid-sparing agents for AIBD are summarized. Clinicians must be familiar with this information to optimally manage patients with AIBD.

Autoimmune blistering disease (AIBD) in pregnancy raises several complex management issues associated with underlying pathogenesis and treatment options. This article considers the effects of the disease as well as its treatment for both mother and fetus. All AIBDs can occur in pregnancy but are relatively rare. Pemphigoid gestationis is a rare AIBD that is specific to pregnancy. The article considers each AIBD in turn and then looks at treatment options for the group as a whole, as there are many issues common to all.

Infection contributes to considerable morbidity and mortality in patients treated for autoimmune bullous disorders because of the impaired cutaneous barrier, alteration of the protective normal flora, and host immunosuppression (inherent and iatrogenic). Prevention of cutaneous impetiginization and infection starts with excellent wound care. In patients to be started on immunosuppressive medications, consideration should be given to vaccination status and possible need for pneumocystis pneumonia prevention. Patients should be educated on the signs and symptoms of early infection and the need to seek early medical intervention as needed.

before remitting. It typically presents with papulovesicles and blisters configured in an arcuate pattern on an urticated base, with 2 peaks of onset. The first peak is in young prepubescent children, called chronic bullous disease of childhood, and the second peak affects patients older than 60 years of age. In this article, the management of linear IgA in adults is considered.

dermatologists and other specialists in their area who are experts in autoimmune bullous disease. The IPPF hosts the largest worldwide registry of pemphigus/pemphigoid patients with biospecimen collection opportunities are planned. Twice a year the IPPF hosts formal meetings with invited speakers.

Dermatologic Clinics

THE CLINICS ARE NOW AVAILABLE ONLINE!

Access your subscription at:
www.theclinics.com

Preface

Autoimmune Blistering Diseases Part II—Diagnosis and Management

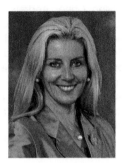

Dédée F. Murrell, MA, BMBCh, FAAD, MD, FACD
Guest Editor

When invited to edit a special issue of *Dermatologic Clinics* on Autoimmune Blistering Diseases by Bruce Thiers, I was delighted and honored to accept. I had just finished editing two issues on the genetic blistering disease, Epidermolysis Bullosa, for *Dermatologic Clinics* and found that the scientific and dermatologic community were keen to contribute to these theme-based issues. There have been a few excellent textbooks devoted to autoimmune blistering diseases (AIBD), with some focusing on the pathology and others on management, but the field is advancing rapidly. There was so much to cover about AIBD that it was decided to cover clinical features, diagnostic testing, and pathogenesis in the first issue and follow it with this issue on management.

Unlike a textbook, where the articles may be over a year or two out of date by the time the book is published, these articles have been written in the last 6 months and by respected leaders in the particular aspects of AIBD. The issue has been organized such that the drugs that are commonly used to treat AIBD are discussed in detail first by dermatologists familiar in their use for AIBD, including Stefan Beissert on azathioprine, Daniel Mimouni on mycophenolate mofetil, Vicky Werth on dapsone, and Pascal Joly on rituximab. This is followed by specific sections on the complications that can result from these treatments and how to manage them, overall by Amit Pandya and specifically on preventing infections

by Julia Lehman, Michael Camilleri, and Amer Kalaaji. There is a special article devoted to issues of management of AIBD in pregnancy by Tess McPherson and Vanessa Venning. This is important because the major morbidity and mortality these patients have (apart from risk of blindness in mucous membrane pemphigoid) stem from the treatments themselves. It is not merely a matter of writing a prescription for oral steroids without considering what can be done from baseline to reduce the risks of significant side effects from corticosteroids.

Subsequently, a leading AIBD clinician or team has written about the practical aspects of treating each AIBD, including pemphigus vulgaris and foliaceus, paraneoplastic pemphigus, bullous pemphigoid, mucous membrane pemphigoid, pemphigoid gestationes, linear IgA disease, epidermolysis bullosa acquisita, bullous lupus, and dermatitis herpetiformis. These leaders include Luca Borradori, Russell Hall, Pascal Joly, Sarolta Karpati, Vanessa Venning, and Kim Yancey.

As AIBD are relatively rare skin diseases, it has been difficult to perform randomized controlled trials with sufficient power to demonstrate a statistically significant difference between treatments. To address this, an international group of AIBD experts has developed consensus definitions of the stages in the management of the AIBD and severity scoring systems which have been validated, so that even small clinical trials as well as

Dermatol Clin 29 (2011) xv–xvi
doi:10.1016/j.det.2011.07.005

larger ones can be combined using meta-analysis to determine significance. If we all use the same language and outcome measures in our case reports and case series on AIBD, we will be better able to compare the severity of AIBD patients and their responses to treatment. There are articles detailing the outcome measures of disease extent that have been validated so far as well as studies on quality of life.

Last, we have a section about the services and management of AIBD in various countries and the patient support group, the International Pemphigus and Pemphigoid Foundation. The countries where I could recruit experts willing and able to write about this include Australia, Austria (Martin Laimer, Gabi Pohla-Gubo, Johann Bauer, Helmut Hintner, and colleagues), Croatia (Branka Marinovich and Jasna Lipozencic), France (Nicolas Meyer, Carle Paul, and Pascal Joly), Germany (Enno Schmidt and Detlef Zillikens), Iran (Cheyda Chams Davatchi), Japan (Masa Amagai), and Spain (Ricardo Suárez, Agustín España, and José Mascaró Jr).

Unlike a textbook, these articles can be found on Medline and PubMed and are accessible online. The individual issues of the journal may be purchased for much less cost than either buying a textbook or the articles individually.

The contributors deserve many thanks for their time and effort in writing these articles at relatively short notice and in a succinct manner with excellent color photographs and figures. Inevitably, there are topics and experts whose contributions I would have liked to include but it is difficult for busy clinicians to find extra time to write these articles. On that note, I would particularly like to acknowledge and thank my current and former fellows, Benjamin Daniel, Lizbeth Intong, Linda Martin, and Supriya Venugopal, as well as my former research medical students, Shien-Ning Chee, Andrew Dermawan, John Frew, and Deshan Sebaratnam, who have all been doing projects on AIBD and who have written many of these articles with me. It is good for patients with AIBD if more young dermatologists take an interest in their condition.

Hopefully these two issues will be educational not only for dermatologists but also for all clinicians who interact with patients with AIBD, as well as scientists, family members, and the patients themselves. Understanding what is known so far about a disease leads to improved clinical practice, better research, and improved compliance with therapy.

Dédée F. Murrell, MA, BMBCh, FAAD, MD, FACD
Department of Dermatology
St George Hospital
University of New South Wales
Kogarah, Sydney, NSW 2217, Australia

E-mail address:
d.murrell@unsw.edu.au

Corticosteroid Use in Autoimmune Blistering Diseases

John W. Frew, MBBS, MMed (Clin Epi)[a,b],
Dédée F. Murrell, MA, BMBCh, FAAD, MD, FACD[c],*

KEYWORDS

- Pemphigus • Pemphigoid • Linear IgA dermatosis
- Autoimmune blistering diseases • Corticosteroids

Corticosteroids have been used in the management of autoimmune blistering diseases (AIBD) for more than 50 years, and are an essential component in the pharmacologic management of these conditions. While providing rapid remission and ongoing control of the symptoms of AIBD, they come with a variety of potentially serious acute and long-term side effects. The advent of immunomodulating and immunosuppressive therapies has complemented the use of corticosteroids but have not usurped its pivotal role. The advent of evidence-based medicine (EBM) has reevaluated the various types of corticosteroids and forms of corticosteroid delivery in AIBD to ascertain whether any advantages of specific delivery systems or regimens exist. With rare diseases such as those that comprise AIBD, large randomized controlled trials are difficult to coordinate and accomplish, meaning a paucity of high-level evidence exists as to the best methods of corticosteroid use in these conditions. Experience and evidence from cross-discipline use of corticosteroids shows that careful monitoring of patients and simple preventive measures are effective in minimizing the adverse outcomes associated with their use. This article attempts to outline the current level of evidence for corticosteroid use in a variety of AIBDs, and discusses appropriate investigations and interventions to minimize or prevent the associated adverse effects.

PHARMACOLOGY OF CORTICOSTEROIDS

Corticosteroids are based around the cyclopentanopenanthrane nucleus, a conjoined series of three 6-carbon rings and one 5-carbon ring, a base structure shared by cholesterol and sex hormones.[1] All corticosteroids exhibit a double bond between carbon atoms 4 and 5, as well as two ketone groups, attached to carbon atoms 3 and 20, which distinguish them from other cholesterol-based compounds. Different corticosteroids differ by their differing functional groups attached to the core ring structure as well as the oxidation state of the carbon atoms comprising the rings. General additions that increase corticosteroid potency include the insertion of a double bond between carbon atoms 1 and 2 (as in prednisone); the fluorination of carbon atoms 6 or 9 (as in clobetasol or dexamethasone); and the addition of a hydroxyl group at carbon atom 11 (as in clobetasol).[1]

Corticosteroids act through binding to glucocorticoid-specific receptors and altering transcription factors as well as diffusing through the cell membrane and acting directly on the cell nucleus.[2] Inflammatory inhibition is mainly achieved through the interaction with and inhibition of nuclear factor κB transcription factor, suppressing the production of chemokines and cytokines. Suppressed mediators include cyclooxygenases (COX), interleukins (IL) 1 through 6, tumor necrosis

[a] St George Hospital, Kogarah, Sydney, NSW 2217, Australia
[b] Faculty of Medicine, University of Sydney, Sydney, NSW 2006, Australia
[c] Department of Dermatology, St George Hospital, University of New South Wales, Gray Street, Kogarah, Sydney, NSW 2217, Australia
* Corresponding author.
E-mail address: d.murrell@unsw.edu.au

Dermatol Clin 29 (2011) 535–544
doi:10.1016/j.det.2011.06.004
0733-8635/11/$ – see front matter © 2011 Elsevier Inc. All rights reserved.

derm.theclinics.com

factor (TNF)-α, and macrophage colony stimulating factor. Although all of the exact mechanisms controlling the plethora of side effects of corticosteroids have not yet been elucidated, it is believed the majority of them are controlled through cyclic adenosine monophosphate–mediated pathways.[2] The end result is cytokine suppression, eosinopenia, lymphopenia, and monocytopenia. Neutrophilia is also observed. However, this is thought to be indirectly attributable to the decreased ability of neutrophils to migrate to the sites of inflammation due to cytokine suppression; neutrophil apoptosis is delayed as a result, contributing further to neutrophilia.[2]

Regarding the pharmacokinetics of corticosteroids, when prednisone is consumed orally it must be reduced enzymatically in the liver to prednisolone (the active product); this is done through reduction of a ketone group by the enzyme 11β-hydroxysteroidiesterase. Consequently, patients with hepatic dysfunction may have impaired conversion of prednisone to active prednisolone.[3] In these circumstances, administration of prednisolone would be more beneficial than prednisone in achieving the desired serum concentrations necessary for treatment. In patients with otherwise normal hepatic function, prednisone and prednisolone are drugs of equivalency. A table of steroid equivalencies for those drugs used in AIBDs is presented in **Table 1**.[1–4] With regard to conversion rates, serum concentrations for systemic steroids are roughly consistent. Measurements of equivalency for topical steroids have a much wider range than systemic steroids because, dependent on the site of measurement in the skin of the active ingredient, concentrations differ.[3] The measurements presented in **Table 1** are taken from studies wherein concentrations were measured in the dermis or at the dermoepidermal junction—the site of activity of disease and immune suppression. Consequently, concentrations in the epidermis would be much higher for topical steroids.

RESPONSIVENESS OF AIBD TO CORTICOSTEROIDS
Pemphigus Vulgaris/Pemphigus Foliaceus

Steroids have been used as the cornerstone of pemphigus management for more than 50 years.[5] The different types of corticosteroids used in pemphigus include oral prednisone/prednisolone as a continuous dosage for remission or maintenance therapy, and dexamethasone as used in oral pulsed dosage for remission and topical application for local or mucosal disease.[6] **Table 2** presents the current recommendations and levels of evidence available for corticosteroid use in AIBD.

A recent systematic review and meta-analysis[5] examined a randomized controlled trial (RCT) of 22 participants comparing low-dose (45–60 mg/d) with high-dose (120–180 mg/d) oral prednisolone in a cohort of newly diagnosed pemphigus vulgaris (PV) and pemphigus foliaceus (PF) patients.[7] Although the low number of participants made the study underpowered, no significant difference in the time to disease control was demonstrated.[7] All patients achieved remission in a time ranging from 5 to 42 days for the high-dose steroids and 7 to 42 days for the low-dose steroids. Rates of remission as recorded over a 5-year period were also not statistically significant ($P = .30$).[7]

Regarding pulsed corticosteroid use, an RCT of 22 participants[8] compared the efficacy of adjuvant pulsed oral dexamethasone (300 mg/d for 3 consecutive days, monthly) versus placebo in newly diagnosed patients concurrently treated with prednisolone and azathioprine. Although the small number of patients in the cohort contributed to the poor power of the study, no significant differences in the rates of remission or relapse were identified. Of importance, the rates of adverse outcomes or side effects were significantly higher among the pulsed-corticosteroid cohort when compared with the continuous-dosage cohort ($P<.01$).[8] It must be noted, however, that the patients enrolled in this particular study did not have severe or refractory disease, and that pulsed corticosteroids may have a useful role in those particular subgroups of patients.[6] At present no double-blinded placebo-controlled RCTs are available that evaluate pulsed corticosteroids in severe or refractory pemphigus, so the evidence supporting this stems from expert recommendation.[6] As the power of the study by Mentink and colleagues[8] was low, there is no evidence supporting the use of one intervention (dexamethasone or the control regimen) over the other. The study also commented that pulsed dexamethasone was associated with higher rates of corticosteroid-associated adverse effects.[8] These findings again highlight the importance of a dynamic corticosteroid regimen individualized for each patient depending on their individual disease severity, treatment response, and degree of adverse effects from therapy.

Topical corticosteroid use in PV and PF has been documented in several case reports,[9,10] and expert recommendations state that it may be useful in localized or mild disease.[6] No controlled trials exist to formally evaluate its efficacy, but strong corticosteroids such as betamethasone or clobetasol are typically used. For mucosal lesions, topical clobetasol propionate is typically used in mild disease, although mostly as an adjunct to systemic treatment.[6,11]

Table 1
Equivalence table of different forms of corticosteroids used in AIBDs

Steroid Used		Converting To:					
		Prednisone/ Prednisolone[a]	Oral Dexamethasone	Intravenous Dexamethasone	Intravenous Hydrocortisone	Topical Betamethasone Valerate (0.1%)[b]	Topical Clobetasol Propionate (0.05%)[b]
Converting from:	Prednisone/ prednisolone[a]	Multiply by 1 mg/kg/d	Multiply by 0.12 mg/kg/d	Multiply by 0.196 mg/kg/d	Multiply by 16 mg/kg/d	Multiply by 0.48 mg/kg/d	Multiply by 360 mg/kg/d
	Oral dexamethasone	Divide by 0.12 mg/kg/d	Multiply by 1 mg/kg/d	Multiply by 0.61 mg/kg/d	Multiply by 133 mg/kg/d		
	Intravenous dexamethasone	Divide by 0.196 mg/kg/d	Divide by 0.61 mg/kg/d	Multiply by 1 mg/kg/d			
	Intravenous hydrocortisone	Divide by 16 mg/kg/d	Divide by 133.3 mg/kg/d		Multiply by 1 mg/kg/d		
	Topical betamethasone valerate (0.1%)[b]	Divide by 0.48 mg/kg/d				Multiply by 1 mg/kg/d	
	Topical clobetasol propionate (0.05%)[b]	Divide by 360 mg/kg/d					Multiply by 1 mg/kg/d

[a] Prednisone and prednisolone are assumed to be equivalent.
[b] Equivalence based on dermal concentrations.
Data from Refs.[1–4]

Table 2
Recommendations and level of evidence for corticosteroid use in autoimmune blistering diseases

Type of Corticosteroid	Recommendations and Level of Evidence				
	Pemphigus	Bullous Pemphigoid	Mucous Membrane Pemphigoid	Linear IgA Dermatoses	Epidermolysis Bullosa Acquisita
Prednisone/ prednisolone (oral)	A (2–3) Basic pillar of therapy. Optimal regimen (high dose vs low dose) unknown with current evidence	C (1) Can be used if topical unfeasible (evidence of deleterious effect compared with topicals in severe disease)	C (3)	I (3)	C (3) Associated with increased mortality and adverse effects
Dexamethasone (intravenous pulsed)	C (2–2) No evidence supporting its use over oral corticosteroids. Experts recommend use in recalcitrant disease	N/A	N/A	N/A	C (3) Use in intractable or severe disease
Dexamethasone (Mouthwash)	N/A	N/A	B (3)	N/A	N/A
Clobetasol propionate (0.05%)	C (3) Localized or mild disease	A (1) Recommended for severe disease over systemic corticosteroids based on 12-mo mortality rates	C (3)	I (3)	N/A
Betamethasone (topical)	C (3)	N/A	I (3)	I (3)	N/A

Key to Recommendations and Level of Evidence

Recommendations:

Level A: Good scientific evidence suggests that the benefits of the clinical service substantially outweigh the potential risks

Level B: At least fair scientific evidence suggests that the benefits of the clinical service outweigh the potential risks

Level C: At least fair scientific evidence suggests that there are benefits provided by the clinical service, but the balance between benefits and risks are too close for making general recommendations

Level D: At least fair scientific evidence suggests that the risks of the clinical service outweigh potential benefits

Level I: Scientific evidence is lacking, of poor quality, or conflicting, such that the risk-versus-benefit balance cannot be assessed

Levels of Evidence:

Level 1: Evidence obtained from at least one properly designed randomized controlled trial

Level 2-1: Evidence obtained from well-designed controlled trials without randomization

Level 2-2: Evidence obtained from well-designed cohort or case-control analytical studies, preferably from more than one center or research group

Level 2-3: Evidence obtained from multiple time series with or without the intervention. Dramatic results in uncontrolled trials might also be regarded as this type of evidence

Level 3: Opinions of respected authorities, based on clinical experience, descriptive studies, or reports of expert committees

Abbreviation: N/A, data not available.

Bullous Pemphigoid

Corticosteroids, both oral and topical, are used widely in the management of bullous pemphigoid (BP), with topical preparations of high-potency steroids (such as clobetasol propionate) being used for mild to moderate disease and systemic corticosteroids used for more severe disease.[12] As BP is a disease of the elderly, mortality of those diagnosed with BP is relatively high, and despite the introduction of corticosteroids and other immunosuppressive and immunomodulating agents has not improved since the 1950s.[12,13] Debate is ongoing as to whether this is indicative of the underlying comorbidities inherent in the patient population and if the role of treatment actually improves mortality rates. Recent research by Parker and MacKelfresh[13] indicates that as the natural history of the disease is usually self limiting and the majority of patients succumb to causes unrelated to their BP, adverse effects primarily from systemic corticosteroids may actually increase the risk of mortality.[13]

A recent Cochrane systematic review and meta-analysis[12] examined an RCT of 26 participants comparing high-dose (1.25 mg/kg) and low-dose (0.75 mg/kg) oral prednisolone in patients with newly diagnosed BP.[14] Fifty-one percent of patients in the low-dose cohort patients achieved remission by day 21 compared with 64% of high-dose cohort patients. Power was limited by the small sample size of the study, and no significant difference between time to remission or overall mortality was revealed. A second study comparing oral prednisolone with methylprednisolone comprised 57 participants, monitored for 10 days. No significant difference in rates of remission or decrease in the number of bullous lesions was seen between the two treatment groups.[15] Self-reported pruritus scores were found to be significantly more improved in the methylprednisolone cohort than in the prednisolone cohort.[15] Examination of the methodology of the study shows that randomization and blinding were adequate, although the degree of allocation concealment is questionable, thus querying the reliability of this result.

The 2002 RCT by Joly and colleagues[16] comparing topical clobetasol propionate (0.05%) with oral prednisone demonstrated a significant advantage of topical clobetasol propionate (0.05%, 40 g/d) over oral prednisone (1 mg/kg/d) in individuals with severe BP (defined as more than 10 new blisters per day) in regard of overall mortality within 1 year of initiation of treatment. The significance of this finding increased when multiple regression analysis took into account age and functional status. Of importance, this study[16] also had adequate power to detect a decrease in the 1-year mortality rate in both severe and moderate disease groups. This result lends credence to the suggestion that in severe BP, systemic corticosteroids may have a deleterious effect on mortality rates when compared with topical high-potency corticosteroids. A follow-on study with 309 participants[17] found that lower doses of clobetasol propionate (0.05%, 10–30 g/d) had noninferior mortality rates than the standard regimen of 40 g/d in both severe and moderate disease. When adjusted for age and functional status, the investigators concluded that the lower doses were more beneficial to patients with both moderate and severe disease, with lower rates of mortality or life-threatening adverse effects (including sepsis and diabetes mellitus) than the original 2002 study.[12,17] Although the evidence may suggest that twice-daily topical corticosteroids more beneficial than oral dosing, the practicalities of application by elderly patients with multiple comorbidities is a significant barrier to the implementation of these recommendations.

Mucous Membrane Pemphigoid

Therapies for AIBD that involve mucous membranes are targeted at topical applications as well as the consideration of systemic corticosteroids in severe disease.

There is a paucity of evidence from RCTs regarding treatments for mucous membrane pemphigoid (MMP), cicatricial pemphigoid (CP), and other subtypes of AIBD that contain mucous membrane involvement. Expert recommendations cite topical therapies such as clobetasol propionate, betamethasone valerate, and dexamethasone mouthwashes.[18,19] A Cochrane review confirmed that the only RCT evidence related to MMP regarded the treatment of ocular involvement with dapsone or cyclophosphamide, dependent on disease severity.[19] There were no RCTs of steroid use in either MMP or epidermolysis bullosa acquisita (EBA). Furthermore, to date no reliable evidence sources (such as RCTs) have been found to further elucidate the efficacy of these topical treatments in these conditions.

Linear IgA Disease

Steroid use in linear IgA disease can be separated into topical and systemic regimens. While potent topical steroids such as clobetasol propionate 0.05% has been recommended for mild disease, it can also have a role in symptom control while the offending stimulant is removed in drug-induced disease.[20] No RCTs have been identified to date regarding the efficacy of corticosteroids in linear IgA disease, and expert recommendation quotes dapsone as a first-line agent,[20,21] with other immunosuppressive and immunomodulating agents such as mycophenolate mofetil (MMF) also having reports of successful treatment.[20] In this regard, systemic corticosteroids are only considered a useful adjunctive treatment in the setting of other therapies, and to this end evidence of its usefulness is lacking.

Epidermolysis Bullosa Acquisita

EBA is a recalcitrant AIBD in which treatment is known to be difficult. A recent Cochrane review found no RCTs of treatment modalities in EBA, although a handful of nonrandomized studies were found involving a wide variety of immunosuppressive and immunomodulating therapies.[22,23] Due to the adverse outcomes of the high-dose steroids needed to successfully control EBA, other management strategies such as intravenous immunoglobulins (IVIG) and anti-CD20 monoclonal antibodies (rituximab) have come to the fore as the mainstay of treatment in EBA.[22] While prednisone/prednisolone, 0.5 to 1.0 mg/kg/d is still included in the initial treatment regimen for EBA, recalcitrant or severe disease management concentrates on other immunomodulating therapies such as cyclosporine, plasmapheresis, and colchicine for maintenance therapy. Ishii and colleagues[23] state that pulsed corticosteroids may also be useful in severe disease, although these recommendations have not been borne out in randomized trials. Again, the rarity of the conditions comprising AIBD makes such evidence difficult to compile.

Pemphigoid Gestationis

Although there are no RCTs available assessing the effect of corticosteroids in this condition, as prednisone is relatively safe during the later stages of pregnancy and during breastfeeding as compared with many other systemic immunosuppressants, oral corticosteroids such as prednisone tend to be used.[24]

MINIMIZING THE ADVERSE EFFECTS OF CORTICOSTEROID USE

The side effects or adverse outcomes of corticosteroid use are both acute and chronic.

As outlined in **Table 3**, the adverse effects of corticosteroids range from weight gain and insulin resistance to acute psychopathology. Prevention strategies, ongoing management, and appropriate treatment of adverse effects that do arise are essential aspects of patient care in individuals with AIBD on systemic as well as widespread potent topical corticosteroids.[2] Evidence from studies in pemphigus have suggested that cumulative corticosteroid dose has a significant influence over the rate of adverse effects, again emphasizing the need for titration of steroid use according to individual patient responses.[2]

Metabolic Effects

The most common metabolic effects of corticosteroids include an increase of appetite and salt retention, leading to an increase in eating and drinking with consequent weight gain, hyperglycemia, and insulin resistance, along with hyperlipidemia. Baseline lipids (cholesterol, triglycerides, high-density lipoprotein, low-density lipoprotein, liver function tests) are advised prior to long-term glucocorticoids, with regular monitoring every 4 to 6 weeks, particularly when in combination with hepatotoxic drugs such as methotrexate.[2] Monitoring of weight and blood glucose should also be undertaken alongside lipids, especially in patients with preexisting diabetes or insulin resistance, as well as monitoring for hypertension. The effect of corticosteroids on blood glucose and lipids takes weeks to occur after starting therapy and a similar timeframe to return to normal after cessation of therapy.[2]

Musculoskeletal Effects

One of the most common long-term effects of corticosteroid use is steroid-induced osteoporosis. With the greatest rate of bone mineral density loss occurring in the first 12 months of corticosteroid therapy, assessment and therapy before initiation of therapy or as soon as possible after initiation of therapy is vital.[25–27] Baseline bone mineral density (BMD) testing, along with serum calcium, magnesium, and vitamin D levels are necessary. The test considered most beneficial for BMD is dual x-ray absorption spectrometry (DEXA), due to a combination of its low radiation levels and reproducibility.[25,26] Yearly BMD testing along with ensuring adequate supplementation of calcium (recommended 1500 mg/d) and vitamin D (recommended 800 IU/d) can help minimize osteoporosis.[25,26] Other prophylactic pharmacologic therapies include bisphosphonates such as alendronate and risendronate.[27,28] Rheumatologic guidelines recommend administration of bisphosphonates to all men and postmenopausal women on long-term corticosteroid therapy of greater than 5 mg prednisone per day.[26] Nonpharmacologic methods aimed at maintaining bone mineral density in the setting of long-term

Table 3
Adverse outcomes from corticosteroid use in AIBDs and relevant strategies to prevent and alleviate effects

Adverse Effect	Timeframe of Onset	Prevention Strategies	Treatment Strategies
Weight gain	Weeks to months	Dose minimization	Dose minimization Diuretic therapy
Hyperglycemia/insulin resistance	Weeks	Dose minimization	Endocrinology review Hypoglycemic therapy, insulin therapy
Osteoporosis	Years	Dose minimization Calcium and vitamin D supplementation Bisphosphonates	Calcium and vitamin D supplementation Bisphosphonates Acute management of fracture events
Osteonecrosis	Years	Dose minimization	
Myopathy	Weeks to years	Dose minimization Exercise, physiotherapy	Dose minimization Exercise, physiotherapy
Cataracts	Months	Dose minimization	Ophthalmology review Cataract removal
Glaucoma	Days to weeks	Dose minimization	Ophthalmology review
Psychopathology (Ranging from anxiety to acute psychosis)	Days-Weeks	Dose minimization	Neuropsychiatric review Antipsychotic medications
Hyperlipidemia	Weeks	Dose minimization Dietary modifications	Dietary modifications Statin therapy
Hypertension	Weeks	Dose minimization Dietary modifications (low sodium)	Dietary modifications (low sodium)
Infection/sepsis	Weeks	Dose minimization Prophylactic antibiotics Prophylactic antifungals Prophylactic antivirals	Acute medical management (intravenous antibiotics and supportive care)
Nausea/reflux	Days	Dose minimization Prophylactic proton pump inhibitors	Proton pump inhibitors Histamine-2 receptor antagonists

Data from Refs.[2,25–35]

corticosteroid use include a low sodium diet (to help prevent calcium loss from the renal tubules) and minimizing caffeine and alcohol intake.[25,26] Muscle atrophy and weakness is a delayed complication of systemic steroids, with little that can be done to prevent it; gentle exercise can help to keep the muscles as strong as possible.

Neuropsychiatric Effects

Central nervous system effects of high-dose corticosteroids can include disturbing psychiatric symptoms, which can have rapid onset of several days after initiation of therapy. Affective disturbances including depression and hypomania can be seen at moderate doses, but psychosis and mania are almost exclusively seen at doses above 20 mg/d.[29] One retrospective analysis in patients with multiple sclerosis taking steroids was able to identify individuals at risk by previous episodes of major depression prior to the onset of disease.[29] Factor analysis in a cohort of systemic lupus erythematosus (SLE) patients on systemic glucocorticoids showed that hypoalbuminemia was a significant predisposing factor to corticosteroid-induced psychosis in that patient population.[30] Insomnia is a common complaint present at low doses, and in elderly populations cognitive impairment, particularly memory loss, may manifest.[31] While preventive measures encompass monitoring and education as well as appropriate dosing regimens, treatment of psychosis with various antipsychotic medications has been documented as effective.[30]

Cardiovascular Effects

The risk of ischemic heart disease and cardiac failure is increased in individuals on long-term corticosteroid therapy greater than 7.5 mg of prednisone per day, as per the result of a case-control study of more than 50,000 individuals.[32] The risk as measured by odds ratios was greater for current users of systemic glucocorticoids than for previous users. Although the risk was not as great for cerebrovascular disease as with cardiovascular disease, the results have not been verified in RCTs and, hence, general recommendations on prevention or monitoring of patients on systemic corticosteroids are currently inappropriate.

Gastrointestinal Effects

Corticosteroids have been reported to be associated with an increased risk of peptic ulcer disease, gastritis, and gastroesophageal reflux disease. Several studies have quantified the increased risk as marginally significant for glucocorticoids alone, although in combination with nonsteroidal anti-inflammatory drugs (NSAIDs), a significant elevation in the risk for gastroenterological complications above the level attributable to NSAIDs alone is detectable within the first 3 months of use.[33] Current expert recommendations in other fields do not recommend prophylaxis with proton pump inhibitors (PPIs) in the setting of glucocorticoids alone, but it can be considered for those individuals taking both glucocorticoids and NSAIDs.[33] It is the authors' practice, and that of other dermatologists in the field, to prescribe PPIs to AIBD patients on chronic, high-dose corticosteroids. No information is available as to the effect of COX-2–specific NSAIDs combined with systemic corticosteroids.

Ophthalmologic Effects

Posterior subcapsular cataracts are a well-documented adverse effect of prolonged corticosteroid use. These bilateral, slowly developing cataracts can usually be distinguished clinically from senile cataracts. Findings from rheumatologic research suggests that younger patients, particularly children, are more susceptible to the formation of cataracts, and that doses equivalent to less than 10 mg prednisolone per day can still cause significant increases in the rates of cataract formation when compared with matched controls.[34] Anecdotally, several of the authors' pemphigus patients have had to undergo cataract surgery. Increased intraocular pressure can also occur within months of systemic corticosteroid use, mimicking open-angle glaucoma, although it is much more commonly a risk with ocular use of corticosteroids.[2] Patients with preexisting glaucoma have an increased sensitivity to corticosteroids and risk of disease progression, and regular ophthalmologic reviews are a necessary part of monitoring side effects in these patients.[35]

Risk of Infection

The risk for potentially serious infection in AIBD patients, particularly those on long-term corticosteroid therapy combined with other immunosuppressive therapy, is high. Expert recommendations suggest the consideration of prophylaxis for Candida and/or Pneumocystis infections in patients with high-dose MMP.[2] Although no clear consensus guidelines are available concerning infectious prophylaxis in AIBD, Williams and Nesbitt[2] state that trimethoprim-sulfamethoxasole or dapsone are acceptable options for bacterial prophylaxis, with dapsone having additional anti-inflammatory properties. Valacyclovir can be used for viral prophylaxis for herpes simplex, and chlorhexidine/miconazole mouthwashes are appropriate for oral candidiasis prophylaxis.[2] Concerns over tuberculosis reactivation with individuals on immunosuppressive regimens have led rheumatologic authorities to suggest baseline chest radiographs and tuberculin skin testing prior to long-term immunosuppressive therapies. Opinions vary as to the appropriateness of these investigations in those on glucocorticoids alone, as most concern centers around the use of TNF-α inhibitors, such as infliximab and rituximab.[2] Drugs such as rituximab are being used as first-line treatment for pemphigus patients who have significant contraindications to high-dose corticosteroids.[16] Cost-benefit analyses in the short term may find that oral corticosteroids are cheaper than topical alternatives and biological therapies, but the longer term costs of the sequelae of high-dose steroids, listed above, have yet to be properly evaluated.

EXPERT RECOMMENDATIONS

Corticosteroids are a central tenet in the management of AIBD, and it is unlikely that any ethics committee would permit RCTs of placebos versus systemic steroids in the acute phases of these diseases, because the mortality decreased so dramatically when steroids were introduced for pemphigus. The focus is to minimize side effects with the lowest doses of corticosteroids or an alternative mode of application that is possible for efficacy.

REFERENCES

1. Bikowski J, Pillai R, Shroot B. The position not the presence of the halogen in corticosteroids influences

potency and side effects. J Drugs Dermatol 2006; 5(2):125–30.

2. Williams LC, Nesbitt LT Jr. Update on systemic glucocorticosteroids in dermatology. Dermatol Clin 2001;19(1):63–77.

3. McClain R, Yentzer B, Fledman S. Comparison of skin concentration following topical versus oral corticosteroid treatment: reconsidering the treatment of common inflammatory dermatoses. J Drugs Dermatol 2009;8(12):1076–9.

4. Tóth G, Westerlaken B, Eilders M, et al. Dexamethasone pharmacokinetics after high-dose oral therapy for pemphigus. Ann Pharmacother 2002;36:1109.

5. Martin L, Agero AL, Werth V, et al. Interventions for pemphigus vulgaris and pemphigus foliaceus [review]. Cochrane Database Syst Rev 2009;1:CD006263.

6. Harman KE, Albert S, Black MM. Guidelines for the management of pemphigus vulgaris. Br J Dermatol 2003;149:926–37.

7. Ratnam K, Phay K, Tan C. Pemphigus therapy with oral prednisolone regimens: a five year study. Int J Dermatol 1990;29:363–7.

8. Mentink L, Mackenzie M, Toth G, et al. Randomized control trial of adjuvant oral dexamethasone pulse therapy in pemphigus vulgaris. Arch Dermatol 2007; 143:570–6.

9. Lapiere K, Caers S, Lambert J. A case of long standing pemphigus vulgaris on the scalp. Dermatology 2004;209:162–3.

10. Baykal C, Azizlerli G, Thoma-Uszynski S, et al. Pemphigus vulgaris localized to the nose and cheeks. J Am Acad Dermatol 2002;47:875–8.

11. Dagistan S, Goregen M, Miloglu O, et al. Oral pemphigus vulgaris: a case report with review of the literature. J Oral Sci 2008;50(3):359–62.

12. Kirtschig G, Middleton P, Bennett C. Interventions for bullous pemphigoid. Cochrane Database Syst Rev 2010;10:CD002292.

13. Parker S, MacKelfresh J. Autoimmune blistering diseases in the elderly. Clin Dermatol 2011;29(1):69–79.

14. Morel P, Guillaume JC. Treatment of bullous pemphigoid with prednisolone only: 0.75 mg/kg/day versus 1.25 mg/kg/day. A multicenter randomized study. Ann Dermatol Venereol 1984;111(10):925–8 [in French].

15. Dreno B, Sassolas B, Lacour P, et al. Methylprednisolone versus prednisolone methylsulfobenzoate in pemphigoid: a comparative multicenter study. Ann Dermatol Venereol 1993;120:518–21 [in French].

16. Joly P, Roujeau JC, Benichou J, et al. A comparison of oral and topical corticosteroids in patients with bullous pemphigoid. N Engl J Med 2002;346(5): 321–7.

17. Joly P, Roujeau JC, Benichou J, et al. A comparison of two regimens of topical corticosteroids in the treatment of patients with bullous pemphigoid: a multicenter randomized study. J Invest Dermatol 2009; 129(7):1681–7.

18. Knudson RM, Kalaaj AN, Bruce AJ. The management of mucous membrane pemphigoid and pemphigus. Dermatol Ther 2010;23(3):268–80. Available at: http://onlinelibrary.wiley.com/doi/10.1111/dth.2010. 23.issue-3/issuetoc.

19. Kirtschig G, Murrell D, Wojnarowska F, et al. Interventions for mucous membrane pemphigoid and epidermolysis bullosa acquisita. Cochrane Database Syst Rev 2003;1:CD004056.

20. Korman N. Linear IgA bullous dermatosis. In: Lebwohl M, Heymann W, Berth-Jones J, et al, editors. Treatment of skin disease. Comprehensive therapeutic strategies. 2nd edition. London: Mosby Elsevier Ltd; 2006. p. 358–60.

21. Shimizu S, Natsuga K, Shinkuma S, et al. Localized linear IgA/IgG bullous dermatosis. Acta Derm Venereol 2010;90:621–4.

22. Kirtschig G, Murrell DF, Wojnarowska F, et al. Interventions for mucous membrane pemphigoid and epidermolysis bullosa acquisita. Cochrane Database Syst Rev 2000;4:CD004056.

23. Ishii N, Takahiro Hamada T, Dainichi T, et al. Epidermolysis bullosa acquisita: What's new? J Dermatol 2010;37:220–30.

24. Jenkins RE, Hern S, Black MM. Clinical features and management of 87 patients with pemphigoid gestationis. Clin Exp Dermatol 1999;24(4):255–9.

25. Gulko PS, Mulloy AL. Glucocorticoid-induced osteoporosis: pathogenesis, prevention and treatment. Clin Exp Rheumatol 1996;14:199–206.

26. American College of Rheumatology Ad Hoc Committee on Glucocorticoid-Induced Osteoporosis recommendations for the prevention and treatment of glucocorticoid induced osteoporosis. Arthritis Rheum 2001;44(7):1496–503.

27. Stoch SA, Saag KG, Greenwald M, et al. Once-weekly oral alendronate 70 mg in patients with glucocorticoid induced bone loss: a 12 month randomizes, placebo controlled clinical trial. J Rheumatol 2009;36(8): 1705–14.

28. Cohen S, Levy R, Keller M, et al. Risendronate therapy prevents corticosteroid induced bone loss: a twelve month, multicenter, randomized, double blind placebo controlled parallel group study. Arthritis Rheum 1999;42(11):2309–18.

29. Minden S, Orav J, Schildkraut J. Hypomanic reactions to ACTH and prednisone in treatment for multiple sclerosis. Neurology 1988;38(10):1631–4.

30. Chau SY, Mok CC. Factors predictive of corticosteroid psychosis in patients with systemic lupus erythematosus. Neurology 2003;61(1):104–7.

31. Keenan P, Jacobson M, Soleymani R, et al. The effect on memory of chronic prednisone treatment in patients with systemic disease. Neurology 1996; 47(6):1396–402.

32. Souverein P, Berars A, Van Staa T. Use of oral glucocorticoids and risk of cardiovascular and

cerebrovascular disease in a population based case-control study. Heart 2004;90(8):859–65.

33. Gabriel S, Jaakkimainen L, Bombardier C. Risk for serious gastrointestinal complications related to use of non steroidal anti inflammatory drugs, a meta analysis. Ann Intern Med 1991;115(10): 787–96.

34. McDougall R, Sibley J, Haga M, et al. Outcome in patients with rheumatoid arthritis receiving prednisone compared to matched controls. J Rheumatol 1994;21(7):1207–13.

35. Trikudanathan S, McMahon GT. Optimum management of glucocorticoid treated patients. Nat Rev Endocrinol 2008;4:62–71.

Azathioprine in the Treatment of Autoimmune Blistering Diseases

Volker Meyer, MD, Stefan Beissert, MD*

KEYWORDS

- Azathioprine • Autoimmune blistering diseases
- Pemphigus • Bullous pemphigoid

HISTORY OF AZATHIOPRINE

The pharmaceutical precursor of azathioprine was originally 6-mercaptopurine. 6-Mercaptopurine was synthesized in 1951 by GB Elion and GH Hitchings using techniques reported by Fisher and Traube.[1] 6-Mercaptopurine was first used in 1953 in children with acute lymphatic leukemia.[2] Later, Calne,[3] a young surgeon who later became professor of surgery at Cambridge, successfully treated dogs after renal transplantation with 6-mercaptopurine in 1960, but because of the high toxic potential of the drug it was not found suitable for long-term treatment of humans with solid-organ transplants. Subsequently, it was shown that one of the derivatives of 6-mercaptopurine found by Elion and Hitchings, BW 57-322, presented with less bone marrow toxicity[4] but was as immunosuppressive as 6-mercaptopurine. To protect 6-mercaptopurine from being rapidly metabolized, an imidazole ring had been biochemically connected via the sulfur atom at position 6 of 6-mercaptopurine and thereby azathioprine was finally developed (**Fig. 1**). The first successful allogeneic renal transplant using a combination of azathioprine and corticosteroids was initiated in 1963.[5] Azathioprine is now used in particular for the treatment of autoimmune diseases, such as autoimmune blistering diseases, inflammatory bowel disease, multiple sclerosis, and lupus, to name a few.

STRUCTURE AND METABOLISM

About 88% of azathioprine is ingested and 12% excreted via the gut.[6] Nearly all the incorporated azathioprine is metabolized because only 2% is being excreted unchanged in the urine. The highest serum levels can be found approximately 2 hours after oral application and the half-life is approximately 5 hours. After uptake, azathioprine is nonenzymatically cleaved into its imidazole derivatives (methylnitroimidazole moiety) and 6-mercaptopurine (see **Fig. 1**). Three enzymes have been reported to compete for the cleavage of azathioprine (**Fig. 2**).[7] Thiopurine S-methyltransferase (TPMT) is able to catabolize 6-mercaptopurine into the nontoxic 6-methyl mercaptopurine. Xanthine oxidase (XO) produces the nontoxic inactive metabolite 6-thiouric acid. A lack in one of these enzymes, XO and TPMT, leads to an increased production of toxic metabolites via the hypoxanthine phosphoribosyltransferase (HPRT) pathway. A lack of TPMT activity is normally caused by genetic mutations, whereas XO might be blocked by XO inhibitory drugs such as allopurinol, which is one of the most commonly prescribed drugs in Europe and North America. The enzyme HPRT metabolizes 6-mercaptopurine into 6-thioinosine 5-monophosphate (6-TIMP). This product is processed by TPMT to active methylated metabolites or is phosphorylated to 6-thioinosine triphosphate (6-TITP). 6-TITP is

The authors declare no conflict of interest.
Department of Dermatology, University of Muenster, Von-Esmarch-Str. 58, D-48149 Muenster, Germany
* Corresponding author.
E-mail address: beisser@uni-muenster.de

Dermatol Clin 29 (2011) 545–554
doi:10.1016/j.det.2011.06.009
0733-8635/11/$ – see front matter © 2011 Elsevier Inc. All rights reserved.

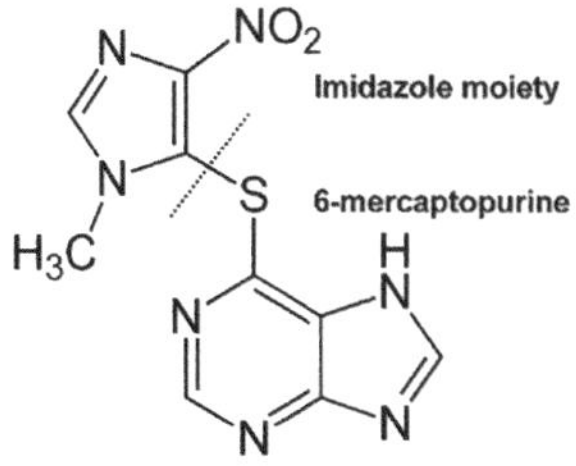

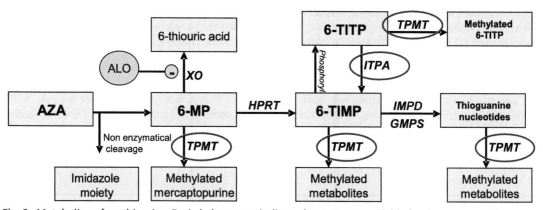

Fig. 1. Structure of azathioprine. The dashed line marks the cleavage site.

converted to 6-TIMP by inosine triphosphate pyrophosphohydrolase (ITPA). A lack of ITPA, often seen in Asian populations,[8] leads to an increase in the level of toxic 6-TITP and induces corresponding side effects, such as leukopenia, gastrointestinal disturbances, or elevated liver function test results (for details concerning side effects see later discussion).

6-TIMP is converted by inosine monophosphate dehydrogenase and guanosine monophosphate synthetase into the principal active 6-thioguanine nucleotides. These nucleotides are converted by TPMT into inactive methylated metabolites.

In patients with Lesch-Nyhan syndrome, reduced expression of HPRT can be detected, which makes these patients less suitable for azathioprine treatment. Although most of the therapeutic effects of azathioprine are dependent on the HPRT pathway, there is experimental evidence that the imidazole derivatives of azathioprine might also be effective.[9]

AZATHIOPRINE IN BULLOUS PEMPHIGOID

In 1971, Greaves and colleagues[10] introduced azathioprine into the treatment of bullous pemphigoid.

Before that, most patients had been treated with systemic corticosteroid monotherapy to prevent recurrent blister formation. It was reported by Greaves and colleagues[10] that in 8 of 10 patients with bullous pemphigoid, no prednisone maintenance therapy was needed for preventing relapses, whereas azathioprine was given at a dose of 2.5 mg/kg body weight per day.

In a small prospective clinical trial in 1978, Burton and colleagues[11] examined azathioprine (2.5 mg/kg/d, n = 12) plus prednisone (30–80 mg/d) versus prednisone alone (n = 13). No significant difference between both groups was found concerning the overall disease control. The prednisone-sparing effect was statistically significant. In the azathioprine group, a cumulative average dose of 3688 mg of prednisone was used for more than 3 years, whereas 6732 mg was used in the prednisone monogroup for the same period. In 1993, Guillaume and colleagues[12] found no significant difference in disease control between prednisone monotherapy (1 mg/kg/d, n = 31) and azathioprine (100–150 mg/d, n = 36) plus prednisone therapy. However, the prednisone-sparing effect has not been investigated in this study.

In a national randomized trial in 2007, Beissert and colleagues[13] compared treatment with methylprednisolone (0.5 mg/kg/d) with either azathioprine (2 mg/kg/d, n = 38) or mycophenolate mofetil (1 g twice a day, n = 35). The results showed no significant differences in the primary outcome (ie, complete healing of skin lesions) and a tendency to faster healing in the azathioprine group (azathioprine 23.8 ± 18.9 days vs mycophenolate mofetil 42.0 ± 55.9 days, P value is nonsignificant). Moreover, similar corticosteroid doses were used to control disease. Mycophenolate

Fig. 2. Metabolism of azathioprine. Encircled enzymes indicate that tests are available for these enzymes for assessment of azathioprine's potential toxicity. ALO, allopurinol; AZA, azathioprine; GMPS, guanosine monophosphate synthetase; HPRT, hypoxanthine phosphoribosyltransferase; IMPD, inosine monophosphate dehydrogenase; ITPA, inosine triphosphate pyrophosphohydrolase; 6-MP, 6-mercaptopurine; 6-TIMP, 6-thioinosine monophosphatase; 6-TITP, 6-thioinosine triphosphatase; TPMT, thiopurine S-methyltransferase; XO, xanthine oxidase.

mofetil was significantly less liver toxic compared with azathioprine, which can be an advantage especially in elderly patients.

A Cochrane review concluded from the available study results that the addition of azathioprine in the treatment of bullous pemphigoid had not been established.[14] The results of several studies concerning the treatment of bullous pemphigoid with azathioprine are summarized in **Table 1**.

AZATHIOPRINE IN PEMPHIGUS

The treatment of pemphigus vulgaris and pemphigus foliaceus usually does not differ significantly. Most investigators did not specify in their reports whether patients with pemphigus foliaceus or vulgaris had been treated.

The use of azathioprine for the treatment of pemphigus was introduced in 1969, when Krakowski and colleagues[15] presented the first case report of a woman with pemphigus vulgaris treated successfully with azathioprine. At the same time, Aberer and colleagues[16] published a case series of 4 patients describing the use of azathioprine as "steroid saving and beneficial" in patients with pemphigus. In 1977, Lever and Schaumburg-Lever[17] published a retrospective analysis of 63 patients with pemphigus. The investigators treated patients (n = 12) with prednisone monotherapy and the other patients in this cohort (n = 51) with a combination of azathioprine, cyclophosphamide, or methotrexate and prednisone. In this report, azathioprine was described as "steroid saving and effective." The investigators' therapeutic approach is still known as Lever's regime. Initially, patients receive a high dose of prednisone (up to 2 mg/kg body weight) in combination with

azathioprine 2.0 to 2.5 mg/kg. After cessation of new blister formation and reepithelization of erosions, the prednisone dose is reduced to 40 mg/d, while the azathioprine dose remains unchanged. Further proceedings depend on the individual's clinical development. Normally, the prednisone dose is gradually reduced over a period of several months.

There are only a few prospective randomized trials reported on pemphigus. Beissert and colleagues[18] examined 38 patients with pemphigus vulgaris or pemphigus foliaceus and found no significant differences between treatment with azathioprine and mycophenolate mofetil, both in combination with methylprednisolone, concerning remission of disease and corticosteroid-sparing effects. The patients treated with azathioprine received a median methylprednisolone dose of 8.916 ± 29.844 mg. In the mycophenolate mofetil–treated group, patients received a median of 9.334 ± 13.280 mg methylprednisolone (n = nonsignificant). The mean duration of follow-up was 438 days in both groups. However, the time needed to achieve disease control in 50% of the patients was about 30 days in the azathioprine group compared with 75 days in the mycophenolate mofetil group. Perhaps the inhibition of at least 3 enzymatic pathways by azathioprine (see **Fig. 2**) is able to induce a faster response in comparison with mycophenolate mofetil, which inhibits primarily 1 signaling pathway. Nevertheless, after 200 days of treatment, the patients in the mycophenolate mofetil group had a remission rate of 90%, whereas those who were treated with azathioprine had a remission rate of 75%. After 600 days, this trend persisted because 20% of patients with pemphigus were still not achieving effective control

Table 1
Use of azathioprine in bullous pemphigoid (case reports are not included)

Investigators	Year	N	AZA Dose	Main Outcome
Greaves et al[10]	1971	10	2.5 mg/kg/d	8/10 symptom free, no prednisone needed
van Dijk & van Velde[44]	1973	5	75–250 mg/d	4/5 excellent response
Burton & Greaves[45]	1974	12	2.5 mg/kg/d	12/12 excellent response
Ahmed et al[46]	1977	15	1.5 mg/kg/d	Reduces duration of maintenance, steroid sparing
Burton et al[11]	1978	12	2.5 mg/kg/d	Steroid sparing, but control of disease not significantly different from steroid alone
Guillaume et al[12]	1993	36	100–150 mg/d	No significant difference to steroid monotherapy concerning disease control
Beissert et al[13]	2007	73	2 mg/kg/d	No significant differences in primary outcome between AZA + MP and MMF + MP, tendency of faster healing in AZA-treated patients

Abbreviations: AZA, azathioprine; MMF, mycophenolate mofetil; MP, methylprednisolone; N, number of patients treated with azathioprine.

with azathioprine compared with 10% of patients using mycophenolate. The recurrence rate was similar in both groups.

In another study with 120 patients analyzed, Chams-Davatchi and colleagues[19] found no significant difference concerning disease remission between azathioprine and mycophenolate mofetil, but the patients treated with azathioprine showed significantly less steroid consumption. These findings indicate that azathioprine is well suited for first-line treatment of pemphigus. Rose and colleagues[20] compared dexamethasone-cyclophosphamide pulse therapy with oral methylprednisolone/azathioprine therapy in pemphigus. A tendency was found in favor of methylprednisolone/azathioprine concerning complete remissions.

In IgA pemphigus, azathioprine showed no considerable effect. Dapsone is usually the first-line treatment.[21] For pemphigus vegetans, azathioprine seems to work in individual cases.[22] For treatment of refractory patients, disease control has been reported under the corticosteroid/azathioprine regimen using additionally photopheresis or retinoids.[23,24]

In paraneoplastic pemphigus, therapy for the underlying malignancy is essential. Concomitant treatment with azathioprine and other immunomodulatory drugs has been reported, but it is difficult to conclude whether any of them will reliably affect the prognosis of the disease because its mortality approaches 90%.[25] Lam and colleagues[26] presented a case of a 77-year-old man with chronic conjunctivitis, acanthosis nigricans, and pemphigus-like mucocutaneous lesions. Further examinations revealed an underlying bronchogenic squamous cell carcinoma (SCC). Although skin lesions resolved with oral prednisone and azathioprine (100 mg/d) therapy, the conjunctivitis and mucous membrane erosions persisted. Verrini and colleagues[27] described another patient with paraneoplastic pemphigus who showed good response to azathioprine (100 mg/d) but died after a short time after initiation of treatment.

The importance of systemic corticosteroids in the treatment of pemphigus is clearly documented. Because the reports show a tendency in favor of azathioprine concerning corticosteroid-sparing effects and no significant differences regarding disease control, the authors suggest using azathioprine as first-line therapy in mild to moderate cases of pemphigus. Mycophenolate mofetil seems to be a valid second-line choice. In severe and rapidly progressing cases, dexamethasone/cyclophosphamide pulse therapy should be considered.

Because pemphigus is a chronic disease, long-term follow-up studies (>3 years) are clearly needed. A Cochrane review concluded from the available study results that the optimal immunomodulatory agent in the treatment of pemphigus has not yet been found. Although azathioprine and cyclophosphamide did show advantages concerning the steroid-sparing effect, mycophenolate showed superior disease control.[28]

The results of several studies concerning the treatment of pemphigus with azathioprine are shown in **Table 2**.

AZATHIOPRINE IN OTHER AUTOIMMUNE BLISTERING DISEASES

Several case reports show that azathioprine can be effective in cicatricial pemphigoid. These reports demonstrate that azathioprine is able to control disease and prevent progression. However, azathioprine showed no beneficial effect on already existing scars and cicatrizing vegetation. Unfortunately, there are no randomized or blinded trials available. The results of relevant case reports concerning the treatment of cicatricial pemphigoid are shown in **Table 3**.

Pemphigus can also develop in children, which is a rare event in Europe and North America. Some reports center around therapy for juvenile pemphigus with azathioprine and demonstrate the efficiency of azathioprine in children with pemphigus.[29] The results of important case reports concerning the use of azathioprine in juvenile pemphigus are shown in **Table 4**.

AZATHIOPRINE DURING PREGNANCY

The use of immunomodulatory agents during pregnancy should always be extremely well considered. Azathioprine is able to cross the human placenta.[30] The fetal liver does not possess the enzymes to convert azathioprine into its active metabolites, suggesting that the fetus might have a certain protection against azathioprine-induced cellular toxicity.[31] Most large studies have shown that azathioprine during pregnancy is tolerated, although the rate of congenital malformations seems to be 3% to 9% in infants exposed antenatally.[32] Reported malformations include myelomeningocele, preaxial polydactyly, microcephaly, thymic atrophy, hypospadias, and adrenal hypoplasia.[31,32]

SIDE EFFECTS OF AZATHIOPRINE

Azathioprine is generally well tolerated. In a study of Japanese patients (n = 114) treated with azathioprine 50 mg/d for inflammatory bowel disease, 33% developed side effects over a period of 48 months of investigation.[33] The most common

Table 2
Use of azathioprine in pemphigus (most case reports are not included)

Investigators	Year	N	AZA Dose	Main Outcome
Krakowski et al[15]	1969	1	75–150 mg	Control of disease after 4 mo
Aberer et al[16]	1969	4	1–3 mg/kg/d	Steroid saving and beneficial
Burton et al[47]	1970	4	2.5 mg/kg/d	3 of 4 with excellent response, but relapse after discontinuation of AZA; 1 patient dropped out because of severe side effects
Roenigk & Deodhar[48]	1973	10	50–250 mg/d	7, excellent; 2, good; 1, fair
van Dijk & van Velde[44]	1973	5	50–200 mg/d	5/5 excellent response
Lever & Schaumburg-Lever[17]	1977	6	50–150 mg/d	Steroid saving and effective
Lever & Schaumburg-Lever[49]	1984	21	100 mg/d	Safe and effective, disease control in 21
Aberer et al[16]	1987	27	1–3 mg/kg/d	45% free of disease; 38% clinically free of disease, but with raised antibody titers; 17% with controlled disease
Tan-Lim & Bystryn[50]	1990	12	50–150 mg/d	AZA in combination with plasmapheresis decreased antibodies faster than without plasmapheresis
Mourellou et al[51]	1995	15	100 mg/d	Remission in 14 patients, less mortality compared with steroid monotreatment
Carson et al[52]	1996	72	50–250 mg/d	AZA significantly reduced mortality, steroid sparing, 37% remission, 33% stable disease
Scully et al[53]	1999	17	1–3 mg/kg/d	Not pointed out clearly. 2 deaths reported under treatment with AZA
Ljubojevic et al[54]	2002	129	100–150 mg/d	Reduction of mortality compared with patients with steroid monotherapy
Beissert et al[18]	2006	18	2 mg/kg/d	Steroid-sparing effect of AZA similar to that of MMF. Quicker response to therapy with AZA than with MMF. No significant differences in overall outcome
Rose et al[20]	2005	11	2–2.5 mg/kg/d	Tendency in favor of AZA concerning complete remissions compared with cyclophosphamide pulse therapy
Chams-Davatchi et al[19]	2007	30	2.5 mg/kg/d	AZA most effective compared with CYP and MMF or cortisone monotherapy, but no significant differences in complete remission
Chaidemenos et al[55]	2011	19	100 mg/d	Notable steroid-sparing effect of AZA; high dose of prednisone leads significantly faster to remission than low dose of prednisone combined with AZA

Abbreviations: AZA, azathioprine; CYP, cyclophosphamide; MMF, mycophenolate mofetil; N, number of patients treated with azathioprine.

side effect of azathioprine is leukopenia (white blood cells $\leq$3000/μl), with 18 (15.8%) affected patients. Of these patients, 15 experienced mild leukopenia with no necessary change of dosage. Two patients (1.8%) had severe leukopenia (<1000/μl), followed by a decrease in the dose of azathioprine. Although the mild forms of leukopenia occurred after an average treatment period of 13.7 months (mean; range 1–47 months), the severe forms of leukopenia occurred in less than 1 month.

The next common side effects were gastrointestinal disturbances, including vomiting, nausea, and diarrhea. Eleven patients (9.6%) experienced such symptoms, which occurred shortly (<1 month)

Table 3
Use of azathioprine in cicatricial pemphigoid

Investigators	Year	N	AZA Dose	Main Outcome
Dantzig[56]	1973	1	150 mg/d	Remission of disease
Braun-Falco et al[57]	1981	1	100 mg/d	Among several trials of treatment, only AZA effective
Mondino & Brown[58]	1983	9	1.5 mg/kg/d	10 of 18 eyes showed no progress
Pawlofsky et al[59]	1985	1	150 mg/d	Successful treatment
Tauber et al[60]	1991	11	2 mg/kg/d	AZA failed to control disease in 9% of cases, diaminodiphenylsulfone recommended for treatment
Lugovic et al[61]	2007	1	2 mg/kg/d	AZA effective for treatment of inflammation and blistering, but no effect on scaring

Abbreviations: AZA, azathioprine; N, number of patients treated with azathioprine.

after initiation of therapy and were all self-limited after a few days. Further side effects were elevated liver function test results. One patient (0.9%) had a severe increase in liver enzyme levels with more than 20-fold increase of transaminases levels compared to normal levels after 2 weeks of treatment. After azathioprine had been discontinued, liver enzymes returned to normal levels. Three patients (2.6%) had flulike symptoms (ie, fever, headache, rash, arthralgia, myalgia, and malaise) that were self-limited after discontinuation of azathioprine. Two more patients showed mild loss of hair that did not lead to discontinuation of therapy.

The side effects observed in the Japanese patients were identical to those observed in white patients but developed after half the azathioprine dose that leads to similar side effects in white patients. Japanese patients showed TPMT gene polymorphisms less frequently compared with white patients or Africans. Although, for instance, TPMT activity–reducing *TPMT*3A* alleles were detected in 4.5% of British white patients, Kumagai and colleagues[34] could not find any individual in a cohort of 522 Japanese patients who carried

that allele. **Table 5** shows the frequency of variant TPMT alleles in different ethnic populations. The most frequent TPMT gene polymorphisms can be found in Africans and white patients, whereas Asians have a low prevalence of TPMT gene polymorphisms. In white patients, approximately 1 in 300 patients has a distinctly reduced TPMT activity, and about 11% of white patients show a moderately reduced activity, resulting in increased production of toxic metabolites (eg, thioinosine monophosphates) when taking azathioprine.[35] Myelosuppression in patients with reduced TPMT activity develops more rapidly.[36] Uchiyama and colleagues[8] examined the relationship between the incidence of azathioprine-associated adverse effects and either the incidence of TPMT or ITPA gene polymorphisms (for the metabolic mechanism of ITPA see **Fig. 2**). In 5 of 6 patients who had developed an acute bone marrow toxicity, a mutation (*94C>A*) of the ITPA gene was detectable. About 75% of patients with agranulocytosis had the *94C>A* allele. In red blood cells of patients with the homozygous *94C>A* missense mutation, ITPA activity was below detectable levels. The frequency of *94C>A* alleles was 31 of 200 in

Table 4
Use of azathioprine in juvenile pemphigus

Investigators	Year	Patients' Age (y)	N	AZA Dose	Main Outcome
Harrington et al[62]	1978	15	1	50–100 mg/d	Good response
Lynde et al[63]	1984	15	1	50–125 mg/d	Complete remission after 2.5 y
Fine et al[64]	1988	13	1	50–125 mg/d	Complete remission in combination with plasmapheresis after 12 mo
Wananukul & Pongprasit[65]	1999	11–14	3	2 mg/kg/d	2 patients, controlled disease; 1 patient, complete remission
Harangi et al[66]	2001	10	1	2 mg/kg/d	After 4.5 y of treatment, complete remission

Abbreviations: AZA, azathioprine; N, number of patients treated with azathioprine.

Table 5
Frequency of variant TPMT alleles in different ethnic populations

Population	n	TPMT*2 (%)	TPMT*3A (%)	TPMT*3C (%)
British	398	0.5	4.5	0.3
French	382	0.5	5.7	0.8
Americans	282	0.2	3.2	0.2
South-west Asians	198	0	1	0
African Americans	248	0.4	0.8	2.4
Kenyans	202	0	0	5.4
Ghanaians	434	0	0	7.6
Chinese	384	0	0	2.3
Japanese	1044	0	0	1.6

Abbreviation: n, number of alleles.
Adapted from Kumagai K, Hiyama K, Ishioka S, et al. Allelotype frequency of the thiopurine methyltransferase (TPMT) gene in Japanese. Pharmacogenetics 2001;11(3):277.

Japanese individuals (15.5%), which is 2.6-fold higher than in white patients.[8,37] Because of the high correlation between the side effects of azathioprine therapy and the prevalence of ITPA polymorphism genes in Japanese, it is suggested that in Japanese patients, instead of determination of TPMT gene polymorphisms or activity, a screen for ITPA gene mutations or activity should be introduced.[8] In white patients and Africans, monitoring for deficiency in TPMT activity is recommended before azathioprine is introduced.

With regard to the observed side effects of azathioprine, laboratory monitoring, including blood cell counts and serum analysis (especially liver enzymes), is recommended weekly for the first 8 weeks of treatment. After 8 weeks of treatment, the interval of laboratory monitoring can be extended to once per month.

The acute toxicity of azathioprine is low. A renal transplant patient who received a massive single overdose of azathioprine of 7500 mg experienced nausea, vomiting, and diarrhea followed by mild leukopenia, mild abnormalities in liver functions, as well as improved renal function.[38]

Like all immunosuppressive drugs, long-term intake of azathioprine raises the risk of immunosuppression-induced malignancies. In a large 20-year follow-up study, patients with rheumatoid arthritis receiving azathioprine had a 10-fold increased risk for developing immunosuppression-associated myeloproliferative disorders compared with the general population. Patients with rheumatoid arthritis without a history of azathioprine treatment had only a 5-fold increased risk of developing myeloproliferative disorders.[39] The risk of developing nonmelanoma skin cancers ([NMSCs]; SCCs and basal cell carcinomas

[BCCs]) was 2-fold increased in the azathioprine-treated group with rheumatoid arthritis compared with the general population. There was a significant increase in cancer development in relation to the cumulative lifetime intake of azathioprine. In 8.6% of the patients with a lifetime intake of up to 50 g azathioprine, different kinds of cancer developed within 20 years. In patients with a cumulative dose of 200 g azathioprine, different kinds of cancer developed in more than 20% of cases within 20 years.[39]

There is strong evidence for an additive carcinogenic effect of UV radiation, especially UV-A (320–400 nm), in combination with azathioprine treatment concerning the development of NMSCs. Ramsay and colleagues[40] examined transplant recipients of Fitzpatrick skin types I to IV. From 361 patients, 187 (51.8%) developed histologically diagnosed NMSCs. The ratio of SCC to BCC was reversed in these patients from 1:3.7 before transplantation to 2:1 after transplantation.[40] NMSC increased with the duration of medical immunosuppression. Among the transplant recipients, 29.1% developed 1 or more NMSCs when immunosuppression did not exceed 5 years, but immunosuppression for 10 to 20 years led to an incidence of 72.4% of NMSCs in the treated patients. However, the patients received not only azathioprine (on average 100 mg daily) but also 225 mg of cyclosporine and 7 mg of prednisone daily (follow-up 7.1 years).

Most of the observed NMSCs in immunosuppressed transplant recipients developed on sun-exposed areas (80% of SCCs, 71% of BCCs, and 64% of keratoacanthomata). One of the active metabolites of azathioprine is thioguanine nucleotides. These nucleotides are precursors for

6-thioguanine, which can be incorporated into DNA on replication. Normally, DNA does not significantly absorb UV-A wavelengths (320–400 nm), whereas thiopurines do. 6-Thioguanine nucleotides have an absorbance maximum at 342 nm.[41] Moreover, 6-mercaptopurine as a metabolite of azathioprine generates reactive oxygen species (ROS) when exposed to UV-A.[42] O'Donovan and colleagues[41] demonstrated that biologically relevant doses of UV-A generate ROS in cultured cells with 6-thioguanine–substituted DNA. In experimental cell lines (HCT116, human colorectal carcinoma cells) containing about 0.01% 6-thioguanine–substituted DNA, irradiation with a nontoxic dose of 1 kJ/m^2 UV-A led to a 3-fold increase in adenine phosphoribosyltransferase (aprt) mutation frequencies compared with nonsubstituted DNA. Neither 6-thioguanine nor UV-A alone was detectably mutagenic. In normal DNA without substitutes, 500 kJ/m^2 of UV-A irradiation was required to induce a similar increase in aprt mutation frequency. O'Donovan and colleagues[41] measured the amount of 6-thioguanine in DNA extracted from clinically normal skin of 3 azathioprine-treated patients. Around 0.02% of 6-thioguanine–substituted DNA was found. In a control group of patients who did not receive azathioprine, no substituted DNA was detectable. Furthermore, azathioprine-treated patients showed a reduction of the minimal erythema dose for UV-A but not for UV-B. These findings indicate that the mutagenic effect of UV radiation is increased under azathioprine treatment. UV-A seems to play a more important role for photocarcinogenesis in these patients than UV-B.

In a mouse model, Reeve and colleagues[43] showed that azathioprine but not cyclophosphamide increased the incidence of skin tumors significantly after UV irradiation. Based on these results, it is recommended that patients undergoing therapy with azathioprine should use effective sunscreens and avoid unnecessary long-term exposure to the sun. Patients who require long-term treatment with azathioprine should undergo a clinical examination of the skin twice a year.

SUMMARY

Although there are still no standard guidelines for the treatment of autoimmune blistering diseases, azathioprine has shown good efficacy in acquired autoimmune blistering diseases. Azathioprine is normally well tolerated. Side effects of azathioprine normally occur in mild variants. Severe reactions are often caused by reduced TPMT or ITPA activity. Therefore, screening for the activity of TPMT should be conducted in white patients and Africans, whereas the Japanese should be screened for the activity of ITPA before therapy with azathioprine is started. Due to its potential steroid-sparing effect and the relatively rare side effects, azathioprine is clinically meaningful for the treatment of pemphigus, and recent developments in targeting B cells in autoimmune blistering disorders must prove their superiority against azathioprine.

REFERENCES

1. Elion GB. The purine path to chemotherapy. Science 1989;244(4900):41–7.
2. Burchenal JH, Murphy ML, Ellison RR, et al. Clinical evaluation of a new antimetabolite, 6-mercaptopurine, in the treatment of leukemia and allied diseases. Blood 1953;8(11):965–99.
3. Calne RY. The rejection of renal homografts. Inhibition in dogs by 6-mercaptopurine. Lancet 1960;1(7121):417–8.
4. Calne RY, Murray JE. Inhibition of the rejection of renal homografts in dogs by Burroughs Wellcome 57–322. Surg Forum 1961;12:118–20.
5. Calne RY, Loughridge LW, Pryse-Davies J, et al. Renal transplantation in man: a report of five cases, using cadaveric donors. BMJ 1963;2(5358):645–51.
6. Berlit P. Azathioprin, internist. Praxis 1995;35:661–5.
7. Karran P, Attard N. Thiopurines in current medical practice: molecular mechanisms and contributions to therapy-related cancer. Nat Rev Cancer 2008;8(1):24–36.
8. Uchiyama K, Nakamura M, Kubota T, et al. Thiopurine S-methyltransferase and inosine triphosphate pyrophosphohydrolase genes in Japanese patients with inflammatory bowel disease in whom adverse drug reactions were induced by azathioprine/6-mercaptopurine treatment. J Gastroenterol 2009;44(3):197–203.
9. Szawlowski PW, Al-Safi SA, Dooley T, et al. Azathioprine suppresses the mixed lymphocyte reaction of patients with Lesch-Nyhan syndrome. Br J Clin Pharmacol 1985;20(5):489–91.
10. Greaves MW, Burton JL, Marks J, et al. Azathioprine in treatment of bullous pemphigoid. BMJ 1971;1(5741):144–5.
11. Burton JL, Harman RR, Peachey RD, et al. Azathioprine plus prednisone in treatment of pemphigoid. BMJ 1978;2(6146):1190–1.
12. Guillaume JC, Vaillant L, Bernard P, et al. Controlled trial of azathioprine and plasma exchange in addition to prednisolone in the treatment of bullous pemphigoid. Arch Dermatol 1993;129(1):49–53.
13. Beissert S, Werfel T, Frieling U, et al. A comparison of oral methylprednisolone plus azathioprine or mycophenolate mofetil for the treatment of bullous pemphigoid. Arch Dermatol 2007;143(12):1536–42.

14. Kirtschig G, Middleton P, Bennett C, et al. Interventions for bullous pemphigoid [review]. Cochrane Database Syst Rev 2010;10:CD002292.

15. Krakowski A, Covo J, Rozanski Z. Pemphigus vulgaris. Arch Dermatol 1969;100(1):117.

16. Aberer W, Wolff-Schreiner EC, Stingl G, et al. Azathioprine in the treatment of pemphigus vulgaris. A long-term follow-up. J Am Acad Dermatol 1987;16(3 Pt 1): 527–33.

17. Lever WF, Schaumburg-Lever G. Immunosuppressants and prednisone in pemphigus vulgaris: therapeutic results obtained in 63 patients between 1961 and 1975. Arch Dermatol 1977;113(9):1236–41.

18. Beissert S, Werfel T, Frieling U, et al. A comparison of oral methylprednisolone plus azathioprine or mycophenolate mofetil for the treatment of pemphigus. Arch Dermatol 2006;142(11):1447–54.

19. Chams-Davatchi C, Esmaili N, Daneshpazhooh M, et al. Randomized controlled open-label trial of four treatment regimens for pemphigus vulgaris. J Am Acad Dermatol 2007;57(4):622–8.

20. Rose E, Wever S, Zilliken D, et al. Intravenous dexamethasone-cyclophosphamide pulse therapy in comparison with oral methylprednisolone-azathioprine therapy in patients with pemphigus: results of a multicenter prospectively randomized study. J Dtsch Dermatol Ges 2005;3(3):200–6.

21. Zillikens D, Miller K, Hartmann AA, et al. IgA pemphigus foliaceus: a case report. Dermatologica 1990;181(4):304–7.

22. Monshi B, Marker M, Feichtinger H, et al. Pemphigus vegetans–immunopathological findings in a rare variant of pemphigus v vulgaris. J Dtsch Dermatol Ges 2010;8(3):179–83.

23. Faulde MK, Sorhage B, Ksoll A, et al. Complete remission of drug resistant Pemphigus vegetans treated by extracorporeal photopheresis. J Eur Acad Dermatol Venereol 2007;21:822–49.

24. Ichimiya M, Yamamoto K, Muto M. Successful treatment of pemphigus vegetans by addition of etretinate to systemic steroids. Clin Exp Dermatol 1998; 23(4):178–80.

25. Kimyai-Asadi A, Jih MH. Paraneoplastic pemphigus. Int J Dermatol 2001;40(6):367–72.

26. Lam S, Stone MS, Goeken JA, et al. Paraneoplastic pemphigus, cicatricial conjunctivitis, and acanthosis nigricans with pachydermatoglyphy in a patient with bronchogenic squamous cell carcinoma. Ophthalmology 1992;99(1):108–13.

27. Verrini A, Cannata G, Cozzani E, et al. A patient with immunological features of paraneoplastic pemphigus in the absence of a detectable malignancy. Acta Derm Venereol 2002;82(5):382–4.

28. Martin LK, Agero AL, Werth V, et al. Interventions for pemphigus vulgaris and pemphigus foliaceus. Cochrane Database Syst Rev 2009;1:CD006263. DOI: 10.1002/14651858.CD006263.pub2.

29. Mensing H, Brehm H, Nasemann T. Bullöses Pemphigoid im Kindesalter. Hautarzt 1984;35:254–8 [in German].

30. Ostensen M. Treatment with immunosuppressive and disease modifying drugs during pregnancy and lactation [review]. Am J Reprod Immunol 1992;28(3–4):148–52.

31. Janssen NM, Genta MS. The effects of immunosuppressive and anti-inflammatory medications on fertility, pregnancy, and lactation. Arch Intern Med 2000;160(5):610–9.

32. Tendron A, Gouyon JB, Decramer S. In utero exposure to immunosuppressive drugs: experimental and clinical studies. Pediatr Nephrol 2002;17(2):121–30.

33. Takatsu N, Matsui T, Murakami Y, et al. Adverse reactions to azathioprine cannot be predicted by thiopurine S-methyltransferase genotype in Japanese patients with inflammatory bowel disease. J Gastroenterol Hepatol 2009;24(7):1258–64.

34. Kumagai K, Hiyama K, Ishioka S, et al. Allelotype frequency of the thiopurine methyltransferase (TPMT) gene in Japanese. Pharmacogenetics 2001; 11(3):275–8.

35. Lennard L, Van Loon JA, Weinshilboum RM. Pharmacogenetics of acute azathioprine toxicity: relationship to thiopurine methyltransferase genetic polymorphism. Clin Pharmacol Ther 1989;46(2):149–54.

36. Anstey A, Lennard L, Mayou SC, et al. Pancytopenia related to azathioprine–an enzyme deficiency caused by a common genetic polymorphism: a review. J R Soc Med 1992;85(12):752–6.

37. Sumi S, Marinaki AM, Arenas M, et al. Genetic basis of inosine triphosphate pyrophosphohydrolase deficiency. Hum Genet 2002;111(4–5):360–7.

38. Carney DM, Zukoski CF, Ogden DA. Massive azathioprine overdose. Case report and review of the literature. Am J Med 1974;56(1):133–6.

39. Silman AJ, Petrie J, Hazleman B, et al. Lymphoproliferative cancer and other malignancy in patients with rheumatoid arthritis treated with azathioprine: a 20 year follow up study. Ann Rheum Dis 1988; 47(12):988–92.

40. Ramsay HM, Fryer AA, Hawley CM, et al. Non-melanoma skin cancer risk in the Queensland renal transplant population. Br J Dermatol 2002;147(5): 950–6.

41. O'Donovan P, Perrett CM, Zhang X, et al. Azathioprine and UVA light generate mutagenic oxidative DNA damage. Science 2005;309:1871–4.

42. Hemmens VJ, Moore DE. Photochemical sensitization by azathioprine and its metabolites–I. 6-Mercaptopurine. Photochem Photobiol 1986;43(3): 247–55.

43. Reeve VE, Greenoak GE, Gallagher CH, et al. Effect of immunosuppressive agents and sunscreens on UV carcinogenesis in the hairless mouse. Aust J Exp Biol Med Sci 1985;63(Pt 6):655–65.

44. van Dijk TJ, van Velde JL. Treatment of pemphigus and pemphigoid with azathioprine. Dermatologica 1973;147(3):179–85.

45. Burton JL, Greaves MW. Azathioprine for pemphigus and pemphigoid–a 4 year follow-up. Br J Dermatol 1974;91(1):103–9.

46. Ahmed AR, Maize JC, Provost TT. Bullous pemphigoid. Clinical and immunologic follow-up after successful therapy. Arch Dermatol 1977;113(8):1043–6.

47. Burton JL, Greaves MW, Marks J, et al. Azathioprine in pemphigus vulgaris. BMJ 1970;3(5714):84–6.

48. Roenigk HH Jr, Deodhar S. Pemphigus treatment with azathioprine. Clinical and immunologic correlation. Arch Dermatol 1973;107(3):353–7.

49. Lever WF, Schaumburg-Lever G. Treatment of pemphigus vulgaris. Results obtained in 84 patients between 1961 and 1982. Arch Dermatol 1984;120(1):44–7.

50. Tan-Lim R, Bystryn JC. Effect of plasmapheresis therapy on circulating levels of pemphigus antibodies. J Am Acad Dermatol 1990;22(1):35–40.

51. Mourellou O, Chaidemenos GC, Koussidou T, et al. The treatment of pemphigus vulgaris. Experience with 48 patients seen over an 11-year period. Br J Dermatol 1995;133(1):83–7.

52. Carson PJ, Hameed A, Ahmed AR. Influence of treatment on the clinical course of pemphigus vulgaris. J Am Acad Dermatol 1996;34(4):645–52.

53. Scully C, Paes De Almeida O, Porter SR, et al. Pemphigus vulgaris: the manifestations and long-term management of 55 patients with oral lesions. Br J Dermatol 1999;140(1):84–9.

54. Ljubojević S, Lipozencić J, Brenner S, et al. Pemphigus vulgaris: a review of treatment over a 19-year period. J Eur Acad Dermatol Venereol 2002;16(6):599–603.

55. Chaidemenos G, Apalla Z, Koussidou T, et al. High dose oral prednisone vs. prednisone plus azathioprine for the treatment of oral pemphigus: a retrospective, bi-centre, comparative study. J Eur Acad Dermatol Venereol 2011;25(2):206–10.

56. Dantzig P. Circulating antibodies in cicatricial pemphigoid. Arch Dermatol 1973;108(2):264–6.

57. Braun-Falco O, Wolff HH, Ponce E. Disseminated cicatricial pemphigoid. Hautarzt 1981;32(5):233–9.

58. Mondino BJ, Brown SI. Immunosuppressive therapy in ocular cicatricial pemphigoid. Am J Ophthalmol 1983;96(4):453–9.

59. Pawlofsky C, Simon M Jr, Fartasch M, et al. Disseminated cicatricial pemphigoid. Dermatologica 1985;171(4):259–63.

60. Tauber J, Sainz de la Maza M, Foster CS. Systemic chemotherapy for ocular cicatricial pemphigoid. Cornea 1991;10(3):185–95.

61. Lugović L, Buljan M, Situm M, et al. Unrecognized cicatricial pemphigoid with oral manifestations and ocular complications. A case report. Acta Dermatovenerol Croat 2007;15(4):236–42.

62. Harrington I, Sneddon IB, Walker AE. Pemphigus vulgaris in a 15-year-old girl. Acta Derm Venereol 1978;58(3):277–9.

63. Lynde CW, Ongley RC, Rigg JM. Juvenile pemphigus vulgaris. Arch Dermatol 1984;120(8):1098–9.

64. Fine JD, Appell ML, Green LK, et al. Pemphigus vulgaris. Combined treatment with intravenous corticosteroid pulse therapy, plasmapheresis, and azathioprine. Arch Dermatol 1988;124(2):236–9.

65. Wananukul S, Pongprasit P. Childhood pemphigus. Int J Dermatol 1999;38(1):29–35.

66. Harangi F, Várszegi D, Schneider I, et al. Complete recovery from juvenile pemphigus vulgaris. Pediatr Dermatol 2001;18(1):51–3.

Mycophenolate Mofetil for the Management of Autoimmune Bullous Diseases

Marina Eskin-Schwartz, MD, PhD[a,b], Michael David, MD[a,b], Daniel Mimouni, MD[a,b],*

KEYWORDS

- Mycophenolate mofetil • Autoimmune bullous diseases
- Immunosuppression • Mycophenolic acid

Mycophenolate mofetil (MMF) is the 2-morpholinoethyl ester of mycophenolic acid (MPA), one of the several phenol compounds first described by Alsberg and Black in 1913 in cultures of *Penicillium stoloniferum*. MPA has been found to inhibit DNA synthesis by selectively inhibiting inosine monophosphate dehydrogenase (IMPDH), an enzyme that catalyzes the rate-limiting step in the de novo biosynthesis of guanine nucleotides (reviewed in Ref.[1]). MPA targets mainly T and B lymphocytes which, unlike other cell types, are dependent almost exclusively on the de novo guanine nucleotide synthesis pathway for proliferation and differentiation.[2] MPA is a fivefold more potent inhibitor of the IMPDH II isoform specific to lymphocytes than of the housekeeping IMPDH I isoform, found in most cell types.[3] MMF inhibits T and B cell proliferation,[4] induces apoptosis of T cells,[5] and inhibits antibody production by B cells.[6]

Besides its antiproliferative effect on lymphocytes, MMF has several other mechanisms of action. Guanosine triphosphate (GTP) depletion caused by MMF impairs fucosylation and surface expression of adhesion molecules of lymphocytes and monocytes, preventing their attachment to endothelial cells during their recruitment to inflammation sites.[7,8] As monocytes and macrophages are major producers of proinflammatory cytokines causing fibroblast recruitment and proliferation at the inflammation site (such as tumor necrosis factor α and interleukin-1), their depletion reduces production of these cytokines, inhibiting fibroblast proliferation and tissue fibrosis.[9] MPA was shown to inhibit the surface expression of antigens responsible for maturation and efficient antigen presentation by dendritic cells, thereby suppressing immune responses.[10,11] GTP depletion also impairs inducible nitric oxide synthase (iNOS) activity, which leads to a reduction of the oxidative stress caused by activated monocytes, macrophages, and endothelial cells.[12]

MMF has 94% oral bioavailability.[13] Following absorption MMF is converted to its active metabolite, MPA, by plasma, liver, and kidney esterases. MPA is almost completely inactivated in the liver by glucuronyl transferase,[14] and a significant portion of MPA-glucuronide (MPAG) is secreted into the bile and recycled via enterohepatic

Disclosure: The authors have no financial interest in this article.
[a] Department of Dermatology, Rabin Medical Center, Beilinson Campus, Jabotinski Street 39, Petah Tiqwa 49100, Israel
[b] Department of Dermatology, Sackler Faculty of Medicine, Tel Aviv University, PO Box 39040, Tel Aviv 69978, Israel
* Corresponding author. Department of Dermatology, Rabin Medical Center, Beilinson Campus, Jabotinski Street 39, Petah Tiqwa 49100, Israel.
E-mail address: mimouni@post.tau.ac.il

recirculation. MPAG is converted back to MPA by β-glucuronidase, found mainly in the epidermis and the gastrointestinal tract. The peak plasma level of the drug is reached in less than 1 hour; the elimination rate is 18 hours. A secondary MPA peak occurs at 6 to 12 hours, due to the enterohepatic circulation.[15] Ninety-seven percent of MPA is albumin bound. Most of the drug is excreted as MPAG in the urine.[13]

The most common side effects of MMF are nausea, vomiting, abdominal cramps, and diarrhea, reported in 12% to 36% of patients.[16] All are dose dependent. Hematologic side effects, also dose dependent and reversible upon discontinuation of the drug, include leukopenia, neutropenia, and thrombocytopenia. There are reports of genitourinary side effects of urgency, frequency, dysuria, and sterile pyuria, which generally resolve with continued drug use.[17] Neurologic complaints (headache, tinnitus, and insomnia), rash, and cardiovascular effects (peripheral edema and hypertension) have also been described. MPA/MMF treatment has been associated with an increased incidence of both bacterial and viral infections (especially herpes zoster[17,18] and cytomegalovirus[19–21]). Of importance, a risk of cytomegalovirus infection has been reported in organ transplant patients given MPA/MMF, concomitantly treated with other immunosuppressive agents. The ability of MMF to induce malignancy is controversial. MMF is expected to be less carcinogenic than azathioprine because it is not incorporated into the DNA and does not cause chromosomal breaks.[22] Some studies reported a dose-dependent increase in the risk of lymphoproliferative malignancy in MMF-treated organ transplant patients,[23–25] but this finding was not supported in a comparative study of MMF-based and other immunosuppressive regimens in renal transplant patients.[26] In dermatologic literature an early report described 3 cases of malignancy during MMF treatment in psoriatic patients.[27] Subsequently, Epinette and colleagues[17] found no increase in the incidence of cancer in psoriatic patients treated with MMF.

A limited number of cases reports suggested MMF could cause fetal malformations in humans.[27,28] MMF is classified as pregnancy category D (ie, there is positive evidence of human fetal risk based on adverse reaction data from investigational or marketing experience or studies in humans, but potential benefits may warrant use of the drug in pregnant women despite potential risks), and therefore it is recommended to use two different reliable methods of birth control 4 weeks before starting and during MMF therapy, and continue birth control for 6 weeks after stopping MMF.

Several drugs are known to interact with MMF via mechanisms of absorption inhibition (antacids), disruption of enterohepatic recirculation (antibiotics, cholestyramine), albumin binding (phenytoin, salicylic acid), and prevention of kidney tubular secretion of MPA (acyclovir, gancyclovir, probenecid).[29,30]

MPA was first used in dermatology in the 1970s as an anti-inflammatory agent to treat moderate to severe psoriasis.[31,32] However, by the end of the decade its use was discontinued owing to its gastrointestinal side effects, increased risk of latent viral infections, and possible carcinogenicity.[27] A decade later MMF, the 2-morpholinoethyl ester of MPA, received approval from the from the Food and Drug Administration as an immunosuppressive agent in renal transplant patients, with studies showing that it had better oral bioavailability than MPA and caused fewer gastrointestinal side effects. Owing to its long-term safety and tolerability, it began to be applied in other fields, including dermatology.

Autoimmune bullous diseases are a group of blistering disorders that share a pathogenetic mechanism of autoantibody production against different epidermal and dermoepidermal junction proteins. High-dose steroids are the traditional first-line treatment, but their multiple and potentially severe side effects with prolonged use have prompted dermatologists to seek alternative or steroid-sparing agents. Today, immunosuppressive agents such as azathioprine, cyclophosphamide, and MMF are widely used in the treatment of these diseases.

The initial evidence of the benefit of MMF for pemphigus stems from several case series, reporting the efficacy of MMF as a steroid-sparing agent.

Enk and Knop[33] combined MMF (2 g/d) with prednisolone (2 mg/kg/d) in 12 patients with pemphigus vulgaris, who had relapsed during azathioprine and prednisolone therapy. Eleven patients responded to this therapy, with no relapses during the 9- to 12-month follow-up period. A similar regimen was applied by Chams-Davatchi and colleagues[34] in 10 patients with pemphigus vulgaris with severe resistant/recurrent disease. The lesions completely cleared in 9 patients by 6 to 16 weeks. Five patients relapsed after MMF discontinuation at 6 months' follow-up, suggesting MMF should be administered for a longer period to sustain remission. Several years later, a large historical prospective trial was conducted that included 31 patients with pemphigus vulgaris and 11 patients with pemphigus foliaceus, who had relapsed on prednisone therapy or had had adverse effects from previous drug therapy.[35] Treatment with MMF (35–45 mg/kg) combined with prednisone led to complete remission in 71% of the pemphigus vulgaris group and 45% of the pemphigus foliaceus group. Mean time to remission was 9 months, and the remission was maintained throughout the 22 months of follow-up.

Powell and colleagues[36] reported treating 16 refractory pemphigus vulgaris and pemphigus foliaceus patients with MMF (starting at 500 mg/d and increasing as tolerated) and prednisone. Clinically inactive disease was achieved in 7 patients. The much lower doses of prednisone at the time of MMF initiation in this study are noteworthy, and may explain the relatively low rate of clinical remission.

In a prospective study of MMF as first-line treatment, Esmaili and colleagues[37] administered MMF (2 g/d) and prednisolone (2 mg/kg/d) to 31 patients with pemphigus vulgaris, with a 12-month follow-up. MMF was beneficial in 21 patients (67.7%), and its addition made it possible to taper down the prednisolone, suggesting its value as a steroid-sparing agent. A more recent prospective controlled trial was conducted by Beissert and colleagues,[38] who randomized 96 patients with mild to moderate pemphigus vulgaris to receive MMF (2–3 g/d) plus prednisolone or placebo plus prednisolone. At the end of the 52-week follow-up, a similar treatment response rate was observed in the two groups. The patients given MMF showed faster and more durable responses, but this difference may have been attributable to the milder disease of the placebo group, which may not have needed the additional immunosuppressive therapy. In all the aforementioned studies the MMF therapy was well tolerated. The most common side effects were gastrointestinal complaints, lymphopenia, and bacterial and viral infections.[33–38]

MMF/mycophenolate sodium monotherapy for pemphigus vulgaris has shown variable success in several case series.[39,40]

Several randomized open-label trials compared the efficacy of MMF as a steroid-sparing agent with other immunosuppressive drugs in patients with pemphigus. Beissert and colleagues[41] treated 40 patients with pemphigus vulgaris or pemphigus foliaceus with methylprednisolone and azathioprine or methylprednisolone and MMF. There was no difference between MMF and azathioprine in efficacy, steroid-sparing effect, or safety profile.

In a random controlled study Chams-Davatchi and colleagues[42] compared 4 treatment regimens in 120 patients with pemphigus vulgaris: prednisolone only, prednisolone and azathioprine, prednisolone and MMF, and prednisolone and intravenous cyclophosphamide pulse therapy. There was no difference in complete remission rate between the groups (70%–80% of patients).

All immunosuppressive drugs had a steroid-sparing effect; the most efficacious was azathioprine, followed by pulse cyclophosphamide and then MMF.

A few patients with paraneoplastic pemphigus were reported to benefit from combined immunosuppressive regimens, including MMF and corticosteroids[36] or MMF, corticosteroids, and azathioprine.[43]

Several case reports suggested that MMF, alone or combined with corticosteroids, is effective for the treatment of bullous pemphigoid.[39,44,45]

A large, prospective, randomized trial of 73 patients with bullous pemphigoid found MMF to be equally efficacious to azathioprine in inducing disease remission (100%) when combined with corticosteroids.[46] Although the average time to complete remission was shorter in the azathioprine-treated group, the MMF group had less liver toxicity.

Enteric-coated mycophenolate sodium (EC-MPS)/ MMF has also been used as a steroid-sparing agent[47,48] or in combination with dapsone[49] for the treatment of cicatricial pemphigoid. Two retrospective studies addressed the role of MMF in the treatment of ocular cicatricial pemphigoid. Daniel and colleagues[50] reported successful control of eye inflammation at 1 year in 70% of 18 patients treated with MMF and prednisone. Saw and colleagues[51] retrospectively compared various immunosuppressive drugs in 115 patients with ocular cicatricial pemphigoid, and found cyclophosphamide to be more successful (69%) than mycophenolate (59%) in controlling the inflammation. However, mycophenolate had the fewest side effects of all the drugs used in the study.

MMF has shown variable success in individual patients with epidermolysis bullosa acquisita.[52–54] Similarly, several case reports suggested that MMF and EC-MPS were effective for the treatment of refractory linear IgA disease[55–57] and linear IgA bullous dermatosis of childhood.[58]

In summary, MMF is an immunosuppressive drug widely used today in multiple fields of medicine, including dermatology. Advantages of MMF include its wide therapeutic index, mild side effects, and lack of major end-organ toxicity. MMF has been successfully applied for the treatment of various autoimmune blistering diseases, including pemphigus, bullous pemphigoid, and cicatricial pemphigoid, mostly as a steroid-sparing agent. According to numerous case series, MMF could be of value in treating refractory disease. The few randomized clinical trials conducted to date of patients with pemphigus and bullous pemphigoid report a similar efficacy for MMF to other immunosuppressants. Large-scale clinical trials are needed to further delineate the value of MMF in this setting.

REFERENCES

1. Allison AC. Mechanisms of action of mycophenolate mofetil. Lupus 2005;14(Suppl 1):s2–8.
2. Allison AC, Eugui EM. Immunosuppressive and other effects of mycophenolic acid and an ester pro-drug, mycophenolate mofetil. Immunol Rev 1993; 136:5–28.
3. Carr SF, Papp E, Wu JC, et al. Characterization of human type I and type II IMP dehydrogenases. J Biol Chem 1993;268:27286–90.
4. Allison AC, Eugui EM. Mycophenolate mofetil and its mechanisms of action. Immunopharmacology 2000; 47:85–118.
5. Cohn RG, Mirkovich A, Dunlap B, et al. Mycophenolic acid increases apoptosis, lysosomes and lipid droplets in human lymphoid and monocytic cell lines. Transplantation 1999;68:411–8.
6. Allison AC, Almquist SJ, Muller CD, et al. In vitro immunosuppressive effects of mycophenolic acid and an ester pro-drug, RS-61443. Transplant Proc 1991;23:10–4.
7. Allison AC, Kowalski WJ, Muller CJ, et al. Mycophenolic acid and brequinar, inhibitors of purine and pyrimidine synthesis, block the glycosylation of adhesion molecules. Transplant Proc 1993;25: 67–70.
8. Blaheta RA, Leckel K, Wittig B, et al. Mycophenolate mofetil impairs transendothelial migration of allogeneic CD4 and CD8 T-cells. Transplant Proc 1999; 31:1250–2.
9. Morath C, Schwenger V, Beimler J, et al. Antifibrotic actions of mycophenolic acid. Clin Transplant 2006; 20(Suppl 17):25–9.
10. Colic M, Stojic-Vukanic Z, Pavlovic B, et al. Mycophenolate mofetil inhibits differentiation, maturation and allostimulatory function of human monocyte-derived dendritic cells. Clin Exp Immunol 2003; 134:63–9.
11. Lagaraine C, Lebranchu Y. Effects of immunosuppressive drugs on dendritic cells and tolerance induction. Transplantation 2003;75:37S–42S.
12. Senda M, DeLustro B, Eugui E, et al. Mycophenolic acid, an inhibitor of IMP dehydrogenase that is also an immunosuppressive agent, suppresses the cytokine-induced nitric oxide production in mouse and rat vascular endothelial cells. Transplantation 1995;60:1143–8.
13. Bullingham RE, Nicholls AJ, Kamm BR. Clinical pharmacokinetics of mycophenolate mofetil. Clin Pharm 1998;34:429–55.
14. Sweeney MJ. Mycophenolic acid and its mechanism of action in cancer and psoriasis. Jpn J Antibiot 1977;30(Suppl):85–92.
15. Bullingham R, Monroe S, Nicholls A, et al. Pharmacokinetics and bioavailability of mycophenolate mofetil in healthy subjects after single-dose oral and intravenous administration. J Clin Pharmacol 1996; 36:315–24.
16. Hoffman-La Roche Ltd. Cellcept (mycophenolate mofetil); 1997 [package insert]. Available at: http://www.gene.com/gene/products/information/cellcept/pdf/pi.pdf. Accessed June 24, 2011.
17. Epinette WW, Parker CM, Jones EL, et al. Mycophenolic acid for psoriasis. A review of pharmacology, long-term efficacy, and safety. J Am Acad Dermatol 1987;17:962–71.
18. Simmons WD, Rayhill SC, Sollinger HW. Preliminary risk-benefit assessment of mycophenolate mofetil in transplant rejection. Drug Saf 1997;17:75–92.
19. Hambach L, Stadler M, Dammann E, et al. Increased risk of complicated CMV infection with the use of mycophenolate mofetil in allogeneic stem cell transplantation. Bone Marrow Transplant 2002;29:903–6.
20. Sarmiento JM, Dockrell DH, Schwab TR, et al. Mycophenolate mofetil increases cytomegalovirus invasive organ disease in renal transplant patients. Clin Transplant 2000;14:136–8.
21. ter Meulen CG, Wetzels JF, Hilbrands LB. The influence of mycophenolate mofetil on the incidence and severity of primary cytomegalovirus infections and disease after renal transplantation. Nephrol Dial Transplant 2000;15:711–4.
22. Kitchin JE, Pomeranz MK, Pak G, et al. Rediscovering mycophenolic acid: a review of its mechanism, side effects, and potential uses. J Am Acad Dermatol 1997;37:445–9.
23. Mycophenolate mofetil in cadaveric renal transplantation. US Renal Transplant Mycophenolate Mofetil Study Group. Am J Kidney Dis 1999;34:296–303.
24. Mathew TH. A blinded, long-term, randomized multi-center study of mycophenolate mofetil in cadaveric renal transplantation: results at three years. Tricontinental Mycophenolate Mofetil Renal Transplantation Study Group. Transplantation 1998;65:1450–4.
25. Mycophenolate mofetil in renal transplantation: 3-year results from the placebo-controlled trial. European Mycophenolate Mofetil Cooperative Study Group. Transplantation 1999;68:391–6.
26. Robson R, Cecka JM, Opelz G, et al. Prospective registry-based observational cohort study of the long-term risk of malignancies in renal transplant patients treated with mycophenolate mofetil. Am J Transplant 2005;5:2954–60.
27. Lynch WS, Roenigk HH Jr. Mycophenolic acid for psoriasis. Arch Dermatol 1977;113:1203–8.
28. Anderka MT, Lin AE, Abuelo DN, et al. Reviewing the evidence for mycophenolate mofetil as a new teratogen: case report and review of the literature. Am J Med Genet A 2009;149A:1241–8.
29. Perlis C, Pan T, McDonald C. Cytotoxic agents. In: Wolverton S, editor. Comprehensive dermatologic drug therapy. Philadelphia: Elsevier; 2007. p. 1099.

30. Gimenez F, Foeillet E, Bourdon O, et al. Evaluation of pharmacokinetic interactions after oral administration of mycophenolate mofetil and valaciclovir or aciclovir to healthy subjects. Clin Pharm 2004; 43:685–92.

31. Jones EL, Epinette WW, Hackney VC, et al. Treatment of psoriasis with oral mycophenolic acid. J Invest Dermatol 1975;65:537–42.

32. Gomez EC, Menendez L, Frost P. Efficacy of mycophenolic acid for the treatment of psoriasis. J Am Acad Dermatol 1979;1:531–7.

33. Enk AH, Knop J. Mycophenolate is effective in the treatment of pemphigus vulgaris. Arch Dermatol 1999;135:54–6.

34. Chams-Davatchi C, Nonahal Azar R, Daneshpazooh M, et al. Open trial of mycophenolate mofetil in the treatment of resistant pemphigus vulgaris. Ann Dermatol Venereol 2002;129:23–5 [in French].

35. Mimouni D, Anhalt GJ, Cummins DL, et al. Treatment of pemphigus vulgaris and pemphigus foliaceus with mycophenolate mofetil. Arch Dermatol 2003; 139:739–42.

36. Powell AM, Albert S, Al Fares S, et al. An evaluation of the usefulness of mycophenolate mofetil in pemphigus. Br J Dermatol 2003;149:138–45.

37. Esmaili N, Chams-Davatchi C, Valikhani M, et al. Treatment of pemphigus vulgaris with mycophenolate mofetil as a steroid-sparing agent. Eur J Dermatol 2008;18:159–64.

38. Beissert S, Mimouni D, Kanwar AJ, et al. Treating pemphigus vulgaris with prednisone and mycophenolate mofetil: a multicenter, randomized, placebo-controlled trial. J Invest Dermatol 2010; 130:2041–8.

39. Grundmann-Kollmann M, Korting HC, Behrens S, et al. Mycophenolate mofetil: a new therapeutic option in the treatment of blistering autoimmune diseases. J Am Acad Dermatol 1999;40:957–60.

40. Baskan EB, Yilmaz M, Tunali S, et al. Efficacy and safety of long-term mycophenolate sodium therapy in pemphigus vulgaris. J Eur Acad Dermatol Venereol 2009;23:1432–4.

41. Beissert S, Werfel T, Frieling U, et al. A comparison of oral methylprednisolone plus azathioprine or mycophenolate mofetil for the treatment of pemphigus. Arch Dermatol 2006;142:1447–54.

42. Chams-Davatchi C, Esmaili N, Daneshpazhooh M, et al. Randomized controlled open-label trial of four treatment regimens for pemphigus vulgaris. J Am Acad Dermatol 2007;57:622–8.

43. Williams JV, Marks JG Jr, Billingsley EM. Use of mycophenolate mofetil in the treatment of paraneoplastic pemphigus. Br J Dermatol 2000;142: 506–8.

44. Bohm M, Beissert S, Schwarz T, et al. Bullous pemphigoid treated with mycophenolate mofetil. Lancet 1997;349:541.

45. Nousari HC, Griffin WA, Anhalt GJ. Successful therapy for bullous pemphigoid with mycophenolate mofetil. J Am Acad Dermatol 1998;39:497–8.

46. Beissert S, Werfel T, Frieling U, et al. A comparison of oral methylprednisolone plus azathioprine or mycophenolate mofetil for the treatment of bullous pemphigoid. Arch Dermatol 2007;143:1536–42.

47. Megahed M, Schmiedeberg S, Becker J, et al. Treatment of cicatricial pemphigoid with mycophenolate mofetil as a steroid-sparing agent. J Am Acad Dermatol 2001;45:256–9.

48. Marzano AV, Dassoni F, Caputo R. Treatment of refractory blistering autoimmune diseases with mycophenolic acid. J Dermatolog Treat 2006;17:370–6.

49. Ingen-Housz-Oro S, Prost-Squarcioni C, Pascal F, et al. Cicatricial pemphigoid: treatment with mycophenolate mofetil. Ann Dermatol Venereol 2005; 132:13–6 [in French].

50. Daniel E, Thorne JE, Newcomb CW, et al. Mycophenolate mofetil for ocular inflammation. Am J Ophthalmol 2010;149:423–32.

51. Saw VP, Dart JK, Rauz S, et al. Immunosuppressive therapy for ocular mucous membrane pemphigoid strategies and outcomes. Ophthalmology 2008;115: 253–61.

52. Schattenkirchner S, Eming S, Hunzelmann N, et al. Treatment of epidermolysis bullosa acquisita with mycophenolate mofetil and autologous keratinocyte grafting. Br J Dermatol 1999;141:932–3.

53. Kowalzick L, Suckow S, Ziegler H, et al. Mycophenolate mofetil in epidermolysis bullosa acquisita. Dermatology 2003;207:332–4.

54. Tran MM, Anhalt GJ, Barrett T, et al. Childhood IgA-mediated epidermolysis bullosa acquisita responding to mycophenolate mofetil as a corticosteroid-sparing agent. J Am Acad Dermatol 2006;54:734–6.

55. Talhari C, Mahnke N, Ruzicka T, et al. Successful treatment of linear IgA disease with mycophenolate mofetil as a corticosteroid sparing agent. Clin Exp Dermatol 2005;30:297–8.

56. Lewis MA, Yaqoob NA, Emanuel C, et al. Successful treatment of oral linear IgA disease using mycophenolate. Oral Surg Oral Med Oral Pathol Oral Radiol Endod 2007;103:483–6.

57. Marzano AV, Ramoni S, Spinelli D, et al. Refractory linear IgA bullous dermatosis successfully treated with mycophenolate sodium. J Dermatolog Treat 2008;19:364–7.

58. Farley-Li J, Mancini AJ. Treatment of linear IgA bullous dermatosis of childhood with mycophenolate mofetil. Arch Dermatol 2003;139:1121–4.

Dapsone in the Management of Autoimmune Bullous Diseases

Evan W. Piette, MD[a], Victoria P. Werth, MD[a,b],*

KEYWORDS
• Dapsone • Autoimmune bullous disease • Review

Dapsone is a sulfone-derived medication that was first used in humans to treat leprosy in the 1940s.[1] Since then, it has been used as an antimicrobial agent and has been found to have antiinflammatory properties. Dapsone is used in several dermatologic conditions, particularly those with neutrophil predominance because it inhibits neutrophil activation and recruitment through several different pathways.[1] Dapsone has also been used in the treatment of the autoimmune bullous diseases (AIBD), a group of disorders resulting from autoimmunity directed against basement membrane and/or intercellular adhesion molecules on cutaneous and mucosal surfaces.[2] This review summarizes the published data evaluating dapsone as a therapy for AIBD. Common adverse effects of this medication include methemoglobinemia and anemia, particularly in patients who are glucose-6-phosphate dehydrogenase deficient. There are also several additional rare adverse effects associated with dapsone use, notably agranulocytosis and a hypersensitivity reaction known as the dapsone syndrome.[1,2]

PEMPHIGUS

Pemphigus is an antibody-mediated blistering disease that primarily affects the elderly and is associated with high morbidity and, when untreated, mortality. Two subtypes of pemphigus are reviewed here: pemphigus vulgaris (PV) and pemphigus foliaceus (PF). Immunosuppressives are the mainstay of treatment of PV, and dapsone was first reported as an adjunct to therapy in the 1960s.[3] There has been 1 randomized, double-blind, placebo-controlled trial evaluating the use of dapsone for PV.[4,5] In this study by Werth and colleagues,[4] 19 patients receiving systemic immunosuppressive therapy for PV were randomized to 2 groups treated with the addition of either dapsone or placebo. Success was defined by the ability to taper systemic glucocorticoids to at least 7.5 mg/d within 1 year of reaching the maximum dose of dapsone (200 mg/d). Of the 9 patients receiving dapsone, 5 (56%) were successfully treated, 3 failed treatment, and 1 dropped out of the study. Of the 10 patients receiving placebo, 3 (30%) were successfully treated and 7 failed treatment. Although the difference between groups was not significant ($P = .37$), the trend favored the dapsone-treated group. In addition, 4 patients in the placebo group failed treatment and were switched to treatment with dapsone. Of these, 3 (75%) were successfully treated after initiating dapsone. Overall, 8 of 11 patients (73%) receiving dapsone versus 3 of 10 (30%) receiving placebo reached the primary outcome measure of 7.5 mg/d or less of prednisone. No adverse events requiring the discontinuation of dapsone were noted.[4]

The remaining published data on dapsone for pemphigus stem from case reports and series,

Funding: National Institutes of Health, including NIH K24-AR 02207 (V.P.W.).
[a] Department of Dermatology, Perelman Center for Advanced Medicine, Suite 1-330A, 3400 Civic Center Boulevard, Philadelphia, PA 19104, USA
[b] Division of Dermatology, Philadelphia V.A. Medical Center, Philadelphia, PA, USA
* Corresponding author. Department of Dermatology, Perelman Center for Advanced Medicine, Suite 1-330A, 3400 Civic Center Boulevard, Philadelphia, PA 19104.
E-mail address: werth@mail.med.upenn.edu

nicely summarized in a 2009 review by Gürcan and Ahmed.[6] In their review, the investigators found 12 reports, in addition to the trial by Werth and colleagues[4] discussed earlier, describing an additional 26 patients who received dapsone for treatment of their PV.[6] In these additional cases, at dosages varying between 50 and 200 mg/d, 24 of the 26 (92%) patients responded to dapsone alone or in addition to other systemic immunomodulators. In 16 of these reported cases, dapsone was added to prednisone presumably as a steroid-sparing agent, although this was not explicitly stated in every study. In 10 of these 16 patients (63%), prednisone doses were reduced after initiation of dapsone. In 6 of 16 patients (38%), prednisone dosages could not be decreased because of either continued disease or adverse events associated with dapsone. Overall, dapsone was discontinued because of adverse effects in only 4 of the 26 (15%) patients, 3 secondary to hemolysis and 1 secondary to dapsone syndrome.[6]

PF causes disease similar to PV, with the key clinical difference being that mucosal surfaces are spared in PF. Of the 10 published reports summarized by Gürcan and colleagues,[6] 9 are reports of dapsone use in only a single patient. Basset and colleagues[7] reported 9 additional patients with PF treated with dapsone in a case series published in 1987. Of the total 18 patients reported in the literature, 14 (78%) responded to dapsone at doses of 25 to 300 mg/d alone or in combination with systemic prednisone.[6] Of the 18 patients, 6 had adverse events (33%) and 2 (11%) required discontinuation of dapsone therapy (one patient because of peripheral neuropathy and the other because of dapsone-induced hypersensitivity).[6]

PEMPHIGOID

Bullous pemphigoid (BP) affects both mucosal and cutaneous surfaces. In contrast to PV, BP may remit spontaneously and can often be treated with lower doses of immunosuppressives.[2] A Cochrane review published in 2010 did not identify any randomized controlled trials evaluating dapsone as a therapy for BP.[8] The 2009 review by Gürcan and Ahmed[6] summarized the available case series and concluded that there are at least 6 published studies encompassing 170 patients with BP who received dapsone. Of these patients, 139 (81%) showed clinical improvement with 50 to 300 mg/d of dapsone alone or in combination with immunosuppressives. Adverse effects developed in 63 patients (37%), and 9 (5%) required discontinuation of the drug.[6]

Mucous membrane pemphigoid (MMP) differs from BP in that it is limited to mucosal surfaces. A randomized, double-blind, non–placebo-controlled trial published in 1986 compared 40 patients with ocular MMP treated for 6 months with either dapsone (2 mg/kg/d) or cyclophosphamide (2 mg/kg/d).[9,10] Cyclophosphamide was found to be superior to dapsone in this group of patients because all 20 patients (100%) treated with cyclophosphamide responded to the drug compared with 14 of 20 (70%) in the dapsone group.[9,10] The remaining data investigating dapsone for MMP are from nonrandomized studies and reports. In the Gürcan review, 6 additional publications encompassing 182 patients with MMP treated with dapsone are discussed.[6] Of the 182 patients, 156 (86%) showed improvement with dapsone therapy. Twenty patients (11%) developed adverse effects that required discontinuation of dapsone.[6]

BULLOUS LUPUS ERYTHEMATOSUS

Bullous lupus erythematosus is a subtype of acute cutaneous lupus erythematosus (ACLE) characterized by subepidermal vesiculobullous skin lesions. Dapsone is occasionally used as an adjunctive treatment of cutaneous lupus erythematosus and is thought to be particularly useful in patients with bullous disease.[11] However, there is a dearth of studies in the literature evaluating its use, and published data are largely anecdotal. There are at least 19 patients with bullous ACLE reported in 12 case reports and series, and 17 (89%) showed improvement in their bullous lesions within days to weeks of initiation of 50 to 100 mg/d of dapsone therapy.[12–23] One of the 2 patients reported as a nonresponder had progression of disease after a week of dapsone 50 mg/d, but developed abnormal liver enzymes when the dose was increased to 100 mg/d requiring discontinuation of therapy.[18] Thus, it is difficult to determine whether dapsone may have been effective in this patient at a higher dose. Of the 17 patients reported as improving with dapsone, at least 8 (42%) had failed systemic glucocorticoid therapy, which prompted the addition of dapsone.[12,15,16,21,23]

EPIDERMOLYSIS BULLOSA ACQUISTA

Epidermolysis bullosa acquista (EBA) is an autoimmune blistering disease characterized by IgG autoantibodies that target type VII collagen. It is a rare disease without sex or racial predilection and has a prevalence of approximately 0.2 per million people.[24] EBA is a notoriously difficult disease to treat and typically requires therapy with glucocorticoids and additional immunosuppressives such as methotrexate, mycophenolate, or azathioprine.[24] Dapsone is occasionally used as an adjunctive treatment; although similar to bullous ACLE, published reports regarding dapsone's effectiveness in adults are sparse.[10] Hughes and Callen[25] reported a patient who responded to dapsone 150 mg/d, after failing treatment with niacinamide, tetracycline, and systemic prednisone. Two single-patient case reports note improvement with the use of dapsone in combination with systemic steroids.[26,27] A report published from Vienna in 1988 noted improvement with dapsone and corticosteroids in 2 of 3 patients,[28] and a German study from 1994 reported a patient successfully treated with colchicine after failing to respond to dapsone.[29] Cunningham and colleagues[30] reported on a patient partially treated with colchicine who showed complete improvement after the addition of dapsone 50 mg/d. Overall, 6 of the 8 (75%) reported patients with EBA treated with dapsone responded to the medication.

DERMATITIS HERPETIFORMIS

Dermatitis herpetiformis (DH) is an inflammatory skin condition associated with celiac disease. It is primarily a disease of white skin, with a multifactorial cause involving both genetics and environmental triggers.[31] Because of the association with celiac disease, the definitive treatment of DH is a gluten-free diet,[32] with pharmacologic therapy used as an adjunct until the diet becomes effective. Dapsone has long been used as the first-line therapy in this capacity.[31,33,34] Like most of the blistering diseases discussed in this review, randomized controlled trials evaluating the efficacy of dapsone in DH are lacking, and currently published data are limited to small case series.[33–35] Nonetheless, there is strong expert consensus that dapsone is highly efficacious for the treatment of DH, and it remains the only medication approved by the US Food and Drug Administration for use in this disease.[31,36]

LINEAR IgA BULLOUS DERMATOSIS

Linear IgA bullous dermatosis (LABD) is an immunobullous disease that has been recognized as a unique entity since the 1980s.[37] Classically, LABD has features similar to BP and DH and can be distinguished by linear IgA deposition on direct immunofluorescence. Dapsone is regarded as the first-line therapy for LABD, but, as with DH, the evidence in adults is largely based on small case reports, case series, and anecdotal evidence.[37–41]

Treatment is generally started at low doses and is slowly titrated to a maintenance dose of 100 to 200 mg/d in adults.[37,41]

SUMMARY

Although dapsone is regularly used in the treatment of the AIBD, large studies evaluating its effectiveness and safety are lacking. Smaller studies and isolated reports do indicate that dapsone is effective, but, to truly determine the benefits and risks of using this medication, larger studies are needed. The best data available seem to be in MMP and PV because evidence from randomized controlled trials has been published. In addition, there seems to be wide consensus that dapsone should be the first-line pharmacologic therapy for DH and LABD. When used, the lowest effective dose should be prescribed up to a maximum of 200 mg/d, although doses up to 300 mg/d have been reported.[6] Before initiation of dapsone therapy, patients should be screened for glucose-6-phosphate dehydrogenase deficiency because patients with decreased activity of this enzyme show an approximately 2-fold increased sensitivity toward development of hemolysis.[1] In addition, a complete blood cell count with reticulocyte count should be checked weekly during the initial titration of dapsone dose, then every 2 weeks for the first 3 months, and then every 3 months after that for the development of hemolytic anemia and agranulocytosis. Liver enzymes, electrolytes, and urinalysis should also be monitored when using dapsone. Peripheral neuropathy, although rare, is a well-described adverse effect of dapsone, and periodic screening for both motor and sensory neuropathy is warranted.[1]

REFERENCES

1. Zhu YI, Stiller MJ. Dapsone and sulfones in dermatology: overview and update. J Am Acad Dermatol 2001;45(3):420–34.
2. Mutasim DF. Therapy of autoimmune bullous diseases. Ther Clin Risk Manag 2007;3(1):29–40.
3. Winkelmann RK, Roth HL. Dermatitis herpetiformis with acantholysis or pemphigus with response to sulfonamides: report of two cases. Arch Dermatol 1960;82:385–90.
4. Werth VP, Fivenson D, Pandya AG, et al. Multicenter randomized, double-blind, placebo-controlled, clinical trial of dapsone as a glucocorticoid-sparing agent in maintenance-phase pemphigus vulgaris. Arch Dermatol 2008;144(1):25–32.
5. Martin LK, Werth V, Villanueva E, et al. Interventions for pemphigus vulgaris and pemphigus foliaceus. Cochrane Database Syst Rev 2009;1:CD006263.

6. Gürcan HM, Ahmed AR. Efficacy of dapsone in the treatment of pemphigus and pemphigoid: analysis of current data. Am J Clin Dermatol 2009;10(6):383–96.

7. Basset N, Guillot B, Michel B, et al. Dapsone as initial treatment in superficial pemphigus. Report of nine cases. Arch Dermatol Jun 1987;123(6):783–5.

8. Kirtschig G, Middleton P, Bennett C, et al. Interventions for bullous pemphigoid. Cochrane Database Syst Rev 2010;10:CD002292.

9. Foster CS. Cicatricial pemphigoid. Trans Am Ophthalmol Soc 1986;84:527–663.

10. Kirtschig G, Murrell D, Wojnarowska F, et al. Interventions for mucous membrane pemphigoid/cicatricial pemphigoid and epidermolysis bullosa acquisita: a systematic literature review. Arch Dermatol 2002;138(3):380–4.

11. Walling HW, Sontheimer RD. Cutaneous lupus erythematosus: issues in diagnosis and treatment. Am J Clin Dermatol 2009;10(6):365–81.

12. Aboobaker J, Ramsaroop R, Abramowitz I, et al. Bullous systemic erythematosus. A case report. S Afr Med J 1986;69(1):49–51.

13. Alarcon GS, Sams WM Jr, Barton DD, et al. Bullous lupus erythematosus rash worsened by dapsone. Arthritis Rheum 1984;27(9):1071–2.

14. Burrows NP, Bhogal BS, Black MM, et al. Bullous eruption of systemic lupus erythematosus: a clinico-pathological study of four cases. Br J Dermatol 1993;128(3):332–8.

15. Fujimoto W, Hamada T, Yamada J, et al. Bullous systemic lupus erythematosus as an initial manifestation of SLE. J Dermatol 2005;32(12):1021–7.

16. Hall RP, Lawley TJ, Smith HR, et al. Bullous eruption of systemic lupus erythematosus. Dramatic response to dapsone therapy. Ann Intern Med 1982;97(2):165–70.

17. Ludgate MW, Greig DE. Bullous systemic lupus erythematosus responding to dapsone. Australas J Dermatol 2008;49(2):91–3.

18. Prystowsky JH, Finkel L, Tar L, et al. Bullous eruption in a woman with lupus erythematosus. Bullous systemic lupus erythematosus (SLE). Arch Dermatol 1988;124(4):571, 574–5.

19. Shirahama S, Yagi H, Furukawa F, et al. A case of bullous systemic lupus erythematosus. Dermatology 1994;189(Suppl 1):95–6.

20. Sirka CS, Padhi T, Mohanty P, et al. Bullous systemic lupus erythematosus: response to dapsone in two patients. Indian J Dermatol Venereol Leprol 2005; 71(1):54–6.

21. Tani M, Shimizu R, Ban M, et al. Systemic lupus erythematosus with vesiculobullous lesions. Immunoelectron microscopic studies. Arch Dermatol 1984; 120(11):1497–501.

22. Tay YK, Wong SN, Tan T. Bullous systemic lupus erythematosus—a case report and review. Ann Acad Med Singapore 1995;24(6):879–82.

23. Yung A, Oakley A. Bullous systemic lupus erythematosus. Australas J Dermatol 2000;41(4):234–7.

24. Ishii N, Hamada T, Dainichi T, et al. Epidermolysis bullosa acquisita: what's new? J Dermatol 2010; 37(3):220–30.

25. Hughes AP, Callen JP. Epidermolysis bullosa acquisita responsive to dapsone therapy. J Cutan Med Surg 2001;5(5):397–9.

26. Luke MC, Darling TN, Hsu R, et al. Mucosal morbidity in patients with epidermolysis bullosa acquisita. Arch Dermatol 1999;135(8):954–9.

27. Taniuchi K, Inaoki M, Nishimura Y, et al. Nonscarring inflammatory epidermolysis bullosa acquisita with esophageal involvement and linear IgG deposits. J Am Acad Dermatol 1997;36(2 Pt 2):320–2.

28. Rappersberger K, Konrad K, Schenk P, et al. Acquired epidermolysis bullosa. A clinico-pathologic study. Hautarzt 1988;39(6):355–62 [in German].

29. Megahed M, Scharffetter-Kochanek K. Epidermolysis bullosa acquisita—successful treatment with colchicine. Arch Dermatol Res 1994;286(1):35–46.

30. Cunningham BB, Kirchmann TT, Woodley D. Colchicine for epidermolysis bullosa acquisita. J Am Acad Dermatol 1996;34(5 Pt 1):781–4.

31. Caproni M, Antiga E, Melani L, et al. Guidelines for the diagnosis and treatment of dermatitis herpetiformis. J Eur Acad Dermatol Venereol 2009;23(6): 633–8.

32. Garioch JJ, Lewis HM, Sargent SA, et al. 25 years' experience of a gluten-free diet in the treatment of dermatitis herpetiformis. Br J Dermatol 1994;131(4): 541–5.

33. Alexander JO. Dapsone in the treatment of dermatitis herpetiformis. Lancet 1955;268(6876):1201–2.

34. Morgan JK, Marsden CW, Coburn JG, et al. Dapsone in dermatitis herpetiformis. Lancet 1955; 268(6876):1197–200.

35. DeMento FJ, Grover RW. Acantholytic herpetiform dermatitis. Arch Dermatol 1973;107(6):883–7.

36. Junkins-Hopkins JM. Dermatitis herpetiformis: pearls and pitfalls in diagnosis and management. J Am Acad Dermatol 2010;63(3):526–8.

37. Egan CA, Zone JJ. Linear IgA bullous dermatosis. Int J Dermatol 1999;38(11):818–27.

38. Provost TT, Maize JC, Ahmed AR, et al. Unusual subepidermal bullous diseases with immunologic features of bullous pemphigoid. Arch Dermatol 1979;115(2):156–60.

39. Wojnarowska F. Linear IgA dapsone responsive bullous dermatosis. J R Soc Med 1980;73(5): 371–3.

40. Long SA, Argenyi ZB, Piette WW. Arciform blistering in an elderly woman. Linear IgA dermatosis (LAD). Arch Dermatol 1988;124(11):1705, 1708.

41. Patricio P, Ferreira C, Gomes MM, et al. Autoimmune bullous dermatoses: a review. Ann N Y Acad Sci 2009;1173:203–10.

The Use of Intravenous Immunoglobulin in Autoimmune Bullous Diseases

Shien-Ning Chee, MBBS (UNSW)[a,b],
Dédée F. Murrell, MA, BMBCh, FAAD, MD, FACD[c],*

KEYWORDS

- Intravenous immunoglobulin • Pemphigus
- Autoimmune bullous disease • Inflammatory disease

Autoimmune blistering diseases (AIBD) are a rare group of diseases that affects the skin and mucous membranes. They tend to be chronic remitting conditions, which have implications on best treatment and quality of life. AIBD includes pemphigus and its subtypes: bullous pemphigoid (BP), linear IgA bullous dermatosis, mucous membrane pemphigoid (MMP), and epidermolysis bullosa acquisita (EBA). There are two major categories dependent of whether the blistering is intraepidermal (pemphigus) or subepidermal (BP).

The mainstay of treatment of AIBD is corticosteroids, with doses and route of administration dependant on the type of AIBD. With exacerbations and relapses of blistering, the dose of prednisone is increased and, later, slowly tapered according to clinical response. Other immunosuppressive agents are used for a steroid-sparing effect because corticosteroids cause a significant number of side effects, including immune suppression, diabetes mellitus, osteoporosis, myopathy, cataracts, hypertension, mood changes, and peptic ulcer disease, all of which add to disease burden. Immunosuppressive agents often used include azathioprine and mycophenolate. However, these in turn have their own side effects, including bone marrow suppression, which may lead to anemia, leucopenia and thrombocytopenia, and liver function abnormalities. Intravenous immunoglobulin (IVIG) is a third-line adjunctive approach to treat AIBD unresponsive to conventional therapy.[1]

INTRODUCTION TO IVIG

IVIG is made of IgG fractionated from pooled plasma, via whole blood donors or by plasmapheresis. Since its introduction in the 1950s in subcutaneous or intramuscular form, and its availability in intravenous (IV) form in the 1980s, administration has increased dramatically for a wide variety of diseases. It is used mainly in two situations. First, as replacement therapy in patients with antibody deficiency diseases—these are usually genetic conditions that have onset in early childhood. The second use is in autoimmune or inflammatory diseases.[2]

Each plasma pool of IVIG ranges from 4000 to 50,000 L, preferably from more than 1000 donors per lot. IVIG lots are not identical, with each containing varying amounts of IgG subclasses and other proteins and immunoglobulins such as albumin, IgA, IgE, and IgM.[3] Each step in production (fractionation, purification, stabilization, viral inactivation, formulation) and the varying plasma sources can

a Department of Dermatology, St George Hospital, Gray Street, Kogarah, Sydney, NSW 2217, Australia
b Faculty of Medicine, University of New South Wales, High Street, Kensington, Sydney, NSW 2052, Australia
c Department of Dermatology, St George Hospital, University of New South Wales, Gray Street, Kogarah, Sydney, NSW 2217, Australia
* Corresponding author.
E-mail address: d.murrell@unsw.edu.au

Dermatol Clin 29 (2011) 565–570
doi:10.1016/j.det.2011.06.010
0733-8635/11/$ – see front matter © 2011 Elsevier Inc. All rights reserved.

exert an influence on the final product, including an effect on the biologic activity of the IgG molecule.[3]

The majority of side effects, including headache, nausea, fever, and cough, are transient and do not require discontinuation of therapy. Most of these are preventable by the administration of oral antihistamines before the infusion or slowing of the infusion rate. However, rare and potentially fatal adverse events include anaphylactic reactions, aseptic meningitis, acute renal failure, cardiovascular compromise from fluid overload, and thromboembolic events such as cerebral infraction and pulmonary emboli. Adverse effects may be related to factors such as concentration of the IVIG (thus affected volume load) and osmolality (mostly due to sodium and sugar content, possibly affecting thromboembolic events).[3,4] There are also social problems related to the use of IVIG. It is a very expensive drug, with laboratory tests, infusion equipment, and facility fees adding to the cost. It is also time consuming, with patients having to travel and take time from their normal activities for infusions.[5] The concentration of IVIG is usually 5% to 6%.[6] A higher concentration allows for smaller volumes, which is useful in patients who have conditions such as heart failure where fluid balance is a concern. Most are delivered by IV infusions, but it may also be given subcutaneously. Subcutaneous administration is helpful in patients who experience severe rate-related adverse reactions, have poor venous access, or want the convenience of self-administration. The monthly IV dose is converted into grams, then milliliters, for weekly subcutaneous administration. A subcutaneous dose of 137% of the IV dose may be needed to achieve a comparable metabolic rate. Adults usually tolerate 15 to 20 mL per infusion site.[7]

Pemphigus

Pemphigus is characterized by loss of adhesion between keratinocytes, giving rise to blister formation. This loss of adhesion is due to auto-antibodies directed against intercellular adhesion structures (acantholysis). The subtypes of pemphigus may be distinguished by the specificity of the auto-antibodies for different targets or by the location of blister formation. In the most common form, pemphigus vulgaris (PV), blisters are located just above the basal skin layer. The hallmark is flaccid blisters that easily rupture to leave denuded painful erosions, often with oral involvement. With pemphigus foliaceus (PF), blisters occur within the granular layer of the epidermis. There are superficial blisters that easily rupture to leave superficial erosions. Cutaneous involvement is often more extensive than in PV, but mucous

membrane involvement is uncommon. Other pemphigus variants include paraneoplastic and drug-induced pemphigus. The titer of autoantibodies detected by indirect immunofluorescence microscopy and ELISA against desmogleins 1 and 3 in pemphigus is related to disease activity.[1,8]

IVIG is believed to work by rapidly and selectively lowering serum levels of these pathogenic antibodies that mediate pemphigus. This may be achieved by increasing catabolism of the immunoglobulin molecules. Cytotoxic agents given in conjunction with IVIG may reduce the rebound increase in levels of the depleted antibody after administration of IVIG.[9] Typically, pemphigus patients commenced on IVIG as a third-line treatment are given IVIG in addition to their oral corticosteroid and oral adjunctive agent, to which they were not responding adequately.

There have been numerous small studies, investigating the use of IVIG in PV and PF. In general, these studies show that IVIG is effective, even more so when administered concurrently with a cytotoxic drug such as cyclophosphamide or azathioprine. The addition of a cytotoxic drug is thought to offset the rebound in the level of antibodies that occurs after IVIG treatment.[9–11] However, these studies were not all placebo-controlled, randomized, or double-blinded.

The first placebo-controlled study investigating the use of IVIG in PV involved a single patient who had multiple relapses of PV despite treatment with steroids and adjunctive immunosuppressants. The patient was never disease-free and had many complications related to steroid use, including diabetes, osteopenia, ruptured tendons, and cutaneous infections secondary to immunosuppression. In 2004, all adjuvant therapies except azathioprine were discontinued, and he was placed on 140 g (2 g/kg) IVIG fortnightly for eight infusions, which led to dramatic improvement and allowed for a reduction in prednisolone from 45 to 30 mg daily. He was maintained on 80 g (1 g/kg) of IVIG monthly for 16 months. Thereafter, a formal randomized, double-blind, placebo-controlled, crossover trial was commenced. There were two phases of the trial, each consisting of 6 consecutive months of either IVIG 1 g/kg or placebo infusion. Prednisolone was continued during the trial with instructions given to the patient to taper the dose by 5 mg decrements at fortnightly intervals when lesions became quiescent and azathioprine was continued throughout at an unchanged dose. The mean subjective patient disease scores were much improved with IVIG compared with placebo (mean overall score of 11.6 vs 20.6). Also improved were pemphigus autoantibody titers (1:20 on placebo vs 1:80 with

IVIG), desmoglein 3 antibody levels (79 vs 126), and desmoglein 1 antibody levels (94 vs 126). On placebo, the mean dose of prednisolone was 33.7 compared with 35.8 mg on IVIG, which is of questionable significance because there was no attempt in the protocol to taper the steroid using a standard method during the 6-month periods.[10]

There has been only one multicenter, randomized, placebo-controlled, double-blinded trial conducted in pemphigus vulgaris that were unresponsive to standard treatments or relapsing. This study was based in Japan, using patients who were unresponsive to prednisone doses over 20 mg/day. It investigated the effect of a single 5-day cycle of IVIG. Twenty-one patients were given 400 mg IVIG daily (2 g over 5 days; for a 70 kg patient equivalent to 2.5 mg/kg), 20 were given 200 mg IVIG daily, and 20 were given a placebo identical solution. There was a significant difference between the 400 mg and placebo groups in terms of therapeutic endpoint, defined as time to escape from the protocol (a novel efficacy indicator). There was also improvement with 200 mg versus placebo, but this did not reach statistical significance. Clinical severity improved significantly with both 400 mg and 200 mg compared with placebo, though the 200 mg group needed an additional 42 days to reach the same level of improvement as the 400 mg group. Anti-desmoglein 3 IgG autoantibodies decreased significantly with 400 mg, decreased slightly with 200 mg, and not at all with placebo. Unlike most previous studies that suggest efficacy of IVIG for treatment of pemphigus with multiple treatment cycles, Amagai and colleagues[12] (2009) show that a single 5-day cycle has therapeutic benefits.

BP

IVIG has been reported only in uncontrolled studies of BP and found to be somewhat effective. One study investigated 15 patients who had with relapsing BP despite treatment with prednisone or systemic therapies. Data was collated regarding prednisone regimes, side effects from treatment, hospital admissions, disease activity, and quality of life as measured on a five-point Likert scale. IVIG was then initiated at 2 g/kg over 3 days every 4 weeks and prednisone and adjuvant treatments were tapered. However, patients had twice daily baths or normal saline compresses to remove skin debris followed by medium-strength topical corticosteroid cream applied to improve healing and any lesions unresponsive to topical therapy were treated with sublesional injections of 15 to 20 mg/ml of triamcinolone acetonide. This practice could have compounded the assessment of the IVIG, because topical steroids have since been shown to be effective for BP. Hence, the conclusions on demonstration of efficacy are limited from this study.[13]

Another study, coordinated by Ahmed and colleagues (2003),[14] involved 10 patients with severe BP. Serum samples were collected monthly over the study duration of 18 months to measure autoantibody titers. IVIG was administered at 4-week intervals at 2 g/kg per cycle until all lesions had healed. Thereafter the intervals between cycles were gradually increased to 6, 8, 10, 12, and 16 weeks. The mean autoantibody titers before IVIG were 2600 for BP Ag1 and 2380 for BP Ag2. After 3 months of treatment, there was clinical improvement with a statistically significant decrease in mean autoantibody titers. After 11 months, autoantibody tires became nondetectable and lesions had completely healed with no new lesions. Serologic remission was sustained for an average of 7 months with no new blister formation seen for the remainder of the study. Antibody titers to tetanus toxoid were used as controls and no change in tetanus toxoid levels was observed during the study. There was also a control group consisting of seven patients with BP in remission, seven patients with PV, and 15 healthy individuals. Antibody titers to BP Ag1 and Ag2 were nondetectable in the control group. This was the first study demonstrating the serologic response of two autoantibodies to BP when IVIG is administered. It is unknown if the patients were taking steroids or immunosuppressants before or during the study, or if their disease had been refractory to other treatments.[14] The two above studies also originate from the same study center and patient registry numbers are unavailable for tracking.

Bystryn and colleagues (2008)[15] suggest IVIG to be effective only when administered with an immunosuppressive agent. One patient with BP refractory to prednisone and mycophenolate mofetil was commenced on three cycles of IVIG given 3 weeks apart. Serum IgG decreased from 320 to 20, serum IgG4 decreased from 640 to 80 existing lesions completely cleared, and no new lesions developed. Several months later mycophenolate mofetil had been ceased and prednisone tapered to 5 mg/daily. Three cycles of IVIG every 2 weeks was administered with prednisone alone, with no improvement. In fact, serum titers of pemphigoid IgG remained unchanged, levels of IgG4 doubled, and the patient experienced one flare of disease with several new bullae. Azathioprine 150 to 200 mg/day was then added and, after four cycles of IVIG every 2 weeks, serum IgG and IgG4 halved. With another 6 cycles of IVIG, autoantibody levels decreased fourfold. However, disease activity did not correlate because there were several new bullae. Azathioprine was then ceased and IVIG was given with prednisone alone. IgG and IgG4 titers quadrupled over 3 months with an average of one new blister per week. Administration of an immunosuppressive agent with IVIG and prednisone appears to be more effective than IVIG and prednisone alone.[15]

IVIG may also be useful as monotherapy in childhood BP. A 3-month-old boy with BP was unresponsive to prednisone (2.8 mg/kg/day), dexamethasone, erythromycin, and dapsone, with new blisters and erythema over the whole body. After 2 months in hospital trialing the above treatments, a 5-day course of IVIG (300 mg/kg/day) was commenced in addition to dexamethasone 0/75 mg/day, erythromycin, and dapsone. After 4 days, no new skins lesions developed. One week later, skin lesions were much improved allowing for tapering of dexamethasone and discontinuation of erythromycin. A month later there was recurrence of blistering and a second course of IVIG was given, resulting in improvement, which allowed for discontinuation of dapsone and complete tapering of dexamethasone 7 months later. At follow-up 16 months later, there had been no relapse.[16] Another case involved a Chinese, 3-month-old boy with BP and eczema, whose parents refused systemic steroid therapy. IVIG 400 mg/kg/day was given for 4 days with cefaclor. Erythema and most bullae over the body resolved within 1 week. Within the next year, there were several mild relapses of blisters that were controlled with oral antihistamines and topical corticosteroids. In the following 2 years, there were no relapses of bullae.[17]

MMP

MMP affects the mucous membranes of the body, including the oral cavity, ocular membranes, nose, pharynx, larynx, trachea, and genitalia. Ocular involvement can ultimately lead to blindness.[18]

There has been one comparison study involving 18 patients with ocular MMP. Eight patients were treated with IVIG, and then compared with eight other patients on conventional immunosuppressive therapy who had identical disease (duration and severity) and were matched for age and sex. The IVIG group was given 2 g/kg per cycle of 2 to 4 week intervals. Once clinical improvement was observed and disease had stabilized, the previous systemic conventional therapy was discontinued, but the method for tapering was not specified. IVIG continued for 16 weeks. Conventional therapy differed between patients, including agents such as prednisone, diaminodiphenylsulfone (dapsone), methotrexate, azathioprine, or mycophenolate mofetil. All patients in the IVIG group had total control of disease at 24 months with no progression of disease, while the other

group had disease progression despite using conventional therapy at adequate doses for recommended periods of time. IVIG users also had faster control of ocular inflammation and no relapses, unlike patients on conventional therapy. Letko and colleagues[19] (2004) suggest that ocular MMP should be an indication for IVIG treatment.

Another pilot study of six patients with severe ocular involvement unresponsive to conventional therapy also demonstrated the efficacy of IVIG (cycles of 2 g/kg over 3 days), with rapid improvement in symptoms and signs such as conjunctival erythema, photophobia, and discomfort. No patients had a decrease in their disease staging and two patients had an improvement. This study is continuing, investigating the durability of long-term remission.[20]

Three other case studies have found IVIG to be effective in recalcitrant MMP. In these studies, IVIG was given in addition to steroids with or without immunosuppressants. Two studies used IVIG 1 g/kg/daily for 2 to 3 days. One study did not quantify the amount of IVIG given.[21–23]

EBA

EBA is characterized by inflammatory or noninflammatory blisters at sites of trauma that affect the collagen VII under the lamina densa, thus leading to milia and scar formation. There are various types of EBA, some of which resemble BP or MMP.[1] There have been few case studies on the use of IVIG in EBA.

One study involving a 16-year-old boy showed that high-dose IVIG (400 mg/kg/day for 4 days repeated every 2 weeks) led to good clinical improvement when administered with cyclosporin and prednisone. However, there was no decrease in circulating autoantibodies.[24] There have been two studies investigating high-dose IVIG without concomitant use of steroids or immunosuppressants. One of these studies showed improvement after two cycles of IVIG (400 mg/kg/day for 5 days) with healing of most erosions and few new blisters. Six months after the sixth and final cycle, the condition was still in remission.[25] However, the other study showed no improvement in disease either clinically or by measurement of autoantibodies.[26]

Low-dose IVIG is an alternative that allows for reduced costs and side effects. One patient with EBA refractory to steroids, immunosuppressants, colchicine, and plasmapheresis was commenced on IVIG at 40 mg/daily in 3-day cycles repeated every 3 to 4 weeks, coadministered with prednisone. After four cycles, no new blisters appeared and lesions started healing. One year later, prednisone was discontinued and the interval between IVIG infusions was extended to 6 weeks. To the time of publication of the case-study, the patient remained disease-free and continued to receive low-dose IVIG every 6 weeks.[27]

IVIG has also successfully been administered subcutaneously. One patient with EBA resistant to corticosteroids, azathioprine, mycophenolate mofetil, mercaptopurine, minocycline, and plasmapheresis was given two boluses of 1.7 g/kg IVIG at 8 weekly intervals, followed by divided doses every 3 weeks. Treatment was changed to subcutaneous immunoglobulin (SCIG) due to poor venous access and convenience of self-treatment at home. Throughout treatment with both IVIG and SCIG, there was reduction of symptoms and gradual withdrawal of all immunosuppressive therapy. Maintenance was achieved with SCIG at 0.9 g/kg/month given in divided doses on 5 days per week. Circulating autoantibodies reduced from 1:16 to zero on intact skin, and 1:32 to 1:10 on salt split skin testing. Subcutaneous administration may be a good alternative in patients with poor venous access, or those who wish to be able to administer their medication at home.[28]

SUMMARY

IVIG has been shown to be effective in the treatment of AIBD and may be an option if disease is refractory to conventional treatment. Effectiveness of IVIG appears to increase when administered concurrently with a cytotoxic drug. Most reports use multiple treatment cycles, though single cycles may give benefit. Tapering IVIG administration may improve the duration of remission and subcutaneous injections may be an option if IVIG is inconvenient or inappropriate.

There is a need for well-conducted, randomized, placebo-controlled double-blinded trials investigating the use of IVIG in AIBD, particularly in BP, MMP, and EBA, so that patients can receive good, evidence-based care. Issues requiring more investigation include

Optimal IVIG doses and regimens (eg, number of cycles, intervals between cycles, use of tapering of IVIG, when IVIG should be first commenced)
Benefits of adjuvant immunosuppressive agents
Relative benefits of agents
Cost-effectiveness
Effectiveness of IVIG in modification or suppression of the course of disease.

REFERENCES

1. Ahmed A. Use of intravenous immunoglobulin therapy in autoimmune blistering diseases. Int Immunopharmacol 2006;6:557–78.

2. Gelfand E. Differences between IGIV products: impact on clinical outcome. Int Immunopharmacol 2006;6:592–9.

3. Martin T. IGIV: contents, properties, and methods of industrial production—evolving closer to a more physiologic product. Int Immunopharmacol 2006;6: 517–22.

4. Feldmeyer L, Benden C, Haile S, et al. Not all intravenous immunoglobulin preparations are equally well tolerated. Acta Derm Venereol 2010;90(5):494–7.

5. Dahl M, Bridges A. Intravenous immune globulin: fighting antibodies with antibodies. J Am Acad Dermatol 2001;45(5):775–84.

6. Red Cross Australia. Appendix 1 - Comparison of INTRAGAM P, Flebogamma 5% DIF and Octagam. 2011. Available at: http://www.transfusion.com.au/sites/default/files/Comparison%20between%20IVIG%20products%20-%20Final.pdf. Accessed June 24, 2011.

7. Ballow M. Immunoglobulin therapy: methods of delivery. J Allergy Clin Immunol 2008;122(5):1038–9.

8. Nousari H, Anhalt G. Pemphigus and bullous pemphigoid. Lancet 1999;354:667–72.

9. Lolis M, Toosi S, Czernick A, et al. Effect of intravenous immunoglobulin with or without cytotoxic drugs on pemphigus intercellular antibodies. J Am Acad Dermatol 2011;64(3):484–9.

10. Arnold D, Burton J, Shine B, et al. An 'n-of-1' placebo-controlled crossover trial of intravenous immunoglobulin as adjuvant therapy in refractory pemphigus vulgaris. Br J Dermatol 2009;160(5):1098–102.

11. Bystryn J, Jiao D, Natow S. Treatment of pemphigus with intravenous immunoglobulin. J Am Acad Dermatol 2002;47(3):358–63.

12. Amagai M, Ikeda S, Shimizu H, et al. A randomised double-blind trial of intravenous immunoglobulin for pemphigus. J Am Acad Dermatol 2009;60(4): 595–603.

13. Ahmed A. Intravenous immunoglobulin therapy for patients with bullous pemphigoid unresponsive to conventional immunosuppressive treatment. J Am Acad Dermatol 2001;45(6):825–35.

14. Sami N, Ali S, Bhol K, et al. Influence of intravenous immunoglobulin therapy on autoantibody titres to BP Ag1 and BP Ag2 in patients with bullous pemphigoid. J Eur Acad Dermatol Venereol 2003;17:641–5.

15. Czernik A, Bystryn J. Improvement of intravenous immunoglobulin therapy for bullous pemphigoid by adding immunosuppressive agents. Arch Dermatol 2008;144(5):658–61.

16. Sugawara N, Nagai Y, Matsushima Y, et al. Infantile bullous pemphigoid treated with intravenous immunoglobulin therapy. J Am Acad Dermatol 2007; 57(6):1084–9.

17. Xiao T, Li B, Wang Y, et al. Childhood bullous pemphigoid treated by i.v. immunoglobulin. J Dermatol 2007;34:650–3.

18. Chan L, Ahmed A, Anhalt G. The first international consensus on mucous membrane pemphigoid: definition, diagnostic criteria, pathogenic factors, medical treatment and prognostic indicators. Arch Dermatol 2002;138:370–9.

19. Letko E, Miserocchi E, Daoud Y, et al. A nonrandomized comparison of the clinical outcome of ocular involvement in patients with mucous membrane (cicatricial) pemphigoid between conventional immunosuppressive and intravenous immunoglobulin therapies. Clin Immunol 2004;111:303–10.

20. Mignogna M, Leuci S, Piscopo R, et al. Intravenous immunoglobulins and mucous membrane pemphigoid [letter]. Ophthalmology 2008;115(4):752, e751.

21. Galdos M, Etxebarria J. Intravenous immunoglobulin therapy for refractory ocular cicatricial pemphigoid: case report. Cornea 2008;27(8):967–9.

22. Leverkus M, Georgi M, Nie Z, et al. Cicatricial pemphigoid with circulating IgA and IgG autoantibodies to the central portion of the BP180 ectodomain: beneficial effect of adjuvant therapy with high-dose intravenous immunoglobulin. J Am Acad Dermatol 2002;46:116–22.

23. Iaccheri B, Roque M, Fiore T, et al. Ocular cicatricial pemphigoid, keratomycosis, and intravenous immunoglobulin therapy. Cornea 2004;23:819–22.

24. Meier F, Soninichsen K, Schaumburg-Lever G, et al. Epidermolysis bullosa acquisita: efficacy of high-dose intravenous immunoglobulins. J Am Acad Dermatol 1993;29(2):334–7.

25. Gourgiotou K, Exadaktylou D, Aroni K, et al. Epidermolysis bullosa acquisita: treatment with intravenous immunoglobulins. J Eur Acad Dermatol Venereol 2002;16:77–80.

26. Caldwell M, Yancey K, Engler R, et al. Epidermolysis bullosa acquisita: Efficacy of high-dose intravenous immunoglobulins [letter to the editor]. J Am Acad Dermatol 1994;31(5):827–8.

27. Kofler H, Wambacher-Gasser B, Topar G, et al. Intravenous immunoglobulin treatment in therapy-resistant epidermolysis bullosa acquisita. J Am Acad Dermatol 1996;36(2):331–5.

28. Tayal U, Burton J, Chapel H. Subcutaneous immunoglobulin therapy for immunomodulation in a patient with severe epidermolysis bullosa acquisita [letter to the editor]. Clin Immunol 2008;129:518–9.

Rituximab and its Use in Autoimmune Bullous Disorders

Benjamin S. Daniel, BA, BCom, MBBS, MMed (Clin Epi)[a,b],
Dédée F. Murrell, MA, BMBCh, FAAD, MD, FACD[c,*],
Pascal Joly, MD, PhD[d]

KEYWORDS

- CD20 antigen • Autoimmune blistering diseases
- Immunosuppressant • Adverse effects

Rituximab is a chimeric murine-human monoclonal antibody against the CD20 antigen of B lymphocytes[1,2] (anti-CD20 mAb). It is used in multiple medical conditions and its therapeutic role in dermatology has been increasing in the last decade. Initially used in the treatment of non-Hodgkin B-cell lymphoma, the scope of rituximab has been expanded to include autoimmune diseases such as rheumatoid arthritis (RA), systemic lupus erythematosus (SLE), and chronic immune thrombocytopenic purpura syndrome.[3,4] Because the B cells produce immunoglobulins, which in turn have a pathogenic role in autoimmune diseases, their depletion is surmised to result in improved symptoms and disease control. Depleting B cells inevitably decreases the activation of antigen-presenting cells and the transmission of signaling pathways to other key mediators, such as T cells.

MECHANISM OF ACTION

The B-cell antigen CD20 is a transmembrane glycoprotein expressed on nearly all B cells and most B-cell lymphomas.[5,6] However, it is not found on early pre-B cells or stem cells.[5] B cells, originally arising from the bone marrow, mature by migrating through peripheral blood, lymph nodes, and spleen. In bone marrow (BM) they are known as plasma cells. CD20, specific for B cells, is expressed on B cells between the pre-B cell and pre-plasma stages.[7,8] Because rituximab targets CD20, plasma cells in the BM responsible for antibody production[6] are spared. Once rituximab binds to the CD20 protein, transmembrane signals result in altered cell-cycle differentiation and activation. Cell-mediated cytotoxicity, complement system, and direct apoptosis[9] have been implemented in the subsequent reduction in circulating CD20+ B cells in the periphery, lymph nodes, spleen, and bone marrow.[5]

The depletion of B-cell counts occurs within 3 days of rituximab administration and is reported to be reduced by about 90%, although variations occur. It is thought that the variations are due to the underlying disease and polymorphisms of $Fc\gamma RIIIa$ receptors.[8] The B-cell count remains low for 6 months and returns to baseline around 9 to 12 months after receiving 4 weekly doses of 375 mg/m^2.[6,10] In addition to depleting B cells, some data suggest that antigen-specific CD4+ T-cell numbers are reduced after the administration of rituximab,[11] whereas no quantitative change in the different T-cell subpopulations is usually evident.[12]

[a] Department of Dermatology, St George Hospital, Gray Street, Kogarah, Sydney, NSW 2217, Australia
[b] Faculty of Medicine, University of New South Wales, Sydney, NSW 2052, Australia
[c] Department of Dermatology, St George Hospital, University of New South Wales, Gray Street, Kogarah, Sydney, NSW 2217, Australia
[d] Dermatology Department, INSERM U905, Rouen University Hospital, 1 Rue de Germont, 76031 Rouen, France
* Corresponding author.
E-mail address: d.murrell@unsw.edu.au

Dermatol Clin 29 (2011) 571–575
doi:10.1016/j.det.2011.06.023

DOSE AND ROUTE OF ADMINISTRATION

Although rituximab is typically prescribed in weekly infusions of 375 mg/m^2 (approx. 727.5 mg per 75 kg, 1.8 m tall male) for 4 weeks, some advocate 2 intravenous infusions of 1 g, 2 weeks apart.[4] Rituximab is also known as Rituxan or MabThera. Infusions are initially administered over 5 hours and if well tolerated, subsequent infusions can be administered over 3 to 5 hours.[10]

Corticosteroids reduce the intensity of infusion-related adverse effects.[4] Paracetamol and diphenhydramine are recommended before administration to decrease the likelihood and extent of infusion-related adverse events.[10]

Monitoring of B-cell counts does not generally affect treatment because a sharp decline in absolute numbers is expected after the administration of rituximab. The aim of recurrent cycles of rituximab is to maintain circulating B cells at the lowest level for a prolonged period of time. In one report, rituximab was administered every 6 to 9 months for RA without significant adverse effects apart from reduction in serum immunoglobulin M levels.[4] The theoretic risk of increasing the incidence of lymphomas after prolonged B-cell depletion with repeated cycles of rituximab cannot be excluded.

Routine vaccination of all patients should occur several weeks before the commencement of rituximab therapy.[4] Patients should not receive live vaccines while receiving systemic immunosuppressive agents.

ADVERSE EFFECTS

Polymorphisms of the FcγRIIIa receptor may influence the efficacy of rituximab and the extent of associated adverse effects.[9] The most frequent adverse effects are transient, infusion-related, and mild to moderate in severity.[10] They include fever, headache, nausea, chills, orthostatic hypotension, mucocutaneous reactions, and thrombocytopenia.[2,5,9] Severe cytokine release syndrome can occur during the first infusion.[10] It is of major importance not to forget infections, which can be severe. There was 1 case of septicemia leading to death in the series of 21 patients reported by Joly and colleagues,[2] 1 of 7 patients died in the series studied by Hertl,[11–13] and 2 of 17 patients died in the cicatricial pemphigoid series from St Louis,[14] which approximately corresponds to 4 deaths among 44 patients (almost 10%). These severe infections seem favored by older age and the concomitant use of high doses of steroids and/or immunosuppressants. There have been a significant number of reports of progressive multifocal leukoencephalopathy in patients concomitantly treated with rituximab and polychemotherapy for B-cell lymphoma and some reported cases in patients with nondermatologic autoimmune diseases such as SLE, RA, and Wegener granulomatosis.[9]

Although it has been theorized and confirmed by many reports that serum levels of immunoglobulin G (IgG) remain unchanged because stem cells and plasma cells do not contain CD20[15] and are not affected, few case reports have reported reduced levels of immunoglobulins.[14] Anemia, neutropenia, and thrombocytopenia have also been reported in 1% to 7% of patients after the fourth infusion.[10] In the context of these findings, it is important to regularly monitor blood counts in patients treated with rituximab.

USE IN AUTOIMMUNE BLISTERING DISEASES

Autoimmune blistering diseases (AIBD) are a heterogeneous group of blistering diseases affecting the skin and/or mucous membrane. Although these diseases are typically managed with systemic corticosteroids in combination with immunosuppressants or immunomodulators, inefficacy (recalcitrant and relapsing types), contraindications, and adverse effects are reasons for choosing an alternative therapeutic option. This is especially the case with pemphigus and mucous membrane pemphigoid, which often require prolonged administration of systemic corticosteroids and other adjuvant systemic immunosuppressive agents. Rituximab has therefore been used as an alternative and/or adjuvant to other therapies.

Pemphigus

Pemphigus is a rare mucocutaneous disease characterized by antibodies to adhesion protein, desmoglein (Dsg) 1 and 3. Pemphigus vulgaris (PV) and pemphigus foliaceus (PF) are the 2 main types of pemphigus usually managed with systemic corticosteroids. Adjuvant therapies such as mycophenolate, azathioprine, methotrexate cyclophosphamide, and cyclosporine are used with varying degrees of efficacy.[16,17]

The use of rituximab in pemphigus was first reported in 2002 and since then there have been many case reports/series demonstrating favorable results, especially in patients who have not responded to more standard treatments.[18,19] A study assessing the resolution of pemphigus lesions with intravenous immunoglobulin (IVIG) and rituximab was published in 2006.[20] Eleven patients with recalcitrant disease were treated with rituximab (375 mg/m^2) once a week for 3 weeks and with IVIG (2 g/kg) in the fourth week. This cycle was repeated for month 2. During months 3 to 6, these patients were administered one infusion of rituximab and IVIG. By the end of the second cycle, 9 of 11 patients (82%) had resolution of lesions, which was maintained for more than 20 months. The combination of IVIG with rituximab was not compared with rituximab alone, and hence it is uncertain whether IVIG adds any benefit to rituximab alone.

Two patients with recalcitrant PV were successfully treated with 2 courses of rituximab.[21] The 2 reports on these cases implied better outcomes with 2 cycles of rituximab rather than 1 but because these are only isolated case reports, it is difficult to draw any firm conclusions. In 2007, however, a multicenter open-label French trial assessing the effect of a single cycle of rituximab alone in pemphigus was reported.[2] Twenty-one patients (14 with PV, 7 with PF) who failed to respond, be maintained, or had a contraindication to oral corticosteroids were given a single cycle of rituximab. Each patient received 1 infusion (375 mg/m^2) weekly for 4 weeks, with immunologic evaluations at regular intervals. Eighteen of 21 patients (86%) had complete remission at 3 months and 2 of 21 patients (10%) had complete remission by 12 months. Of those who had complete remission, 9 (45%) patients relapsed after a mean of 19 months, 2 of whom required a second cycle of rituximab. This study also demonstrated the corticosteroid-sparing effect of rituximab, with 8 of 21 (38%) patients not requiring any systemic treatment at the end of the study. A relationship between disease activity and antidesmoglein antibody (anti-DSG) levels was evident by the reduction of anti-DSG-1 and, to a lesser degree, anti-DSG-3 titers in patients who had experienced remission at 3 months. Rituximab does not seem to influence the mean IgG levels, which did not change significantly.

In a study in 2006 from Germany, rituximab was administered to 7 patients with AIBD (4 with PV, 2 with bullous pemphigoid (BP), and 1 with mucous membrane pemphigoid [MMP]). Six of 7 patients received weekly infusions (375 mg/m^2) for 4 weeks. Although complete resolution or reduction in lesion size by more than 50% occurred in 6 of 7 patients (86%) at 13 months, 4 of 7 patients (57%) had severe adverse effects including blindness and death secondary to bacterial pneumonia.[22]

Maintenance therapy at a lower dose may be an option in the treatment of pemphigus[21] that requires further evaluation.

MMP/Epidermolysis Bullosa Acquisita

MMP refers to a heterogeneous group of AIBD typically affecting the mucous membranes.[14]

MMP is associated with significant morbidity secondary to scarring and ophthalmologic complications. Typical histologic findings include IgG and C3 depositions in the basement membrane zone.[23] MMP, previously known as cicatricial pemphigoid,[24] is a potentially severe AIBD with an incidence of 1 per 1,000,000 per year with a mean age of 70 years.[25,26] Epidermolysis bullosa acquisita (EBA) has an incidence of 0.2 new cases per 1,000,000 inhabitants per year.[25,26] The use of rituximab in MMP and EBA has been limited to a few case reports.[15,27,28] Combination therapy with IVIG has been reported to be effective in ocular cicatricial pemphigoid.[20,29] In a recent study, 25 patients with severe refractory MMP were treated with 1 to 2 cycles of rituximab (375 mg/m^2) for 4 weeks.[14] Within a median of 12 weeks of having 1 cycle, 17 patients had complete resolution of their lesions. Five of the 8 remaining patients experienced complete resolution after receiving a second cycle of rituximab. Although 22 of 25 patients (88%) had complete resolution of both ocular and extraocular lesions, 10 of 22 patients (45%) had a relapse after a mean of only 4 months. Significant adverse events occurred in this study, with 3 patients experiencing infections, 2 of whom died. Despite the severity of adverse outcomes, it can be argued that in the case of MMP, it is important to quickly achieve disease stabilization and remission as disease progression often leads to blindness, laryngeal, and esophageal complications.[14] The benefits versus the risks must always be considered before administration of rituximab.

Rituximab has been suggested as a potential corticosteroid-sparing agent,[2,18] reducing cumulative doses of systemic corticosteroids, although this has not been demonstrated in a randomized controlled trial.

BP

Although BP is the most common AIBD, the use of rituximab is infrequently reported, probably because BP responds readily to potent topical corticosteroids.[30,31] Typically affecting the elderly with high mortality, BP presents with multiple bullae, erosions, and severe pruritus, and only rarely has mucous membrane involvement. Two female patients with concomitant BP and chronic lymphocytic leukemia were both treated with rituximab (375 mg/m^2 weekly for 4 consecutive weeks) alone after inadequate response to corticosteroids and antihistamines.[32] Maintenance therapy of 1 dose every 2 months was initiated and both patients had complete remission after this treatment, even at the 3-year follow-up.

Successful use of rituximab has been reported in a 5-month old infant who had unsuccessful systemic treatments including corticosteroids, dapsone, IVIG, and cyclosporine.[33] Two doses of rituximab were added to the therapeutic regimen 4 weeks apart (375 mg/m^2 and 187.5 mg/m^2), and improvement was noticed within days.

A retrospective study looking at 7 patients (5 with BP and 2 with MMP) treated with rituximab found that complete and partial remission was achieved in 4 patients with BP and 2 patients with MMP.[34] The main indications for the use of rituximab in BP patients are not clearly defined because of the extremely high efficacy of ultrapotent topical corticosteroids during the acute phase of the disease and the numerous drugs proposed for maintenance therapy (oral corticosteroids, low doses of methotrexate, tetracyclines). Potential indications for the administration of rituximab in BP might be: (1) recalcitrant types of BP (extremely rare) and (2) patients with multiple relapses, who are observed quite frequently.

SUMMARY

In recent years, many clinicians have used rituximab in an off-label way to successfully treat and manage AIBD. Although traditional systemic treatments such as corticosteroids have been effective, they are associated with multiple adverse effects and in some cases fail to adequately control symptoms. Additional therapy in the form of weekly intravenous infusions of rituximab (375 mg/m^2) may benefit patients with recalcitrant disease and allow for tapering and cessation of other systemic agents.

Rituximab induces B-cell depletion and hence a reduction in pathogenic antibodies. Long-term monitoring is advisable, given the possibility of immunocompromise and sepsis. The exact time to initiate rituximab is variable. Due to the cost, potential complications, and lack of data, it is prudent to treat AIBD with rituximab if 2 or more traditional systemic therapies have failed to adequately control symptoms.[33,34] Rituximab is a promising therapeutic agent in AIBD but further research is required.

REFERENCES

1. Carr DR, Heffernan MP. Innovative uses of rituximab in dermatology. Dermatol Clin 2010;28(3):547–57.
2. Joly P, Mouquet H, Roujeau JC, et al. A single cycle of rituximab for the treatment of severe pemphigus. N Engl J Med 2007;357(6):545–52.
3. Looney RJ. B cells as a therapeutic target in autoimmune diseases other than rheumatoid arthritis. Rheumatology (Oxford) 2005;44(Suppl 2):ii13–7.
4. Sanz I. Indications of rituximab in autoimmune diseases. Drug Discov Today Ther Strateg 2009; 6(1):13–9.
5. Maloney DG, Liles TM, Czerwinski DK, et al. Phase I clinical trial using escalating single-dose infusion of chimeric anti-CD20 monoclonal antibody (IDEC-C2B8) in patients with recurrent B cell lymphoma. Blood 1994;84(8):2457–66.
6. Zambruno G, Borradori L. Rituximab immunotherapy in pemphigus: therapeutic effects beyond B cell depletion. J Invest Dermatol 2008;128(12):2745–7.
7. Edwards JC, Cambridge G. B cell targeting in rheumatoid arthritis and other autoimmune diseases. Nat Rev Immunol 2006;6(5):394–403.
8. Schmidt E, Hunzelmann N, Zillikens D, et al. Rituximab in refractory autoimmune bullous diseases. Clin Exp Dermatol 2006;31(4):503–8.
9. McDonald V, Leandro M. Rituximab in non-haematological disorders of adults and its mode of action. Br J Haematol 2009;146(3):233–46.
10. Onrust SV, Lamb HM, Balfour JA. Rituximab. Drugs 1999;58(1):79–88 [discussion: 89–90].
11. Eming R, Nagel A, Wolff-Franke S, et al. Rituximab exerts a dual effect in pemphigus vulgaris. J Invest Dermatol 2008;128(12):2850–8.
12. Mouquet H, Musette P, Gougeon ML, et al. B cell depletion immunotherapy in pemphigus: effects on cellular and humoral immune responses. J Invest Dermatol 2008;128(12):2859–69.
13. Muller R, Hunzelmann N, Baur V, et al. Targeted immunotherapy with rituximab leads to a transient alteration of the IgG autoantibody profile in pemphigus vulgaris. Dermatol Res Pract 2010; 2010:321950.
14. Le Roux-Villet C, Prost-Squarcioni C, Alexandre M, et al. Rituximab for patients with refractory mucous membrane pemphigoid. Arch Dermatol 2011;147:843–9.
15. Sadler E, Schafleitner B, Lanschuetzer C, et al. Treatment-resistant classical epidermolysis bullosa acquisita responding to rituximab. Br J Dermatol 2007;157(2):417–9.
16. Daniel BS, Murrell DF. The actual management of pemphigus. G Ital Dermatol Venereol 2010;145(5):689–702.
17. Martin LK, Werth V, Villanueva E, et al. Interventions for pemphigus vulgaris and pemphigus foliaceus. Cochrane Database Syst Rev 2009;1:CD006263.
18. Fernando SL, O'Connor KS. Treatment of severe pemphigus foliaceus with rituximab. Med J Aust 2008;189(5):289–90.
19. Virgolini L, Marzocchi V. Anti-CD20 monoclonal antibody (rituximab) in the treatment of autoimmune

diseases. Successful result in refractory pemphigus vulgaris: report of a case. Haematologica 2003; 88(7):ELT24.

20. Ahmed AR, Spigelman Z, Cavacini LA, et al. Treatment of pemphigus vulgaris with rituximab and intravenous immune globulin. N Engl J Med 2006; 355(17):1772–9.

21. Faurschou A, Gniadecki R. Two courses of rituximab (anti-CD20 monoclonal antibody) for recalcitrant pemphigus vulgaris. Int J Dermatol 2008;47(3): 292–4.

22. Schmidt E, Seitz CS, Benoit S, et al. Rituximab in autoimmune bullous diseases: mixed responses and adverse effects. Br J Dermatol 2007;156(2):352–6.

23. Kirtschig G, Murrell D, Wojnarowska F, et al. Interventions for mucous membrane pemphigoid/cicatricial pemphigoid and epidermolysis bullosa acquisita: a systematic literature review. Arch Dermatol 2002; 138(3):380–4.

24. Chan LS, Ahmed AR, Anhalt GJ, et al. The first international consensus on mucous membrane pemphigoid: definition, diagnostic criteria, pathogenic factors, medical treatment, and prognostic indicators. Arch Dermatol 2002;138(3):370–9.

25. Zillikens D, Wever S, Roth A, et al. Incidence of autoimmune subepidermal blistering dermatoses in a region of central Germany. Arch Dermatol 1995; 131(8):957–8.

26. Bernard P, Vaillant L, Labeille B, et al. Incidence and distribution of subepidermal autoimmune bullous skin diseases in three French regions. Bullous Diseases French Study Group. Arch Dermatol 1995;131(1):48–52.

27. Niedermeier A, Eming R, Pfütze M, et al. Clinical response of severe mechanobullous epidermolysis bullosa acquisita to combined treatment with immunoadsorption and rituximab (anti-CD20 monoclonal antibodies). Arch Dermatol 2007;143(2):192–8.

28. Crichlow SM, Mortimer NJ, Harman KE. A successful therapeutic trial of rituximab in the treatment of a patient with recalcitrant, high-titer epidermolysis bullosa acquisita. Br J Dermatol 2007; 156(1):194–6.

29. Foster CS, Chang PY, Ahmed AR. Combination of rituximab and intravenous immunoglobulin for recalcitrant ocular cicatricial pemphigoid: a preliminary report. Ophthalmology 2010;117(5):861–9.

30. Joly P, Roujeau JC, Benichou J, et al, Bullous Diseases French Study Group. A comparison of oral and topical corticosteroids in patients with bullous pemphigoid. N Engl J Med 2002;346(5):321–7.

31. Langan SM, Smeeth L, Hubbard R, et al. Bullous pemphigoid and pemphigus vulgaris–incidence and mortality in the UK: population based cohort study. BMJ 2008;337:a180.

32. Saouli Z, Papadopoulos A, Kaiafa G, et al. A new approach on bullous pemphigoid therapy. Ann Oncol 2008;19(4):825–6.

33. Schulze J, Bader P, Henke U, et al. Severe bullous pemphigoid in an infant–successful treatment with rituximab. Pediatr Dermatol 2008;25(4):462–5.

34. Lourari S, Herve C, Doffoel-Hantz V, et al. Bullous and mucous membrane pemphigoid show a mixed response to rituximab: experience in seven patients. J Eur Acad Dermatol Venereol 2010. [Epub ahead of print].

Minimizing Complications in Autoimmune Blistering Diseases

Tiffany Clay, MD[a], Amit G. Pandya, MD[b],*

KEYWORDS

- Corticosteroids • Skin lesions • Emotional impact
- Management

Autoimmune blistering diseases (AIBD) are a group of antibody-mediated disorders that cause painful and disfiguring skin lesions, often leading to significant morbidity and mortality. In addition, complications secondary to the numerous therapies for AIBD contribute significantly to the clinical course of patients with this condition. The side effects of treatment, particularly systemic corticosteroids, may supersede the effects of the disease itself.[1–3]

Bullous diseases affecting the mucous membranes lead to painful oral erosions, which in turn affect the patient's ability to eat or drink. Weight loss, malnutrition, and loss of protein may occur in affected patients over time. Malnutrition leads to increased risk of secondary infection in these exposed areas. Cutaneous erosions compromise the barrier function of the skin and these denuded areas, much like thermal injury, and may lead to volume depletion and infection.[4,5]

Side effects from medications used to treat AIBD can be troublesome. Corticosteroid-related side effects include immunosuppression, diabetes mellitus, osteoporosis, psychological effects, and peptic ulcer disease, to name a few (**Table 1**). The emotional impact of AIBD on affected patients can be profound, including feelings of anxiety, depression, frustration, and fear. Although steroid-sparing agents may prevent steroid-related side effects, they have their own share of adverse effects as well, including bone marrow suppression,

hepatotoxicity, nephrotoxicity, and anaphylaxis. It is vital to collaborate with the patient's primary care physician to aid in the management of these conditions.[1,3,6]

Over the last few decades, morbidity and mortality rates in patients with AIBD have improved for several reasons.[3] New therapeutic modalities have been shown to lower the use of steroids. Earlier recognition and precise diagnosis allow for earlier institution of therapy and milder course of disease. Improved medical and surgical therapy for the numerous complications and more appropriate use of steroids have also lowered the mortality risk.

Patients who present acutely, particularly those with many blisters and erosions, must receive general medical care in addition to skin-directed therapy. Supportive treatment includes oral or parenteral fluids and caloric nutrition. If a patient is unable to swallow because of mucous membrane lesions, a feeding tube or parenteral nutrition may be necessary. Heat loss may lead to chills and thermal dysregulation, requiring the use of blankets and a heated environment. Gentle whirlpool without debridement is helpful to remove necrotic skin. The skin must not be scrubbed to prevent further extension of erosions. Topical bland ointments and pain control are essential for patient comfort. Dressings must avoid tape at all costs because removal of tape frequently

a Meharry Medical College, 1829 Morena Street, Apartment B, Nashville, TN 37208, USA
b Department of Dermatology, University of Texas Southwestern Medical Center, 5323 Harry Hines Boulevard, Dallas, TX 75390-9190, USA
* Corresponding author.
E-mail address: amit.pandya@utsouthwestern.edu

Dermatol Clin 29 (2011) 577–583
doi:10.1016/j.det.2011.06.005

Table 1
Corticosteroid-related side effects and their management

Side Effect	Management
Adrenal insufficiency (weakness, fatigue, myalgias, arthralgias, syncope)	Avoid sudden decrease or discontinuation of corticosteroids; replenish corticosteroids; consultation with endocrinologist
Avascular necrosis of femur or humerus	Monitor for hip and shoulder pain; radiologic studies; consultation with orthopedic surgeon
Cataracts and glaucoma	Review history of visual problems at each visit; consultation with ophthalmologist
Central nervous system toxicity	Monitor for mood swings, psychosis, insomnia, and suicidal thoughts
Delayed wound healing, easy bruising, and thin easily torn skin	Avoidance of trauma; good wound care
Diabetes mellitus	Monitor glucose and hemoglobin A_{1c} levels; may require treatment with oral hypoglycemics or insulin
Electrolyte imbalance (increased sodium level, decreased potassium level)	Monitor electrolytes and replace as necessary
Fluid retention and lower extremity edema	Prevent with low-salt diet, potassium-sparing diuretics, and support hose
Gastrointestinal bleeding	Monitor for anemia; may need to check stool for blood; consultation with gastroenterologist
Hypertension	Antihypertensive agents
Infection (bacterial, fungal, viral, reactivation of tuberculosis)	Culture; PPD (purified protein derivative) testing; quantiferon testing; antimicrobial agents
Menstrual irregularities	May require hormonal therapy if severe
Myopathy and weakness	Adjustment of corticosteroid dose
Osteoporosis, particularly in postmenopausal women	Bone densitometry testing; treatment with bisphosphonates, calcium, vitamin D, and estrogen
PCP (*Pneumocystis carinii* pneumonia) prophylaxis (in those receiving rituximab)	Double-strength trimethoprim/sulfamethoxazole 3 times per wk
Peptic ulcer disease	Oral corticosteroids best if given after meal to prevent ulcers; prevent or treat with H_2 blockers, proton pump inhibitors, and sucralfate
Skin changes (acne, folliculitis, striae, increased growth of unwanted body hair)	Antiacne medications; prevention of weight gain; depilatories; epilation
Weight gain and cushingoid features	Healthy diet; regular exercise

results in new erosions. Nonstick dressings, tube gauze, and rolled bandages are very helpful in correctly dressing affected patients.

CORTICOSTEROID COMPLICATIONS

The impact of the use of steroids in the treatment of AIBD becomes apparent with examination of mortality data. Mortality rates have radically decreased from 60% to 90% in the presteroid era before the 1950s to 5% to 15% since the inception of steroid use.[3] Corticosteroids should be initiated at a high enough dose to control disease (eg, 1 mg/kg/d for pemphigus vulgaris) and tapered slowly over several months when most or all lesions have healed. When doses higher than 30 mg/d of prednisone are given, dividing the dose into a morning and lunchtime or evening dose can reduce some of the side effects. The downside to this therapy is that long-term use for more than a month is associated with side effects that require monitoring and treatment.[7] The team approach, in which a dermatologist and a primary care physician work together to manage such patients, helps to minimize steroid-related side effects. Multiple side effects may occur with the use of chronic steroids, and dermatologists must be aware of these side effects to prevent complications.[8–10]

Immune system suppression may lead to bacterial, fungal, viral, and yeast infections and reactivation of tuberculosis. Topical antibiotics such as mupirocin may limit the development of secondary bacterial infections on eroded skin. Obtaining serology of viral diseases and administering vaccines when indicated helps to prevent severe infection with varicella, zoster, hepatitis, and others. Identification of those at risk of reactivation of tuberculosis is accomplished by tuberculin skin tests and chest radiography, with chemoprophylaxis given to all tuberculin-positive patients.

Diabetes, common in patients who take long-term steroids and gain weight, should be screened for regularly in patients with AIBD through fasting blood glucose testing as well as monitoring of hemoglobin A_{1C} levels. Development of diabetes mellitus often requires temporary treatment with hypoglycemic agents, and when control of blood glucose levels is difficult the patient may require insulin. Patients with preexisting diabetes may require increased treatment intensity because control of blood glucose levels is likely to worsen.

Corticosteroids have also been linked to an increased risk of cardiovascular disease. High doses are particularly associated with heart failure and ischemic heart disease. The evidence for a higher risk of cerebrovascular events is not as strong.

Use of corticosteroids can cause other metabolic abnormalities, including weight gain and a cushingoid appearance, including moon face, buffalo hump, and central obesity (**Figs. 1** and **2**).

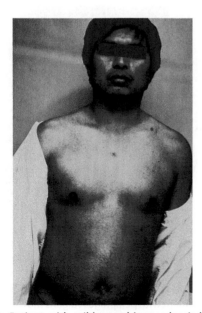

Fig. 1. Patient with mild pemphigus vulgaris before therapy with corticosteroids.

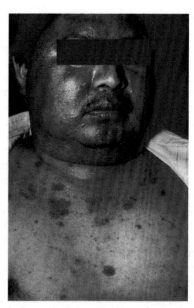

Fig. 2. The same patient as in **Fig. 1** after 18 months of oral corticosteroids in addition to therapeutic trials of azathioprine, dapsone, and intramuscular gold.

Although these changes are difficult to avoid, careful counseling at the outset can help patients in making sure they are eating a healthy diet and getting regular exercise to minimize obesity. Fluid and electrolyte imbalance occurs in the form of sodium and water retention, which may result in the development of hypokalemic alkalosis, hypertension, and lower extremity edema. Patients should be advised to consume a low-sodium potassium-rich diet. Monitoring blood pressure and initiation of potassium-sparing diuretics, if necessary, can help prevent the complications of hypertension. The use of support hose aids in reducing lower extremity edema.

Osteoporosis may occur in patients on more than 10 mg/d of prednisone, especially postmenopausal women. Bone densitometry testing using dual energy x-ray absorptiometry and treatment with bisphosphonates aid in the reduction of osteoporosis and bone fractures. Concomitant supplementation with calcium, vitamin D, and estrogen must also be considered. Additional measures to consider include weight-bearing exercise, smoking cessation, and avoiding excess alcohol intake. Risk of avascular necrosis of the femur or humerus increases with increased dose of steroids and duration of treatment. Early detection using magnetic resonance imaging is critical in preventing total destruction of a joint.[11] Menstrual irregularities and amenorrhea can occur, and female patients should be made aware of these possibilities.

Gastrointestinal (GI) side effects include peptic ulcer disease and GI bleeding. To prevent ulcers, patients should be advised to take steroids after a meal and prescribed enteric-coated corticosteroids when available. Other preventive and treatment options include proton pump inhibitors, H_2 blockers, and sucralfate. Routine blood tests for anemia and stool tests for occult blood may detect early cases of GI bleeding. Because nonsteroidal antiinflammatory agents can increase the risk of steroid-related peptic ulcer disease, clinicians should use caution when prescribing these medications together.

Exacerbation or development of psychiatric problems can occur with the use of corticosteroids. Previously mentally stable patients may develop mood swings, euphoria, depression, psychosis, suicidal thoughts, and insomnia, which can be very disconcerting to family members. These behavioral changes may occur within 2 weeks of beginning treatment and usually respond to tapering within 3 weeks. Again, counseling patients and their families about these potential side effects and using the assistance of their primary care provider when they develop are helpful in managing such patients.

Cutaneous changes from steroids include easy bruising, thin torn skin, acne, folliculitis, striae, and/or increased growth of unwanted body hair. Meticulously avoiding trauma may limit bruising and thin torn skin, which is also prevented by the use of emollients. Acne and folliculitis may improve with topical or systemic antibiotics. Hypertrichosis can be managed by several methods, including depilation, epilation, or photoepilation, depending on patient preference.

It is obvious from the earlier discussion that a thorough history of the present illness, interim medical and surgical history, and full review of systems must be done at each visit for patients with AIBD on corticosteroids. Obtaining vital signs and performing a physical examination are also important. The dermatologist may be the first health care provider to detect an abnormality from interviewing or examining a patient, ultimately leading to the diagnosis of a complication from steroids.

CORTICOSTEROID-SPARING AGENTS AND THEIR SIDE EFFECTS

Several therapies are available to reduce the dependence on corticosteroids in patients with AIBD, including dapsone, mycophenolate mofetil, azathioprine, oral cyclophosphamide, rituximab, intravenous immunoglobulin (IVIG), and plasmapheresis. Less commonly used therapies are tetracycline and niacinamide, hydroxychloroquine, methotrexate, intramuscular gold, cyclosporine, chlorambucil, and intravenous cyclophosphamide. These agents seem to reduce corticosteroid requirements, and their use can positively affect the outcome of affected patients (**Figs. 3** and **4**). However, these therapies have an array of side effects of their own that must be anticipated, prevented, and managed. In general, all steroid-sparing agents should be monitored carefully by frequent visits and appropriate laboratory testing. In most cases, starting at a low dose and slowly escalating the amount of medication based on tolerance are helpful in minimizing side effects.[1,3]

Dapsone is an antimicrobial agent used in the treatment of leprosy. It competes with p-aminobenzoic acid for incorporation into folic acid and exerts an antiinflammatory effect by inhibiting the neutrophil and eosinophil respiratory burst mechanisms and subsequent tissue damage. In addition to impairing neutrophil chemotaxis, dapsone reduces the release of prostaglandins and leukotrienes and inhibits the adherence of neutrophils to basement membrane zone antibodies in patients with bullous pemphigoid, and IgA dermatoses. Dapsone also interferes with complement activation and deposition. Side effects include headache, lethargy, hemolysis, methemoglobinemia, agranulocytosis, leukopenia, peripheral neuropathy, cutaneous eruptions, psychosis, and GI complications.[12] Avoidance of side effects can be achieved by starting at low doses and slowly increasing the dose while obtaining blood

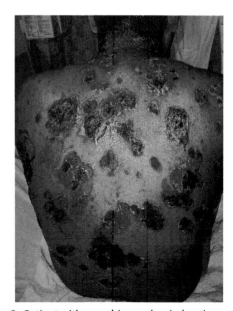

Fig. 3. Patient with pemphigus vulgaris showing active disease despite 1 month of high-dose prednisone, 1 mg/kg/d.

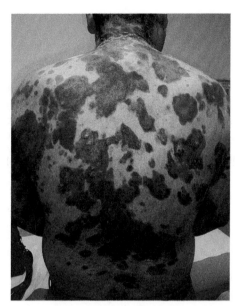

Fig. 4. The same patient as in **Fig. 3** two months after receiving intravenous antibiotics, 4 weekly doses of intravenous rituximab, oral mycophenolate mofetil and corticosteroids. The patient continues on mycophenolate mofetil and oral corticosteroids. Lesions have healed but post-inflammatory pigment changes remain.

tests, particularly a complete blood cell count (CBC) to monitor for anemia. Patients with significant atherosclerotic disease and other conditions in which even mild anemia may not be well tolerated should avoid using dapsone.

Mycophenolate mofetil (Cellcept, Myfortic) is a purine antimetabolite that inhibits the de novo synthesis of purines, particularly in lymphocytes. Mycophenolate mofetil is usually well tolerated, although mild GI distress (diarrhea, nausea) is common. Anemia, leukopenia, and thrombocytopenia may occur, leading to increased incidence of bleeding and infections. These conditions can be monitored with blood counts. Infections, which occur more frequently in patients with mycophenolate mofetil, should be treated with appropriate antimicrobials.[13] Although it is better tolerated than azathioprine, mycophenolate mofetil is more expensive.

Azathioprine, a derivative of mercaptopurine, is a purine analogue. Hepatotoxicity and GI toxicity tend to be the most common side effects. Alopecia, drug fever, and pancreatitis may also occur rarely. Bone marrow suppression with leukopenia or pancytopenia is a rare but serious side effect and responds to discontinuation of azathioprine. Patients should be screened for thiopurine methyltransferase deficiency because 1 in 300 are homozygous for this deficiency, which can lead to severe bone marrow suppression. Those with low normal levels should be monitored

carefully for side effects. Regular laboratory tests such as liver enzyme testing and CBC should be done in patients undergoing azathioprine therapy. If pancreatitis is suspected, amylase and lipase should be monitored as well.[14,15]

Oral cyclophosphamide, an alkylating agent, is most effective in highly proliferative tissues, causing significant toxicity to several tissues and organ systems, including the GI tract, hair follicles, bladder epithelium, and gonads. GI toxicity responds well to antiemetics. Hemorrhagic cystitis and bladder cancer are reported with long-term use, therefore limiting the length of therapy and cumulative dose is essential. Suppression of cellular and humoral immunity, mucosal ulcers, nephrotoxicity, hepatotoxicity, interstitial lung fibrosis, severe myelosuppression, and secondary malignancy may occur and are reversible with discontinuation. With the possibility of sterility, men may consider sperm banking and women oral contraceptives to suppress ovarian function. Hyperpigmentation of the skin, mucous membranes, and nails has been reported with the use of cyclophosphamide.[16–19]

IVIG is prepared from pooled plasma and may contain some IgA. Anaphylaxis may occur in IgA-deficient patients, therefore it is recommended to measure IgA levels before initiating IVIG. Slow intravenous infusion and lower doses usually prevent thrombotic events. Other adverse effects such as myalgia, fevers, chills, tachycardia, and headache are also managed by slowing infusion rates as well as administering antihistamines before infusion. Careful monitoring of patients with cardiac diseases is important to avoid the development of hypertension and congestive heart failure. Association of IVIG with acute renal failure mandates careful evaluation of the benefit/risk ratio in patients with a history of renal disease.[20–22]

Rituximab is a monoclonal antibody against the CD20 antigen on mature B cells. Treatment with this agent is often effective in AIBD. Because rituximab causes a profound long-term reduction of B-cell levels, patients are susceptible to infections after treatment. Pneumocystis infection may occur and can be prevented by prophylactic antimicrobials such as trimethoprim-sulfamethoxazole or dapsone. Because herpes zoster infection is more common in rituximab-treated patients, prophylaxis with oral antiviral agents is also useful. Rare but severe side effects include pyelonephritis, septicemia, toxic epidermal necrolysis, and progressive multifocal leukoencephalopathy. Prescribing physicians should be aware that those patients who are at the extremes of age, have poor general health, or have an underlying

---

Box 1
Sample letter for other physicians participating in the care of patients with autoimmune blistering diseases

Dear Colleague

I have begun high-dose corticosteroids in my patient for a skin disease and anticipate continued treatment for several months. Please help me to monitor the patient for the following:

Infection: bacterial, fungal, viral, yeast, reactivation of tuberculosis

Diabetes mellitus: may require oral hypoglycemics or insulin

Osteoporosis: bone densitometry testing and, if necessary, treatment with bisphosphonates, prophylactic calcium, vitamin D, and estrogen

Avascular necrosis of femur or humerus

Steroid myopathy

Peptic ulcer disease: steroids have been prescribed to be taken after a meal to prevent ulcers; may need H_2 blockers, proton pump inhibitors, or sucralfate

GI bleeding: hemoglobin, hematocrit

Cataracts and glaucoma: will need routine eye examinations

Central nervous system toxicity: mood swings, psychosis, insomnia, suicidal thoughts

Electrolyte imbalance: increased sodium levels, decreased potassium levels

Hypertension: may require treatment with antihypertensives (please avoid angiotensin-converting enzyme inhibitors, angiotensin receptor blockers, and calcium channel blockers, if possible, because they have been associated with the development of AIBD in some patients)

Weight gain and cushingoid appearance (moon face, buffalo hump, and central obesity)

Easy bruising and thin easily torn skin

Fluid retention and edema: low-salt diet, potassium-sparing diuretics

Delayed wound healing

I have asked the patient to follow up with you on a routine basis to monitor their progress. Thank you in advance for your help. I hope that close attention to the patient's health will help to avoid or minimize complications from corticosteroid therapy.

Sincerely
(Name)

---

malignancy are more likely to experience these more severe complications.[23,24]

MINIMIZING COMPLICATIONS IN PREGNANCY

The significance of limiting complications of autoimmune bullous diseases during pregnancy cannot be overemphasized because of the possible risk to the fetus. The disease itself may be harmful to the fetus because pathogenic antibodies may be transmitted transplacentally, causing cutaneous disease in the neonate, placental dysfunction, or stillbirth. Patients should be warned to avoid pregnancy by practicing 2 methods of contraception when being treated for an autoimmune disease with an agent that might harm the fetus. If the patient with active disease does become pregnant, medications should be used only when absolutely necessary, focusing mostly on those with a low incidence of side effects. A good outcome requires close collaboration between a dermatologist and an obstetrician.

Patients may be well controlled with systemic corticosteroids during pregnancy; however, this treatment has been linked with preterm premature rupture of membranes. Addition of azathioprine or intralesional triamcinolone injections to the treatment regimen reduces the required corticosteroid dose and may minimize transplacental transmission of pemphigus vulgaris antibodies. Vaginal delivery is usually chosen because cesarean delivery is not appropriate if there is involvement of the abdomen and corticosteroid therapy may slow wound healing.[25–29]

SUMMARY

Although many treatments have positively affected the outcome of patients with AIBD, each therapeutic approach has its own set of potential adverse effects. Clinicians should proceed with caution when managing such patients and stay up-to-date regarding side effects of these medications and their avoidance. A careful assessment of the benefit/risk ratio should be performed on a case-by-case basis because each patient has unique circumstances. A team approach in which the dermatologist partners with primary care physicians, infectious disease specialists, obstetrician-gynecologists, and other physicians usually results in the best outcomes. A letter to the patient's other physicians at the onset of corticosteroid treatment can help to prevent the many side effects associated with this drug (**Box 1**).

REFERENCES

1. Bystryn JC. Adjuvant therapy of pemphigus. Arch Dermatol 1984;120:941–51.
2. Korman N. Pemphigus. J Am Acad Dermatol 1988; 18:1219–38.
3. Bystryn JC, Steinman NM. The adjuvant therapy of pemphigus. Arch Dermatol 1996;132:203–12.
4. Bean S. Diagnosis and management of chronic oral mucosal bullous diseases. Dermatol Clin 1987;5: 751–60.
5. Mashkilleyson N, Mashkilleyson AL. Mucous membrane manifestations of pemphigus vulgaris. Acta Derm Venereol (Stockh) 1988;68:413–21.
6. Ryan JG. Pemphigus: a 20-year survey of experience with 70 cases. Arch Dermatol 1971;104:14–20.
7. Stanbury RM, Graham EM. Systemic corticosteroid therapy—side effects and their management. Br J Ophthalmol 1998;82:704–8.
8. Moghadam-Kia S, Werth VP. Prevention and treatment of systemic glucocorticoid side effects. Int J Dermatol 2010;49:239–48.
9. Gallant C, Kenny P. Oral glucocorticoids and their complications. J Am Acad Dermatol 1986;14:161–77.
10. DeHoratius DM, Sperber BR, Werth VP. Glucocorticoids in the treatment of bullous diseases. Dermatol Ther 2002;15:298–310.
11. Kamata N, Oshitani N, Sogawa M, et al. Usefulness of magnetic resonance imaging for detection of asymptomatic osteonecrosis of the femoral head in patients with inflammatory bowel disease on long-term corticosteroid treatment. Scand J Gastroenterol 2008;43:308–13.
12. Heaphy MR, Albrecht J, Werth VP. Dapsone as a glucocorticoid-sparing agent in maintenance-phase pemphigus vulgaris. Arch Dermatol 2005;141:699–702.
13. Mimouni D, Anhalt GJ, Cummins DL, et al. Treatment of pemphigus vulgaris and pemphigus foliaceus with mycophenolate mofetil. Arch Dermatol 2003; 139:739–42.
14. Tan BB, Lear JT, Gawkroder JT, et al. Azathioprine in dermatology: a survey of current practice in the U.K. Br J Dermatol 1997;136:351–5.
15. Patel AA, Swerlick RA, McCall CO. Azathioprine in dermatology: the past, the present, and the future. J Am Acad Dermatol 2006;55:369–89.
16. Pandya G, Sontheimer RD. Treatment of pemphigus vulgaris with pulse intravenous cyclophosphamide. Arch Dermatol 1992;128:1626–30.
17. Fleischli ME, Valek RH, Pandya AG. Pulse intravenous cyclophosphamide therapy in pemphigus. Arch Dermatol 1999;135:57–61.
18. Germanas J, Pandya AG. Alkylating agents. Dermatol Ther 2002;15:317–24.
19. Cummins DL, Mimouni D, Anhalt GJ, et al. Oral cyclophosphamide for treatment of pemphigus vulgaris and foliaceus. J Am Acad Dermatol 2003;49:276–80.
20. Jolles S, Hughes J, Whittaker S. Dermatological uses of high-dose intravenous immunoglobulin. Arch Dermatol 1998;134:80–6.
21. Sami N, Qureshi A, Ruocco E, et al. Corticosteroid-sparing effect of intravenous immunoglobulin therapy in patients with pemphigus vulgaris. Arch Dermatol 2002;138:1158–62.
22. Ahmed AR, Dahl MV. Consensus statement on the use of intravenous immunoglobulin therapy in the treatment of autoimmune mucocutaneous blistering diseases. Arch Dermatol 2003;139:1051–9.
23. Joly P, Mouquet H, Roujeau JC, et al. A single cycle of rituximab for the treatment of severe pemphigus. N Engl J Med 2007;357:545–52.
24. Emer JJ, Wolinsky C. Rituximab: a review of dermatological applications. J Clin Aesthet Dermatol 2009; 2:29–37.
25. Goldberg NS, DeFeo C, Kirshenbaum N. Pemphigus vulgaris and pregnancy: risk factors and recommendations. J Am Acad Dermatol 1993;28:877–9.
26. Laskin CA, Bombardier C, Hannah ME, et al. Prednisone and aspirin in women with autoantibodies and unexplained recurrent fetal loss. N Engl J Med 1997; 337:148–53.
27. Fainaru O, Mashiach R, Kupferminc M, et al. Pregnancy and obstetrics. Pemphigus vulgaris in pregnancy: a case report and review of literature. Hum Reprod 2000;15:1195–7.
28. Lehman JS, Mueller KK, Schraith DF. Do safe and effective treatment options exist for patients with active pemphigus vulgaris who plan conception and pregnancy? Arch Dermatol 2008;144:783–5.
29. Kardos M, Levine D, Gurcan HM, et al. Pemphigus vulgaris in pregnancy: analysis of current data on the management and outcomes. Obstet Gynecol Surv 2009;64:739–49.

Management of Autoimmune Blistering Diseases in Pregnancy

Tess McPherson, MD, MRCP*,
Vanessa V. Venning, BMBCh, DM, FRCP

KEYWORDS

- Autoimmune blistering diseases • Pregnancy
- Pemphigoid gestationis • Immunosuppression

Autoimmune blistering disease (AIBD) in pregnancy raises several complex management issues associated with underlying pathogenesis and treatment options. This article considers the effects of the disease as well as treatment for both mother and fetus.

All AIBDs can occur in pregnancy but are relatively rare.[1] There are two distinct clinical situations. The first is a patient with known AIBD who is considering pregnancy or who becomes pregnant. Second is a pregnant woman presenting with a blistering disease that requires diagnosis and management. Pemphigoid gestationis (PG) (formerly called herpes gestationis) is a rare AIBD that is specific to pregnancy.

The authors consider each AIBD in turn and then look at treatment options for the group as a whole, as there are many issues common to all. For each disease the effect of the illness on the pregnant woman is considered as well as the treatments, and the possible effect on the fetus and neonate of maternal illness, maternal antibodies, and maternal treatment.

AUTOIMMUNITY AND IMMUNOLOGY IN PREGNANCY

Tendency to autoimmunity even in the absence of clinically manifest autoimmune disease can affect every aspect of pregnancy beginning with fertilization, and can contribute to maternal complications and adverse fetal outcomes.[2] For this reason, pregnancy in women with preexisting autoimmune conditions, including AIBD, are classified as high risk. However, advances in monitoring and treatment mean that risks can now be managed more effectively, particularly if pregnancy is planned during periods of inactive or stable disease.

Pregnancy is a specific immune state: the mother must maintain tolerance of the fetus while not suppressing her own immune system and exposing herself, and the fetus, to infection. Dramatic hormonal changes occur in pregnancy both in the levels of estrogens and progesterone but also in cortisol, norepinephrine, and dehydroepiandrosterone. At the same time, and partially under the influence of these hormones, profound immunologic changes occur throughout pregnancy and during the postpartum period. These changes are required to accommodate the semi-allogeneic fetus and include immunosuppressive and immune-regulatory processes. Whereas a Th1-dominated milieu is required initially for successful implantation, later gestation requires a predominantly Th2-type pattern of cytokines.[3,4] This situation appears to maintain transient tolerance to paternal antigens in pregnancy. In addition, it seems likely that the generation of specific regulatory T (Treg) cells may play an important role. Treg cells are seen to accumulate in the decidua and are likely to be present in maternal circulation. Tregs are thought to be capable of

Department of Dermatology, Churchill Hospital, Old Road, Oxford OX3 7LJ, UK
* Corresponding author.
E-mail address: tess.mcpherson@imm.ox.ac.uk

Dermatol Clin 29 (2011) 585–590
doi:10.1016/j.det.2011.06.008
0733-8635/11/$ – see front matter © 2011 Elsevier Inc. All rights reserved.

regulating coincidental autoimmune responses through the phenomenon of linked suppression.[3,4] In turn, this suppression may explain why autoantibody levels decline during pregnancy for certain diseases, leading to remission of autoimmune conditions in pregnancy followed by postpartum flares (eg, Graves disease and rheumatoid arthritis).[3] Preexisting AIBD such as pemphigus vulgaris (PV) and linear IgA have been reported to improve during pregnancy, but may flare postpartum.[5] However, not all autoimmune conditions are seen to improve. There are reports of disease flares in most autoimmune disease, and diseases such as systemic lupus erythematosus often worsen, implying that this is a complex process.[2-4]

Maternal autoimmune antibodies cross the placenta and can cause fetal disease both in utero and neonatally.

Bullous Pemphigoid

Bullous pemphigoid is almost never seen in pregnancy, as it affects an older population of people beyond child-bearing age. The rare reports that do exist show the possibility of both flaring and improving in pregnancy.[6]

Pemphigus Vulgaris

PV may improve in pregnancy but often not until the third trimester. A recent review of publications involving 49 pregnant women with PV found that 37% presented with the disease for the first time during pregnancy.[7]

Severe pemphigus in pregnancy may be associated with fetal prematurity and death, but it is difficult to separate the effects of treatment from those of the disease.[8] A recent review found that adverse pregnancy outcomes (ie, neonatal pemphigus and perinatal death) occurred in up to 10% of pregnancies.[7] Adverse outcomes do seem to be correlated more closely with poor maternal disease control, higher maternal serum, and umbilical cord blood antibody titers than with particular medications used to treat maternal PV.[9] Therefore, treatment to cause a decrease in maternal serum autoantibody levels to limit transplacental passage of pathogenic IgG antibodies makes therapeutic sense. However, the effectiveness of such an approach during pregnancy has not been clearly established.[9] It should be remembered that before the advent of systemic steroids PV could cause death, and therefore treatment for some patients will be both necessary and life saving.[10] Additional immunosuppression or plasmapheresis can be used as an adjunct to prednisolone in severe disease.[7,9]

In general, the baby is healthy[11] and although neonatal PV does occur relatively frequently, this tends to be transient disease that is normally mild and treatable topically.[12,13] Differing expression of desmoglein in neonatal skin accounts for the differing clinical manifestations between mother and child.[14,15]

Pemphigus Foliaceus

Pemphigus foliaceus has a variable course in pregnancy. There tends to be no effect on the fetus, and neonatal pemphigus is only seen extremely rarely in the context of exceptionally high antibody titers.[16] Desmoglein 3 is expressed throughout the epidermis including the subcorneal layers in neonatal skin, and may be protective against anti–desmoglein-1 antibodies causing disease.[14,15]

Linear IgA

Linear IgA is seen to improve in pregnancy and commonly remits in the second trimester. For this reason patients may be able to stop dapsone during pregnancy.[17] There is evidence that IgA antibodies become glycosylated during pregnancy, which may explain this remission. There may also be a role for Tregs. However, patients should be counseled about the possibility of a relapse postpartum. Disease may also recur years later even after a prolonged period of remission.[17]

Pemphigoid Gestationis

PG is an autoimmune subepidermal bullous dermatosis uniquely associated with pregnancy. It is an extremely rare condition with an incidence estimated at 1 in 500,000 pregnancies.[18,19] However, a recent review found it was the second most common AIBD diagnosed overall (PG was 9.75% with bullous pemphigoid the most common at 66%[20]), and in a review of pregnant women presenting to dermatology clinics it represented 4.2% of all pregnancy referrals.[1]

PG results from a mismatch between maternal and fetus HLA with paternal antigens, inducing production of antiplacental antibodies that cross-react with the same proteins in skin. The main antigen of PG is BP180 (collagen XVII), present in both skin and placenta, exposed to the maternal immune system through an abnormal expression of major histocompatibility complex class II molecules in the placenta.

Onset of PG is typically late (second to third trimester) but can occur at any point including postpartum.[18] Typical lesions are urticated plaques plus or minus blisters and are initially located around the periumbilicus. Itch can be severe and is the primary symptom. Differentiating from polymorphic eruption of pregnancy (PEP) can be difficult clinically prior to biopsy. However, PEP typically involves striae whereas PG does not. PG can be associated with other autoimmune disease such as Graves disease and vitiligo.[21]

Early onset in pregnancy and presence of blisters does seem to be associated with a worse prognosis, indicating a likely need for more aggressive management. Autoantibody titer has not been shown to correlate with worse disease[22] PG usually resolves within weeks to months after delivery but can recur with subsequent pregnancies (unlike PEP). Recurrence in future pregnancies often occurs earlier (as early as 5 weeks) but may be milder. PG may persist beyond pregnancy, albeit rarely.[23]

PG is associated with fetal morbidity. Several studies have shown an increased risk of preterm birth, small for gestational age, and low birth weight. However, there is no reported increased fetal loss.[18,24–26] Appropriate treatment may decrease this morbidity.[22] BP180 antibodies show transient neonatal disease, which occurs in 2% to 3% of neonates but typically lasts less than 3 weeks, resolving rapidly and causing no permanent harm to the child.[22]

Oral corticosteroids are the therapeutic mainstay both in pregnancy and postpartum, but several other modalities may be tried in recalcitrant disease.[27] Antihistamines can be used for pruritus. No significant associations of adverse pregnancy outcomes with systemic corticosteroid treatment were found in a cohort of 61 women presenting to 3 different tertiary centers.[22]

INVESTIGATIONS IN AIBD IN PREGNANCY

In a patient with known AIBD there may be no need for diagnostic investigation in pregnancy. However, if a pregnant woman presents with a blistering disorder then investigations must be performed to determine diagnosis, just as they would be in a nonpregnant individual. Diagnosis can be made, as in other AIBDs, by skin biopsy and direct and indirect immunofluorescence.

When undertaking a skin biopsy, chlorhexidine can safely be used for disinfection. There is no teratogenic effect described with the use of local anesthetics. However, there is a theoretic risk of prilocaine fetal methemoglobinemia or that adrenaline may reduce uterine blood flow. It is therefore prudent to consider the need for any intervention in pregnancy, including skin biopsy.

TREATMENT OF AIBD IN PREGNANCY

Treatment should be considered for all AIBDs in pregnancy. This strategy is challenging in that all of these diseases are rare and it is difficult to conduct controlled studies. There is limited experience of many drugs in pregnancy, and pregnant women are often excluded from trials. In addition, serious outcomes in pregnancy are rare events and reliable data do not exist. Therefore, most of the treatment options are based on case reports and clinical experience. However, experience of treatments in other diseases gives useful information. As a general rule great care must be taken prescribing in pregnancy, and use of any medication is not recommended unless the potential benefits justify the potential risks to the fetus.

Antihistamines

First-generation H_1 blockers are not associated with an increased risk of major malformations or any other adverse fetal effects.[28] There is a large body of epidemiologic data supporting safety in pregnancy, with a meta-analysis involving more than 200,000 participants concluding that there was no increase in any type of congenital malformation.[29] Although there is less evidence on second-generation H_1 blockers, there is no established link to adverse pregnancy outcomes.[30,31] In addition, none of the antihistamines is excreted in the breast milk in any appreciable amount so as to have any adverse effects on breastfeeding.[32]

Dapsone

Dapsone can be used for its anti-inflammatory effect. It has been used successfully either alone or as an adjunct to corticosteroids in PV and PG.[33] Dapsone has been used widely in the treatment of leprosy and malaria. In this setting there are no reported links to adverse maternal fetal outcomes, and there are no reports of problems if conception occurs while on dapsone.[34] There are rare reports of neonatal hemolysis and neonatal jaundice, and these should be monitored.[35]

Corticosteroids

Although topical corticosteroids are used regularly in pregnancy, a recent systematic review concluded that the evidence is insufficient. Current evidence shows no statistically significant elevated risk of congenital abnormality, preterm delivery, or stillbirth. However, there does appear to be an association between very potent topical corticosteroids and low birth weight.[36]

Systemic corticosteroids are widely used and are effective treatments. Dosage should be tailored to disease control, but a starting dose of 30 to 40 mg is usual for PG.[22] Side effects in pregnant women include all those found in nonpregnant subjects. Increased blood pressure, osteopenia, osteonecrosis, and susceptibility to infection are of particular relevance in pregnancy. Pregnancy induces insulin resistance at later stages, and the resulting glucose intolerance is further enhanced by exogenous glucocorticoids, with an increased risk of gestational diabetes.[37]

Systemic steroids have been reported to cause cleft palate in animal studies, but this is not a consistent finding in human experience.[38,39] On the whole, corticosteroids do not seem to increase the risk of congenital abnormalities in humans.[40] Growth retardation is controversial but has been reported in association with treatment of AIBD.[22] The possible induction of hypertension in adult life by antenatal exposure to corticosteroids has not been proved in humans. Other rare adverse events reported for antenatal exposure to corticosteroids are neonatal cataract and adrenal suppression in children born to women taking high doses of steroids during pregnancy.[37]

There are important differences between classes of steroids. Prednisone and prednisolone are 90% inactivated by the placenta, whereas glucocorticoids with fluorine at the 9α position, such as betamethasone and dexamethasone, are far less inactivated and, therefore, the least dose possible should be used for as short a time as possible for these drugs.

A single course of fluorinated corticosteroids (betamethasone or dexamethasone) given to pregnant women at risk for preterm delivery clearly reduced the risk of death, respiratory distress syndrome, and cerebral hemorrhage in preterm infants.[41] However, evidence has accumulated on the potential harm of repeated courses of fluorinated steroids for the mother and fetus, and these should therefore not be used for disease control.[37]

Other Immunosuppression

Cyclosporine A is an alternative immunosuppressant that seems to be safe in pregnancy. Although not used routinely in pregnancy, it may be preferable to other steroid-sparing medications. Cyclosporine A has been used to treat PG and other pregnancy dermatoses.[9,25] It is known to cross the placenta in high quantities, but is rapidly cleared from the newborn and has not been shown to teratogenic, mutagenic, or myelotoxic in animal models except in very high doses.[42] The data on the safety during pregnancy in humans are primarily derived from transplant recipients. These studies include large series and meta-analyses with cyclosporine in addition to other immunosuppressive agents. Cyclosporine did not appear to increase the rate of malformation frequency, prematurity, or low birth weight.[43–45]

Azathioprine has been shown to have various teratogenic effects at high doses but not at therapeutic doses in animal studies. Available data for larger numbers of patients treated with inflammatory bowel disease suggest that mercaptopurine and the prodrug azathioprine are safe and well tolerated during pregnancy.[46,47] Azathioprine has been successfully used in PV and PG in addition to prednisolone.[9,27]

Mycophenolate mofetil (MMF) and tacrolimus have been shown to be teratogenic in animal studies. There is limited experience of use in pregnant humans, but current advice would be to avoid both topical and systemic tacrolimus and MMF during pregnancy.[47]

Systemic Antibiotics

Antibiotics can be used for an anti-inflammatory effect. Erythromycin and other macrolide antibiotics are considered safe. However, tetracyclines, which are commonly used for combination treatment of AIBD, are contraindicated in pregnancy. Animal studies have revealed evidence of teratogenicity, including toxic effects on skeletal formation. There are no controlled data regarding human pregnancy. However, congenital defects and maternal hepatotoxicity have been reported. When used during tooth development (second half of pregnancy), tetracyclines cause permanent yellow-gray-brown discoloration of the teeth and enamel hypoplasia.[48]

PLANNING FOR PREGNANCY

In patients with established disease, pregnancy is best planned during low disease activity. Medications may have to be changed during pregnancy if current treatment is contraindicated. Steroid-sparing drugs that should be stopped before conception are MMF, cyclophosphamide, and methotrexate. In addition, methotrexate should be avoided in men planning to father a child. There is not sufficient evidence to suggest that changing other medications is essential. However, control with prednisolone is probably advised if possible. If disease cannot be controlled without high doses, azathioprine is probably the best second-line option. Dapsone can be continued if needed for disease control. Cyclosporine is an alternative suitable steroid-sparing drug.[9,17,22,25]

SUMMARY

Management of AIBDs is important in pregnancy for both disease control and symptomatic relief. In PV and PG, treatment may be important to decrease fetal morbidity through reduction of transplacental antibodies. Overall there is more evidence for morbidity following poor disease control than for particular medications used for treatment. However, no drug is safe beyond all doubt in pregnancy. The most well-studied and safest medications in pregnancy are prednisolone, certain antihistamines, certain antibiotics, and cyclosporine. Topical treatments with low absorption should be used if possible, and any systemic treatment should be prescribed with caution and at lowest possible dose for the shortest possible exposure period.

REFERENCES

1. Ambros-Rudolph CM, Müllegger RR, Vaughan-Jones SA, et al. The specific dermatoses of pregnancy revisited and reclassified: results of a retrospective two-center study on 505 pregnant patients. J Am Acad Dermatol 2006;54(3):395–404.

2. Borchers AT, Naguwa SM, Keen CL, et al. The implications of autoimmunity and pregnancy. J Autoimmun 2010;34(3):J287–99.

3. Adams Waldorf KM, Nelson JL. Autoimmune disease during pregnancy and the microchimerism legacy of pregnancy. Immunol Invest 2008;37(5): 631–44.

4. Weetman AP. Immunity, thyroid function and pregnancy: molecular mechanisms. Nat Rev Endocrinol 2010;6(6):311–8.

5. Yip L, McCluskey J, Sinclair R. Immunological aspects of pregnancy. Clin Dermatol 2006;24(2): 84–7.

6. Gee BC, Allen J, Khumalo NP, et al. Bullous pemphigoid in pregnancy: contrasting behaviour in two patients. Br J Dermatol 2001;145(6):994–7.

7. Kardos M, Levine D, Gürcan HM, et al. Pemphigus vulgaris in pregnancy: analysis of current data on the management and outcomes [review]. Obstet Gynecol Surv 2009;64(11):739–49.

8. Goldberg NS, DeFeo C, Kirshenbaum N. Pemphigus vulgaris and pregnancy: risk factors and recommendations. J Am Acad Dermatol 1993; 28:877–9.

9. Lehman JS, Mueller KK, Schraith DF. Do safe and effective treatment options exist for patients with active pemphigus vulgaris who plan conception and pregnancy? Arch Dermatol 2008;144(6):783–5.

10. Ahmed AR, Moy R. Death in pemphigus. J Am Acad Dermatol 1982;7:221–8.

11. Hern S, Vaughan-Jones SA, Setterfield J, et al. Pemphigus vulgaris in pregnancy with favourable foetal prognosis. Clin Exp Dermatol 1998;23:260–3.

12. Chowdhury MM, Natarajan S. Neonatal pemphigus vulgaris associated with mild oral pemphigus vulgaris in the mother during pregnancy. Br J Dermatol 1998;139:500–3.

13. Bjarnason B, Flosadottir E. Childhood, neonatal, and stillborn pemphigus vulgaris. Int J Dermatol 1999; 38:680–8.

14. Wu H, Wang ZH, Yan A, et al. Protection against pemphigus foliaceus by desmoglein 3 in neonates. N Engl J Med 2000;343(1):31–5.

15. Campo-Voegeli A, Muñiz F, Mascaró JM, et al. Neonatal pemphigus vulgaris with extensive mucocutaneous lesions from a mother with oral pemphigus vulgaris. Br J Dermatol 2002;147(4):801–5.

16. Walker DC, Kolar KA, Hebert AA, et al. Neonatal pemphigus foliaceus. Arch Dermatol 1995;131(11): 1308–11.

17. Collier PM, Kelly SE, Wojnarowska F. Linear IgA disease and pregnancy. J Am Acad Dermatol 1994;30(3):407–11.

18. Shornick JK, Bangert JL, Freeman RG, et al. Herpes gestationis: clinical and histologic features of twenty eight cases. J Am Acad Dermatol 1983;8:214–24.

19. Kroumpouzos G, Cohen LM. Specific dermatoses of pregnancy: an evidence-based systematic review. Am J Obstet Gynecol 2003;188(4):1083–92.

20. Bertram F, Bröcker EB, Zillikens D, et al. Prospective analysis of the incidence of autoimmune bullous disorders in Lower Franconia, Germany. J Dtsch Dermatol Ges 2009;7(5):434–40.

21. Shornick JK, Black MM. Secondary autoimmune diseases in herpes gestationis (pemphigoid gestationis). J Am Acad Dermatol 1992;26(4):563–6.

22. Chi CC, Wang SH, Charles-Holmes R, et al. Pemphigoid gestationis: early onset and blister formation are associated with adverse pregnancy outcomes. Br J Dermatol 2009;160(6):1222–8.

23. Holmes RC, Williamson DM, Black MM. Herpes gestationis persisting for 12 years post partum. Arch Dermatol 1986;122(4):375–6.

24. Shornick JK, Black MM. Fetal risks in herpes gestationis. J Am Acad Dermatol 1992;26(1):63–8.

25. Vaughan Jones SA, Hern S, Nelson-Piercy C, et al. A prospective study of 200 women with dermatoses of pregnancy correlating clinical findings with hormonal and immunopathological profiles. Br J Dermatol 1999;141(1):71–81.

26. Mascaró JM Jr, Lecha M, Mascaró JM. Fetal morbidity in herpes gestationis. Arch Dermatol 1995;131(10):1209–10.

27. Semkova K, Black M. Pemphigoid gestationis: current insights into pathogenesis and treatment. Eur J Obstet Gynecol Reprod Biol 2009;145(2):138–44.

28. Gilbert C, Mazzotta P, Loebstein R, et al. Fetal safety of drugs used in the treatment of allergic rhinitis: a critical review. Drug Saf 2005;28(8):707–19.

29. Seto A, Einarson T, Koren G. Pregnancy outcome following first trimester exposure to antihistamines: meta-analysis. Am J Perinatol 1997;14(3):119–24.

30. Einarson A, Bailey B, Jung G, et al. Prospective controlled study of hydroxyzine and cetirizine in

pregnancy. Ann Allergy Asthma Immunol 1997; 78(2):183–6.

31. Källén B. Use of antihistamine drugs in early pregnancy and delivery outcome. J Matern Fetal Neonatal Med 2002;11(3):146–52.

32. Ito S, Blajchman A, Stephenson M, et al. Prospective follow-up of adverse reactions in breast-fed infants exposed to maternal medication. Am J Obstet Gynecol 1993;168(5):1393–9.

33. Armenti VT, Moritz MJ, Davison JM. Drug safety issue in pregnancy following transplantation and immunosuppression: effects and outcomes. Drug Saf 1998;19:219–32.

34. Nosten F, McGready R, d'Alessandro U, et al. Antimalarial drugs in pregnancy: a review [review]. Curr Drug Saf 2006;1(1):1–15.

35. Thornton YS, Bowe ET. Neonatal hyperbilirubinemia after treatment of maternal leprosy. South Med J 1989;82(5):668.

36. Chi CC, Wang SH, Kirtschig G, et al. Systematic review of the safety of topical corticosteroids in pregnancy. J Am Acad Dermatol 2010;62(4): 694–705.

37. Østensen M, Khamashta M, Lockshin M, et al. Anti-inflammatory and immunosuppressive drugs and reproduction. Arthritis Res Ther 2006;8(3):209.

38. Pradat P, Robert-Gnansia E, Di Tanna GL, et al. Contributors to the MADRE database. First trimester exposure to corticosteroids and oral clefts. Birth Defects Res A Clin Mol Teratol 2003;67:968–70.

39. Park-Wyllie L, Mazzotta P, Pastuszak A, et al. Birth defects after maternal exposure to corticosteroids: prospective cohort study and meta-analysis of epidemiological studies. Teratology 2000;62:385–92.

40. Motta M, Tincani A, Meroni PL, et al. Follow-up of children exposed antenatally to immunosuppressive drugs. Rheumatology (Oxford) 2008;47(Suppl 3): iii32–4.

41. National Institutes of Health. Report of the consensus development conference on the effect of corticosteroids for fetal maturation on perinatal outcome. NIH publication no 95-3784. Bethesda (MD): National Institute of Child Health and Human Development; 1994.

42. Ryffel B, Donatsch P, Madorin M, et al. Toxicological evaluation of cyclosporin A. Arch Toxicol 1983;53: 107–41.

43. Armenti VT, Ahlswede KM, Ahlswede BA, et al. National Transplantation Pregnancy Registry—outcomes of 154 pregnancies in cyclosporine-treated female kidney transplant recipients. Transplantation 1994;57:502–6.

44. Armenti VT, Radomski JS, Moritz MJ, et al. Report from the National Transplantation Pregnancy Registry (NTPR): outcomes of pregnancy after transplantation. Clin Transpl 2005;69–83.

45. Bar Oz B, Hackman R, Einarson T, et al. Pregnancy outcome after cyclosporine therapy during pregnancy: a meta-analysis. Transplantation 2001;71:1051–5.

46. Gisbert JP. Safety of immunomodulators and biologics for the treatment of inflammatory bowel disease during pregnancy and breast-feeding [review]. Inflamm Bowel Dis 2010;16(5):881–95.

47. Alstead EM, Nelson-Piercy C. Inflammatory bowel disease in pregnancy. Gut 2003;52(2):159–61.

48. Mylonas I. Antibiotic chemotherapy during pregnancy and lactation period: aspects for consideration. Arch Gynecol Obstet 2011;283(1):7–18.

Infection and Infection Prevention in Patients Treated with Immunosuppressive Medications for Autoimmune Bullous Disorders

Julia S. Lehman, MD[a],
Dédée F. Murrell, MA, BMBCh, FAAD, MD, FACD[b],
Michael J. Camilleri, MD[a], Amer N. Kalaaji, MD[a],*

KEYWORDS

- Immunobullous disease • Immunosuppressive medication
- Infection • Immunization • Vaccination • Wound healing

Infection contributes to considerable morbidity and mortality in patients treated for autoimmune bullous disorders.[1–3] Infection in this population may occur via 3 primary mechanisms. First, when immune-mediated vesicles and bullae rupture, erosions and ulcerations result. Disturbance of the physical, chemical, and biologic barrier provided by the skin (including the keratinocytes with their intercellular scaffolding, acidic lipid secretions of sebaceous glands, antimicrobial peptides, and normal flora) renders hosts increasingly vulnerable to infection.[4] Exudate at eroded cutaneous surfaces nourishes colonizing organisms and potential pathogens. Certain colonizing organisms are capable of forming biofilms, which may contribute to bacterial resistance to topical and systemic antibiotics.[4] Second, most topical or systemic treatments for autoimmune blistering conditions downregulate the immune system, thereby simultaneously compromising the host's ability to fight infection. Third, the very immune dysregulation associated with autoimmunity may increase susceptibility to infection in some patients. For example, complement deficiency associated with systemic lupus erythematosus predisposes patients to infection with encapsulated organisms[5] (eg, Neisseria meningiditis, Streptococcus pneumoniae).

For optimal treatment and prevention of morbidity, it is critical to recognize the increased risk for cutaneous and systemic infection among patients treated for immunobullous disease and to take measures to prevent it. This article reviews localized and systemic bacterial, fungal, viral, and mycobacterial infections associated with immunobullous disease and its treatments. Methods to prevent skin colonization and localized and systemic infection in these patients are also discussed.

No funding sources and no disclosures.
a Department of Dermatology, Mayo Clinic, 200 First Street Southwest, Rochester, MN 55905, USA
b Department of Dermatology, St George Hospital, University of New South Wales, Gray Street, Kogarah, Sydney, NSW 2217, Australia
* Corresponding author.
E-mail address: Kalaaji.amer@mayo.edu

Dermatol Clin 29 (2011) 591–598
doi:10.1016/j.det.2011.06.021

INFECTIONS
Bacterial

Localized
Cutaneous fragility and resultant compromise of the skin barrier associated with autoimmune bullous dermatoses facilitates colonization of the skin (impetiginization) by bacterial organisms, such as *Staphylococcus aureus* and *Staphylococcus epidermidis*. Once bacteria counts achieve a critical level (which, for most species, is 10^5 organisms/gram of tissue[6]), infection and its associated signs (increased localized erythema, tenderness, drainage, edema, and temperature) ensue. Bacterial skin colonization and infection may render the underlying immunobullous disease refractory to treatment by preventing or delaying wound healing (**Figs. 1** and **2**). A study of 30 patients with bullous pemphigoid and cutaneous infection found that 3 had impetiginization and 2 developed erysipelas.[7] Cutaneous infection is significantly associated with increased risk of death in patients with pemphigus.[8]

Distant or systemic
Skin colonization and infection with bacterial organisms can lead to more serious infection of the underlying bone and soft tissue. Once organisms permeate into the vasculature, life-threatening sepsis may ensue. In patients with pemphigus, sepsis is the most common cause of death, with *S aureus* being the most frequently implicated organism.[3] In a study of 30 patients with bullous pemphigoid and cutaneous infection,

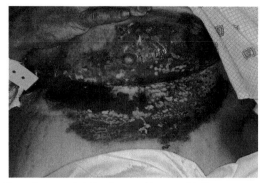

Fig. 2. Impetiginization with methicillin-resistant *S aureus*, *Enterococcus* sp, *Streptococcus viridans*, and *Candida albicans* in a patient taking systemic immunosuppressive medications for pemphigus.

3 developed necrotizing fasciitis and 1 developed sepsis following lymphangiitis.[7] Previously documented rare systemic bacterial infections in patients treated for immunobullous disease include cutaneous and disseminated nocardiosis (**Fig. 3**),[9] *Listeria* meningitis,[10] enterococcal bacteremia,[11] and *Chryseobacterium meningosepticum* cellulitis and sepsis.[12]

Viral

Localized
Viral colonization and infection may complicate immunobullous disease. Some investigators have presented circumstantial evidence that implies a causal association between herpes simplex virus infections and the development of pemphigus.[13] Although herpes simplex virus superinfection is best described in atopic dermatitis (ie, eczema herpeticum), it also occurs in autoimmune bullous conditions (**Fig. 4**).[14,15] In some cases, the presence

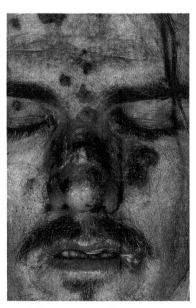

Fig. 1. Staphylococcus impetiginization in a patient taking immunosuppressive medications for pemphigus.

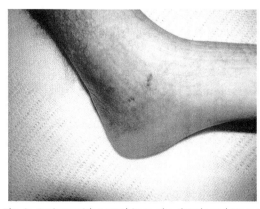

Fig. 3. Patient with pemphigus who developed *Nocardia* infection. (*Courtesy of* Dr D.F. Murrell.)

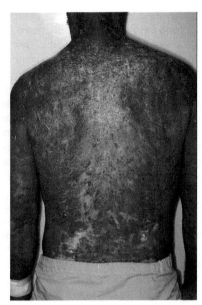

Fig. 4. Herpes simplex virus superinfection in preexisting lesions of pemphigus.

of herpes simplex virus may be clinically occult.[16] Therefore, practitioners must have a high index of suspicion to evaluate for herpes simplex in patients whose immunobullous disease fails to respond to, or worsen on, systemic immunosuppressive medications. Localized Kaposi sarcoma, a low-grade malignant vascular neoplasm caused by human herpesvirus 8 (HHV-8), has been reported in a patient with pemphigus vulgaris.[17] The area of involvement with KS corresponded exactly to the area treated with intralesional corticosteroids. Although HHV-8 has been detected in the skin biopsy specimens of patients with pemphigus vulgaris and pemphigus foliaceus without clinical evidence of Kaposi sarcoma,[18] the clinical and pathogenetic significance of this finding is uncertain.

Distant or systemic

Herpes zoster (HZ; shingles), caused by reactivation of Varicella zoster virus in a dermatomal distribution, usually occurs in the setting of immunosuppression. The risk for HZ in patients treated with systemic immunosuppressive agents for dermatologic conditions is greater than twice that of age-matched control patients (Lehman and Kalaaji, unpublished data, 2010). Specific risk factors for HZ in this population include: advanced age, female sex, underlying solid organ or hematologic malignancy, prednisone use in doses greater than 15 mg per day, lupus, and dermatomyositis (particularly when associated with underlying malignancy). Multifocal Kaposi sarcoma (HHV-8) has occurred in patients treated

for bullous pemphigoid.[19] Patients taking systemic immunosuppressive medications are also at increased risk for reactivation of hepatitis B virus, which may lead to irreversible liver damage.[20]

Fungal

Localized

Superficial cutaneous fungal infections, such as dermatophytosis and candidiasis, may also complicate the course of patients being treated for autoimmune bullous dermatoses (**Fig. 5**).[21,22] The concomitant use of topical corticosteroids could render fungal colonization clinically occult, as with tinea incognito.[23] Therefore, clinicians should adopt an increased index of suspicion for this complicating factor. Whether patients with immunobullous disease have higher rates of onychomycosis is unclear.[24]

Distant or systemic

Pneumocystis pneumonia (PCP), a frequently fatal opportunistic infection caused by the unicellular fungus *Pneumocystis jiroveci*, may occur in patients treated for autoimmune bullous dermatoses. In patients without human immunodeficiency virus infection, mortality from PCP can be high.[25,26] PCP is known to occur in patients taking immunosuppressive medications for dermatologic conditions.[27,28] Particular risk factors for PCP include immunosuppression, advanced age, hypoalbuminemia, underlying pulmonary dysfunction, treatment with prednisone in doses greater than 15 mg per day for greater than 8 weeks, or treatment with cyclophosphamide.[28] Uncommonly reported systemic fungal infections occurring in patients with immunobullous disease include necrotizing fasciitis, cellulitis, or disseminated disease caused by *Cryptococcus neoformans*[29,30] and pulmonary aspergillosis (**Fig. 6**).

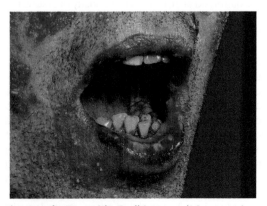

Fig. 5. Infection with *C albicans* and *S aureus* in a patient with pemphigus.

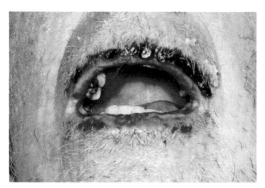

Fig. 6. Patient with paraneoplastic pemphigus who developed pulmonary aspergillosis.

Mycobacterial

Localized
Immunosuppression is a known permissive factor for mycobacterial infections of the skin and soft tissues.[31] This is shown by a case report of cutaneous infection with *Mycobacterium chelonae* in a patient with paraneoplastic pemphigus treated with rituximab.[32]

Distant or systemic
Patients receiving systemic immunosuppression are at increased risk for primary infection with or reactivation of latent tuberculosis by the mycobacterium, *Mycobacterium tuberculosis*. Tuberculosis reactivation in patients with pemphigoid has been reported.[33,34] Moreover, tuberculosis is a well-described risk in patients taking agents that inhibit tumor necrosis factor-α.[35]

PREVENTION
Primary Prevention

Primary prevention of infection should be designed to reduce exposure to potentially pathogenic organisms, improve the barrier function of the damaged skin, reduce the density of colonizing organisms, and optimize factors promoting wound healing in the host.

Measures that can reduce exposure to infectious organisms include avoidance of health care settings, crowded environments, or those with re-circulated air (eg, airplanes), people known to have active infections, travel to places with endemic disease, and other high-risk behaviors, such as getting tattoos. If foreign travel is necessary, it is advisable for patients to be seen by a travel medical specialist familiar with their underlying condition and immunosuppressive medication regimen. Wearing a respiratory mask in high-risk areas (eg, heavily populated areas, doctor's waiting room, airplane) may be considered.

The barrier function of the skin is enhanced with vigilant attention to excellent wound care and the minimization of wound colonization (**Box 1**).[4] In patients with limited mobility or cognitive impairment, the use of a home health nurse or equivalent may be required to assist with personal hygiene regimens and labor-intensive wound dressings. In poorer countries, where infection in the community is a significant risk, patients with autoimmune bullous dermatoses are typically hospitalized for nursing care and dressings. Studies have shown that nursing assistants may also be helpful in identifying early infection in elderly patients.[36]

Gentle cleansing with water and the sparing use of soaps reduces organism counts and thereby reduces the chance for infection. Alkaline soaps, which increase the cutaneous pH and emulsify cutaneous lipids, are to be avoided.[4] The atopic dermatitis literature supports the use of dilute bleach baths in decreasing *S aureus* colonization.[37,38] Moreover, loofah sponges and other fomites making regular contact with the skin should be avoided.[39] When chronic granulation tissue or bacterial biofilms are present, careful manual debridement may be necessary.[40] Wet-to-moist gauze dressings and high-pressure irrigation are reasonable methods for gentle debridement, whereas curettes or a scalpel blade may be used with caution when more extensive debridement is needed. Dressings that maintain an appropriate level of hydration and prevent excessive shearing of the skin should be selected. Silver-containing dressings are nontoxic, have a broad antimicrobial spectrum, and may minimize the development of bacterial resistance.[41]

Box 1
Nonpharmacologic interventions to prevent skin colonization and infection

- Avoid use of alkaline soap or excessive bathing
- Maintain a moist (not overly wet or dry) wound healing environment
- Optimize nutrition and blood glucose levels
- Maintain skin hydration
- Practice regular hand washing/nail cleaning
- Where possible, avoid hospital, group-home settings, or other facilities with high numbers of colonized individuals
- Be educated about early signs and symptoms of infection
- Seek medical interventions early if infection is suspected

In patients known to be colonized with methicillin-resistant *S aureus*, interventions known to be safe and effective include topical mupirocin, chlorhexidine gluconate washes, oral rifampin (with careful attention to potential medication interactions), and doxycycline.[42] Intranasal mupirocin is only marginally effective.[43]

Optimizing other localized and systemic wound healing parameters, such as nutritional status, blood glucose control, lymphedema, and nicotine cessation, is essential.[4] Finding an effective treatment regimen for the underlying immunobullous condition is also important in removing the stimulus for new skin wounds. Patients with autoimmune bullous dermatoses must be educated on signs of infection (eg, fever, increasing skin erythema or drainage) and to seek early medical attention if suspicion for infection exists.

Primary prophylaxis measures for specific infections should be considered in a case-by-case basis. Adult vaccinations for HZ, influenza, and pneumococcal pneumonia are effective methods of disease prevention (www.cdc.gov). Vaccination guidelines have been established for immunosuppressed patients[44] (Table 1) but not specifically for patients taking immunosuppressive medications for immunobullous disease. The organ transplantation literature supports delivery of inactivated vaccinations but not live attenuated vaccinations in iatrogenically immunosuppressed patients,[45] with the recognition that immunosuppression may attenuate vaccination efficacy. However, physician lack of familiarity with vaccine protocols in immunocompromised patients can lead to missed opportunities to immunize these patients.[46–48] Although recent general immunization guidelines have been published,[48] the most up-to-date vaccination information can be found on the Centers for Disease Control Web site (www.cdc.gov).

The HZ vaccination is approved by the US Food and Drug Administration for patients more than 60 years old for the prevention of HZ and is a live, attenuated virus vaccine. It is safe and effective in preventing HZ and postherpetic neuralgia.[49] Although use of high-dose corticosteroids ($\geq$20 mg/d of prednisone or equivalent) for longer than 2 weeks and any use of TNF-α inhibitors represents an absolute contraindication for administration of this vaccination, the vaccine may safely be administered greater than 14 days before initiation of immunosuppressive therapy.[49] Because the trivalent inactivated influenza vaccine is not a live vaccine, immunosuppression is not a contraindication.[48] The pneumococcal vaccination comprises 23 purified capsular polysaccharide antigens of *S pneumonia*.[48] Because it contains no intact virus, this vaccine is encouraged for use in immunocompromised patients.[49]

In patients in whom iatrogenic immunosuppression is anticipated, it is important to consider whether a patient should receive PCP prophylaxis. A recent study estimated the frequency of PCP in a population taking immunosuppressive medications for dermatologic conditions to be 0.5%.[28]

Table 1
Centers for Disease Control recommendations regarding adult vaccinations for immunosuppressed patients

Vaccination	Vaccination Type	Guidelines
Zoster	Live attenuated	Contraindicated during active immunosuppression
Influenza (live)	Live attenuated	Contraindicated during active immunosuppression
Influenza	Inactivated	1 dose recommended
Pneumococcal (polysaccharide)	Inactivated	1 or 2 doses recommended
Tetanus, diphtheria, pertussis (Td/Tdap)	Inactivated	Substitute 1-time dose of Tdap for Td booster; then boost with Td every 10 y
Human papillomavirus	Inactivated	3 doses to age 26 y
Meningococcal	Inactivated	1 or more doses recommended if another risk factor is present
Hepatitis A	Inactivated	2 doses if another risk factor is present
Hepatitis B	Inactivated	Recommended

Abbreviations: Td, tetanus diphtheria toxoid; Tdap, tetanus diphtheria and pertussis vaccine.
Data from Centers for Disease Control and Prevention. Recommended adult immunization schedule – United States. MMWR Morb Mortal Wkly Rep 2011;60(4):1–4. Available at: http://www.cdc.gov/vaccines/recs/schedules/downloads/adult/mmwr-adult-schedule.pdf.

Given this low incidence, and that medications used for PCP prophylaxis have risks, prophylaxis may be reserved for patients with additional risk factors (discussed earlier).[28,50] First-line prophylaxis regimens include trimethoprim-sulfamethoxazole double strength by mouth daily or once 3 times weekly. Alternate regimens include dapsone 50 mg by mouth twice daily or 100 mg by mouth daily, atovaquone 1500 mg by mouth daily, or pentamidine 300 mg aerosol inhaled monthly via nebulizer.[51]

Secondary Prevention

Early antimicrobial intervention with skin infections may serve as secondary prevention of systemic infection. In patients at high risk for cutaneous bacterial infection or a history of cellulitis, it may be reasonable to provide them with a prescription for an appropriate oral antibiotic to start at the first indication of infection to prevent complications. Patients with recurrent herpes simplex infection may be placed on chronic oral suppressive therapy with acyclovir or valacylovir.[52] It is important to screen carefully for and treat latent tuberculosis or viral hepatitis before the initiation of systemic immunosuppressive medications, particularly in patients with known risk factors.[53]

SUMMARY

Patients treated with immunosuppressive medications for immunobullous disease have multifactorial risk factors for developing both cutaneous and systemic infection. Diligent wound care, minimization of exposure to infectious agents, effective treatment of the underlying autoimmune bullous disease, and attention to vaccination status are important in preventing infection and its associated morbidity and mortality.

REFERENCES

1. Langan SM, Hubbard R, Fleming K, et al. A population-based study of acute medical conditions associated with bullous pemphigoid. Br J Dermatol 2009;161(5):1149–52.
2. Savin JA, Noble WC. Immunosuppression and skin infection. Br J Dermatol 1975;93(1):115–20.
3. Ahmed AR, Moy R. Death in pemphigus. J Am Acad Dermatol 1982;7(2):221–8.
4. Wysocki AB. Evaluating and managing open skin wounds: colonization versus infection. AACN Clin Issues 2002;13(3):382–97.
5. Mitchell SR, Nguyen PQ, Katz P. Increased risk of neisserial infections in systemic lupus erythematosus. Semin Arthritis Rheum 1990;20(3):174–84.
6. Robson MC. Wound infection: a failure of wound healing caused by an imbalance of bacteria. Surg Clin North Am 1997;77(3):637–50.
7. Boughrara Z, Ingen-Housz-Oro S, Legrand P, et al. Cutaneous infections in bullous pemphigoid patients treated with topical corticosteroids. Ann Dermatol Venereol 2010;137(5):345–51.
8. Belgnaoui FZ, Senouci K, Chraibi H, et al. Predisposition to infection in patients with pemphigus. Retrospective study of 141 cases. Presse Med 2007; 36(11 Pt 1):1563–9.
9. Asilian A, Yoosefi A, Faghihi G. Cutaneous and pulmonary nocardiosis in pemphigus vulgaris: a rare complication of immunosuppressive therapy. Int J Dermatol 2006;45(10):1204–6.
10. Akyol M, Ozçelik S, Engin A, et al. A case with Listeria meningitis during administration of mycophenolate mofetil for pemphigus vulgaris. J Eur Acad Dermatol Venereol 2007;21(10):1447–8.
11. Garg G, Thami GP. Enterococcal bacteremia complicating pemphigus vulgaris: successful treatment with linezolid. J Dermatol 2004;31(7):580–1.
12. Sood S, Nerurkar V, Malvankar S. Chryseobacterium meningosepticum cellulitis and sepsis in an adult female with pemphigus vulgaris. Indian J Med Microbiol 2010;28(3):268–9.
13. Ruocco V, Wolf R, Ruocco E, et al. Viruses in pemphigus: a casual or causal relationship? Int J Dermatol 1996;35(11):782–4.
14. Feldmeyer L, Trüeb RM, French LE, et al. Pitfall: pemphigus herpeticatus should not be confounded with resistant pemphigus vulgaris. J Dermatolog Treat 2010;21(5):311–3.
15. Marzano AV, Tourlaki A, Merlo V, et al. Herpes simplex virus infection and pemphigus. Int J Immunopathol Pharmacol 2009;22(3):781–6.
16. Nikkels AF, Delvenne P, Herfs M, et al. Occult herpes simplex virus colonization of bullous dermatitides. Am J Clin Dermatol 2008;9(3):163–8.
17. Avalos-Peralta P, Herrera A, Ríos-Martín JJ, et al. Localized Kaposi's sarcoma in a patient with pemphigus vulgaris. J Eur Acad Dermatol Venereol 2006;20(1):79–83.
18. Meibodi NT, Nahidi Y, Mahmoudi M, et al. Evaluation of coexistence of the human herpesvirus type 8 (HHV-8) infection and pemphigus. Int J Dermatol 2010;49(7):780–3.
19. Halpern SM, Parslew R, Cerio R, et al. Kaposi's sarcoma associated with immunosuppression for bullous pemphigoid. Br J Dermatol 1997;137(1):140–3.
20. Yang CH, Wu TS, Chiu CT. Chronic hepatitis B reactivation: a word of caution regarding the use of systemic glucocorticosteroid therapy. Br J Dermatol 2007;157(3):587–90.
21. Hsiao GH, Chiu HC. Dermatophyte infection associated with a local recurrence of bullous pemphigoid. Br J Dermatol 1995;132(5):833–5.

22. Galimberti RL, Flores V, Gonzalez Ramos MC, et al. Cutaneous ulcers due to *Candida albicans* in an immunocompromised patient–response to therapy with itraconazole. Clin Exp Dermatol 1989;14(4): 295–7.

23. Guenova E, Hoetzenecker W, Schaller M, et al. Tinea incognito hidden under apparently treatment-resistant pemphigus foliaceus. Acta Derm Venereol 2008;88(3):276–7.

24. Tuchinda P, Boonchai W, Prukpaisarn P, et al. Prevalence of onychomycosis in patients with autoimmune diseases. J Med Assoc Thai 2006;89(8):1249–52.

25. Green H, Paul M, Vidal L, et al. Prophylaxis of pneumocystis pneumonia in immunocompromised non-HIV-infected patients: systematic review and meta-analysis of randomized controlled trials. Mayo Clin Proc 2007;82(9):1052–9.

26. Yale SH, Limper AH. *Pneumocystis carinii* pneumonia in patients without acquired immunodeficiency syndrome: associated illness and prior corticosteroid therapy. Mayo Clin Proc 1996;71(1): 5–13.

27. Gerhart JL, Kalaaji AN. Development of *Pneumocystis carinii* pneumonia in patients with immunobullous and connective tissue disease receiving immunosuppressive medications. J Am Acad Dermatol 2010;62(6):957–61.

28. Lehman JS, Kalaaji AN. Role of primary prophylaxis for pneumocystis pneumonia in patients treated with systemic corticosteroids or other immunosuppressive agents for immune-mediated dermatologic conditions. J Am Acad Dermatol 2010;63(5):815–23.

29. Adachi M, Tsuruta D, Imanishi H, et al. Necrotizing fasciitis caused by *Cryptococcus neoformans* in a patient with pemphigus vegetans. Clin Exp Dermatol 2009;34(8):e751–3.

30. Yoo SS, Tran M, Anhalt G, et al. Disseminated cellulitic cryptococcosis in the setting of prednisone monotherapy for pemphigus vulgaris. J Dermatol 2003;30(5):405–10.

31. Uslan DZ, Kowalski TJ, Wengenack NL, et al. Skin and soft tissue infections due to rapidly growing mycobacteria: comparison of clinical features, treatment, and susceptibility. Arch Dermatol 2006; 142(10):1287–92.

32. Barnadas M, Roe E, Brunet S, et al. Therapy of paraneoplastic pemphigus with rituximab: a case report and review of literature. J Eur Acad Dermatol Venereol 2006;20(1):69–74.

33. Nanda A, Nanda M, Dvorak R, et al. Bullous pemphigoid (BP) in an infant complicated by tuberculous meningoencephalitis. Int J Dermatol 2007;46(9): 964–6.

34. Kawabata E, Morita K, Matsuyoshi N, et al. Bilateral inguinal scrofuloderma during steroid therapy in a patient with bullous pemphigoid. J Dermatol 1995; 22(8):582–6.

35. Wallis RS. Tumour necrosis factor antagonists: structure, function, and tuberculosis risks. Lancet Infect Dis 2008;8(10):601–11.

36. Tingström P, Milberg A, Sund-Levander M. Early nonspecific signs and symptoms of infection in institutionalized elderly persons: perceptions of nursing assistants. Scand J Caring Sci 2010;24(1):24–31.

37. Huang JT, Rademaker A, Paller AS. Dilute bleach baths for *Staphylococcus aureus* colonization in atopic dermatitis to decrease disease severity. Arch Dermatol 2011;147(2):246–7.

38. Craig FE, Smith EV, Williams HC. Bleach baths to reduce severity of atopic dermatitis colonized by *Staphylococcus*. Arch Dermatol 2010;146(5):541–3.

39. Bottone EJ, Perez AA 2nd, Oeser JL. Loofah sponges as reservoirs and vehicles in the transmission of potentially pathogenic bacterial species to human skin. J Clin Microbiol 1994;32(20):469–72.

40. Wolcott RD, Kennedy JP, Dowd SE. Regular debridement is the main tool for maintaining a healthy wound bed in most chronic wounds. J Wound Care 2009;18(2):54–6.

41. Lipsky BA, Hoey C. Topical antimicrobial therapy for treating chronic wounds. Clin Infect Dis 2009;49(10): 1541–9.

42. Simor AE, Phillips E, McGeer A, et al. Randomized controlled trial of chlorhexidine gluconate for washing, intranasal mupirocin, and rifampin and doxycycline versus no treatment for the eradication of methicillin-resistant *Staphylococcus aureus* colonization. Clin Infect Dis 2007;44(2):178–85.

43. Harbarth S, Dharan S, Liassine N, et al. Randomized, placebo-controlled, double-blind trial to evaluate the efficacy of mupirocin for eradicating carriage of methicillin-resistant *Staphylococcus aureus*. Antimicrob Agents Chemother 1999;43(6):1412–6.

44. Centers for Disease Control and Prevention. Recommended adult immunization schedule – United States. MMWR Morb Mortal Wkly Rep 2011;60(4):1–4. Available at: http://www.cdc.gov/vaccines/recs/schedules/downloads/adult/mmwr-adult-schedule.pdf. Accessed April 20, 2011.

45. Avery RK, Michaels M. Update on immunizations in solid organ transplant recipients: what clinicians need to know. Am J Transplant 2008;8(1):9–14.

46. Haroon M, Adeeb F, Eltahir A, et al. The uptake of influenza and pneumococcal vaccination among immunocompromised patients attending rheumatology outpatient clinics. Joint Bone Spine 2011; 78(4):374–7.

47. Yeung JH, Goodman KJ, Fedorak RN. Inadequate knowledge of immunization guidelines: a missed opportunity for preventing infection in immunocompromised IBD patients. Inflamm Bowel Dis 2011. DOI:10.1002/ibd.21668. [Epub ahead of print].

48. Fiore AE, Uyeki TM, Broder K, et al. General recommendations on immunization – recommendations of

the Advisory Committee on Immunization Practices (ACIP). National Center for Immunization and Respiratory Diseases. MMWR Recomm Rep 2011;60(2): 1–64.

49. Harpaz R, Ortega-Sanchez IR, Seward JF. Advisory Committee on Immunization Practices (ACIP) Centers for Disease Control and Prevention (CDC). Prevention of herpes zoster: recommendations of the Advisory Committee on Immunization Practices (ACIP). MMWR Recomm Rep 2008;57(RR-5): 1–30.

50. Grewal P, Brassard A. Fact or fiction: does the non-HIV/AIDS immunosuppressed patient need *Pneumocystis jiroveci* pneumonia prophylaxis? An updated literature review. J Cutan Med Surg 2009; 13(6):308–12.

51. *Pneumocystis jiroveci* pneumonia treatment and prevention. Medical Letter. Available at: http://dpd.cdc. gov/dpdx/HTML/PDF_Files/MedLetter/Pneumocystis_ jiroveci.pdf. Accessed April 20, 2011.

52. Fillet AM. Prophylaxis of herpesvirus infections in immunocompetent and immunocompromised older patients. Drugs Aging 2002;19(5):343–54.

53. Chan YC, Yosipovitch G. Suggested guidelines for screening and management of tuberculosis in patients taking oral glucocorticoids–an important but often neglected issue. J Am Acad Dermatol 2003;49(1): 91–5.

Evidence-Based Treatments in Pemphigus Vulgaris and Pemphigus Foliaceus

John W. Frew, MBBS, MMed (Clin Epi)[a,b],
Linda K. Martin, MBBS, MMed (Clin Epi)[c],
Dédée F. Murrell, MA, BMBCh, FAAD, MD, FACD[d,*]

KEYWORDS

- Pemphigus • Evidence-based medicine
- Immunosuppressive therapy • Immunomodulating therapy

Treatment modalities in pemphigus vulgaris (PV) and pemphigus foliaceus (PF) are many and varied, although level 1 evidence supporting their use is limited. To date, only 2 systematic reviews exist to support the use of different treatment modalities to control this group of conditions.[1,2] Overall, within the literature, the quality of trials comparing treatment modalities is poor.[3] Cohort sizes are small, methodologies are varied, and standardized outcome measurements are lacking.[1] There is a paucity of high-quality, randomized, double-blind, control clinical trials to accurately assess interventions in pemphigus. The recent development of consensus statements with common definitions and end points will aid in the future by enabling the inclusion of smaller studies, which would otherwise have been underpowered into larger meta-analyses.[4] Although the number of high-quality trials does slowly increase with time, the evidence currently available does allow us to evaluate the efficacy of the more common modalities, such as glucocorticoids, immunomodulating, and antiinflammatory agents. The authors aim to present a comprehensive view of the level 1 evidence that exists for common treatment modalities used in PV and PF.

SYSTEMIC GLUCOCORTICOIDS

Steroids have been used as the baseline treatment and cornerstone of pemphigus management since the 1950s.[1] Although the efficacy of steroids as compared with no intervention is undisputed, the optimal regimen is still unclear. Ratnam's randomized controlled trial (RCT) comparing

This review (Martin L, Agero A-L, Werth V, et al. *Interventions for Pemphigus Vulgaris and Pemphigus Foliaceus (Review)* 2009 Cochrane Database of Systematic Reviews 1: Art No CD006263) is published as a Cochrane Review in the *Cochrane Database of Systematic Reviews* 2009, Issue 1. Cochrane Reviews are regularly updated as new evidence emerges and in response to comments and criticisms, and the *Cochrane Database of Systematic Reviews* should be consulted for the most recent version of the review (http://dx.doi.org/12.1002/14,651,858. CD006263).

[a] St George Hospital, Gray Street, Kogarah, Sydney, NSW 2217, Australia
[b] Faculty of Medicine, University of Sydney, Sydney, NSW 2006, Australia
[c] St John's Institute of Dermatology, St Thomas' Hospital, London SE17EH, England, UK
[d] Department of Dermatology, St George Hospital, University of New South Wales, Gray Street, Kogarah, Sydney, NSW 2217, Australia
* Corresponding author.
E-mail address: d.murrell@unsw.edu.au

Dermatol Clin 29 (2011) 599–606
doi:10.1016/j.det.2011.07.001
0733-8635/11/$ – see front matter © 2011 Elsevier Inc. All rights reserved.

low-dosage (45–60 mg/d) with high-dosage (120–180 mg/d) prednisone did not demonstrate a difference in any outcome, including the time to disease control and relapse rate.[5] All patients achieved remission; however, with only 22 participants, it was inadequately powered. Most expert opinions suggest the initial use of 1 mg/kg/d corticosteroids.[4] The long-term morbidity of glucocorticoids is probably reflected more by the cumulative dose rather than the starting dose, which emphasizes the role of appropriate dose-reduction of steroids when disease control is achieved.[1]

Continuous Versus Pulsed Glucocorticoid Regimens

An RCT of 20 participants was published evaluating the efficacy of adjuvant pulsed oral dexamethasone (300 mg over 3 days monthly) in patients concurrently treated with prednisolone and azathioprine.[5] There was no difference demonstrated in the time to remission (averaging 173 days for the intervention cohort and 176 days for the placebo control cohort), rate of remission or duration of remission.[5] Moreover, the pulsed steroid group experienced considerable adverse events related to the high-dosage steroid. This regimen involved extremely high monthly oral steroid dosages continued for several months after disease control had been achieved, and did not include patients with severe refractory disease for whom pulsed steroids are most likely to be of benefit. These 2 studies both indicate the role for an individual approach to steroid dosage, with dynamic alteration of the dosage according to disease severity and patient response.

SYSTEMIC NONSTEROIDAL IMMUNOMODULATING THERAPIES

Systemic nonsteroidal immunomodulating therapies are typically slow-acting treatments used as maintenance therapies in pemphigus. When combined with systemic glucocorticoids, they often promote disease control while having the added benefit of exerting a steroid-sparing effect caused by the reduction in the amount of glucocorticoid that would have previously been needed to achieve the same level of control. Although the clinical significance of this steroid-sparing effect is still debated in the dermatologic community, the steroid-sparing benefit demonstrated in oncological and transplant medicine is likely to be applicable to pemphigus.

Chams-Davatchi[6] conducted a landmark multi-arm RCT into the steroid-sparing role of adjuvants, comparing prednisolone alone with 3 adjuvant agents: mycophenolate, azathioprine, and pulsed cyclophosphamide. The study demonstrated a significant decrease in the total dose of glucocorticoids when prednisolone was combined with a cytotoxic agent ($P = .047$) using analysis of variance. The average cumulative prednisolone dosages over 12 months were as follows: prednisolone alone 11,631 mg, azathioprine 7712 mg, mycophenolate 9798 mg, and cyclophosphamide 8286 mg. No differences were detected in clinical end points, including time to partial response, complete response, and treatment failure.[6]

Immunosuppressive Therapies

Azathioprine

Azathioprine is a purine synthesis inhibitor originally developed for use in organ transplantation. Azathioprine has been evaluated in 3 RCTs, including comparisons with glucocorticoids alone (prednisolone),[6] cyclophosphamide,[6,7] and mycophenolate.[6,8] Chams-Davatchi's study demonstrated a steroid-sparing benefit of azathioprine compared with prednisolone alone ($P = .047$), although no difference was noted in clinical end points.

In a meta-analysis of 2 studies including 92 patients, Martin and colleagues[1] found a steroid-sparing role for azathioprine compared with mycophenolate (2074 mg prednisone saved, 95% confidence interval [CI] 3543.33 to 608.67, $P = .0056$). In contrast, however, mycophenolate showed superior disease control (relative risk [RR] 0.72, 95% CI 0.52 to 0.99, $P = .043$). Of note, this result was obtained with inclusion of a participant who withdrew after randomization, but before commencement of therapy, and results of the per-protocol analysis performed by the investigators were inconclusive. In light of these disparate findings, there is currently insufficient evidence to draw a conclusion on the relative efficacy of azathioprine compared with mycophenolate.

In their meta-analysis, Martin and colleagues[1] found a superior steroid-sparing role for cyclophosphamide compared with azathioprine (-564.00 mg prednisone 95% CI -1048.54 to -79.46, $P = .023$). However, the statistical analysis conducted by the investigators, which accounted for comparison of multiple groups, found no significant difference ($P = .971$). There was weak evidence of a benefit for azathioprine over cyclophosphamide in disease control (RR 1.80, 95% CI 0.89 to 3.64, $P = .10$)[1]; however, this is based on a study with small patient numbers.[7] The evidence comparing azathioprine with cyclophosphamide is inconclusive. At this stage, selection is advised on an individual basis regarding patient age, fertility, and comorbidities.

Cyclophosphamide

Cyclophosphamide is an alkylating agent that selectively inhibits lymphopoietic cells while sparing hematopoietic cells. It has been shown to be useful in a wide variety of autoimmune conditions by inhibiting cyclical production of antibody-producing B lymphocytes.[8] Martin's systematic review identified 3 studies that included comparisons of cyclophosphamide against glucocorticoids, azathioprine, cyclosporine, and mycophenolate.[1] There was a significant steroid sparing effect when combined as compared with prednisone alone (mean weighted difference [MWD] = -3355 mg; 95% CI -6144 to -566, $P = .018$).[9] The steroid-sparing effect of cyclophosphamide was found to be greater than that of mycophenolate mofetil and lesser than that of azathioprine[9] as shown in **Fig. 1**. It must be noted, however, that reduction in cumulative steroid dose is a surrogate outcome.

Cyclophosphamide can be administered intravenously (IV) or orally. A study of 28 patients was conducted comparing pulsed intravenous dexamethasone-cyclophosphamide plus daily oral cyclophosphamide with pulsed IV cyclophosphamide and daily oral prednisolone.[10] This study demonstrated earlier remission in the pulsed cyclophosphamide/oral prednisolone group (mean 7.3 weeks vs 3.2 weeks, $P = .02$); however, no difference was demonstrated in overall remission or relapse.[10]

When comparing Cyclophosphamide with other immunosuppressive medications, no significant difference was seen in any clinical outcomes when comparing cyclophosphamide and mycophenolate.[11] No difference in any outcome, including time to disease control or relapse, was found when cyclophosphamide was compared with cyclosporine in a small study of 18 participants.[7] The comparison of cyclophosphamide and azathioprine was discussed earlier. A major drawback to the use of cyclophosphamide is its safety profile, which is discussed later.

Mycophenolate

Mycophenolate has been evaluated in 3 RCTs, including comparisons with glucocorticoids, azathioprine, and cyclophosphamide.[9,11] Beissert's[12] recent article comparing mycophenolate with placebo in 96 patients showed no statistically significant difference between the rates of response of glucocorticoids and mycophenolate and glucocorticoids plus placebo. However, the addition of mycophenolate mofetil had a significant impact in hastening the average time to disease control (31.3 weeks in placebo vs 24.1 weeks in mycophenolate) and in delaying the average time to relapse[12] (relapse rate at 24 weeks was 44.5% in the placebo group vs 21.8% in the mycophenolate group [hazard ratio = 0.44, 95% CI 0.2–0.97, $P = .034$]). Beissert and colleagues[12] also found a significant decrease in the total amount of glucocorticoid required from week 12 to week 52 in the mycophenolate group when compared with the placebo group (MWD -1229.50 mg, $P = .028$), although no difference was observed in the total steroid dose when including the initial 12-week taper period. The comparisons of mycophenolate versus azathioprine and mycophenolate versus cyclophosphamide were discussed earlier.

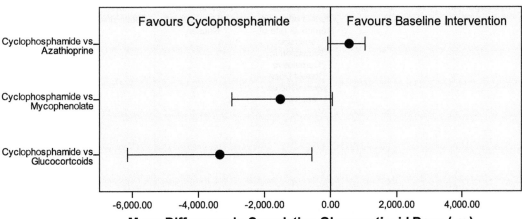

Fig. 1. Steroid-sparing effect of cyclophosphamide compared with baseline intervention (azathioprine, mycophenolate, or glucocorticoids). (*From* Daniel BS, Murrell DF. The actual management of pemphigus. G Ital Dermatol Venerol 2010;145:689–702; with permission.)

Drug	Recommendation and Level of Evidence[26,27]	Evidence	Principal Side Effects	Advantages	Disadvantages
Oral Glucocorticoids	A (2-3)	Basic Pillar of Therapy. Optimal Regimen Unknown	Diabetes; osteoporosis; weight gain; immuno-suppression; mood changes; proximal myopathy;	Oral Administration Effective, Rapid Onset.	Acute and Chronic Side Effect Profile
Pulsed Glucocorticoids	C (3)	No statistical benefit over oral steroids. Expert recommendation in disease recalcitrant to high dose steroids.			Side Effect Profile, Intravenous Administration
Immunosuppressive Adjuvant Therapy					
Azathioprine	C (1)	No statistical benefit over oral steroids in rate of remission. Reduction in Cumulative Steroid Dose when used as adjuvant.	Myelo-suppression, Nausea, Hepatotoxicity	Oral Administration	Slow Onset of Efficacy Side Effect Profile
Cyclo-phosphamide	C (1)	No statistical benefit over oral steroids in rate of remission. Reduction in Cumulative Steroid Dose when used as adjuvant.	Neutropoenia, Nausea, Hepatotoxicity	Oral Administration (Unless Pulsed)	IV Administration (For Pulsed therapy)
Mycophenolate Mofetil	C (1)	No statistical benefit over oral steroids in rate of remission. Reduction in Cumulative Steroid Dose when used as adjuvant.	Neutropenia, Lymphopenia, Thrombocytopenia, Anaemia, Nausea	Oral Administration	Side Effect Profile
Cyclosporine	C (1)	No statistical benefit over oral steroids in rate of remission. Reduction in Cumulative Steroid Dose when used as adjuvant.	Hypertension, Renal Impairment, Nausea	Oral Administration	Side Effect Profile

Fig. 2. Level of evidence for therapeutic modalities in pemphigus. Key to recommendations and level of evidence. (*Data from* Refs.[1,4,9,13,26,27])

Drug	Recommendation	Evidence	Principal Side Effects	Advantages	Disadvantages
Methotrexate	C (2-2)	No statistical benefit over oral steroids in rate of remission	Myelosuppression, Hepatic Toxicity, Pulmonary Fibrosis	Oral Administration	Side Effect Profile
Immunomodulating Adjuvant Therapy					
Dapsone	C (1)	No statistical benefit over oral steroids in rate of remission. Study Underpowered.	Hemolysis, Methemoglobinemia	Oral Administration	Side Effect Profile
Intravenous Immunoglobulin	B (1)	Significant reduction in time to remission for 400mg IVIG	Infusion Reaction (Chills, Pyrexia, Tachycardia) Rarely Anaphylaxis	Rapid Response	Intravenous Administration Labour Intensive
Plasmapheresis	C (1)	No statistical benefit over control	Septicaemia, Electrolyte Disturbances	Rapid Response	Intravenous Administration Labour Intensive
Topical Adjunctive Therapies					
Topical Epidermal Growth Factor	B (1)	Significant improvement in time to healing of cutaneous lesions when used as adjunctive therapy		Topical Administration	
Topical Pimecrolimus	B (1)	Significant improvement in time to healing of cutaneous lesions when used as adjunctive therapy		Topical Administration	
Other Therapies					
Traditional Chinese Medicine	I (1)	One RCT, Poorly Reported	Poorly Reported	Poorly Reported	Poorly Reported
Sulfasalazine and Pentoxifylline	C (1)	One RCT Study.	Hepatotoxicity, Thrombocytopenia, Neutropenia	Low Cost	Side Effect Profile

Fig. 2. (continued)

Safety comparison between azathioprine, mycophenolate, and cyclophosphamide

Comparison of the steroid-sparing capacities of azathioprine, mycophenolate, and cyclophosphamide has shown no significant benefit or detriment of one particular treatment over another with the evidence available at hand. Drug safety is another aspect to take into consideration when choosing an appropriate therapeutic modality. Cyclophosphamide carries significant health risks, including fertility issues and long-term cancer risks (**Fig. 2**).[1,4,9,13] Azathioprine has risks of hepatotoxicity and myelosuppression, which are also side effects shared with mycophenolate mofetil and cyclophosphamide (see **Fig. 2**).[1,4,9,13] In terms of cost, mycophenolate is more expensive than azathioprine and cyclophosphamide.[3,13] This can be a disincentive to the patients who pay for, and the health care providers who may subsidize, these medications. Expert opinion often recommends the avoidance of cyclophosphamide for safety reasons.[3]

Cyclosporine

Cyclosporine has been evaluated in 2 small RCTs, including comparisons with glucocorticoids alone (including prednisone and methylprednisolone)[7,14] and cyclophosphamide.[8] No significant difference was demonstrated for the efficacy of cyclosporine compared with cyclophosphamide or in remission, disease control, or rates of relapse.[7,14] There was no difference observed in the cumulative glucocorticoid dose when compared with placebo control (MWD -51.00 mg; 95% CI -183.38 mg to 81.38 mg).[7] Moreover, there was no difference observed in any clinical outcome, including remission, disease control, or relapse when cyclosporine was compared with glucocorticoids alone.[7]

Antiinflammatory Therapies

Dapsone
Dapsone is a chemotherapeutic agent theorized to function as an antiinflammatory therapy through inhibiting myeloperoxidase resulting in antineutrophilic activity.[15] Martin and colleagues'[1] 2009 systematic review identified 1 placebo-controlled RCT in which the effect of dapsone as a third-line adjuvant agent in pemphigus was examined. It included 19 PV and PF participants who were twice unable to taper their prednisone lower than 15 mg/d using a predefined tapering schedule.[16] The steroid-sparing effect of dapsone was inconclusive because the study was underpowered. The effect of dapsone on the rate of remission and withdrawal caused by adverse events was also inconclusive[1] (remission RR 1.85, 95% CI 0.61–5.63, and withdrawal RR 0.37, 95% CI 0.05–2.95).

Sulfasalazine and pentoxifylline
El-Darouti and colleagues[17] published a RCT in 2009 concerning the efficacy of sulfasalazine and pentoxifylline as low-cost antiinflammatory drugs to control PV. All 64 patients in the study were initiated on 500 mg of an oral glucocorticoid and 100 mg of cyclophosphamide. Forty-two patients also received 500 mg sulfasalazine TDS and 400 mg pentoxifylline TDS with the remaining enrolled patient receiving placebo. The difference between the 2 groups at 8 weeks regarding clinical improvement (as rated by a blinded dermatologist) was statistically significant (P<.001) favoring the intervention group.[17]

Intravenous immunoglobulin
Intravenous immunoglobulin (IVIG) has been used as one component of combined therapy for severe pemphigus since 1989.[18] A recent randomized trial by Amagai and colleagues[18] examined the efficacy of a single-cycle of adjuvant IVIG in the management of pemphigus in 61 participants.

The primary outcome measure reported was time to escape from protocol, which is akin to duration of response. Their results revealed a benefit in duration of response in the 400 mg IVIG treatment group when compared with placebo (P<.001).[18] The comparison between the 200-mg IVIG treatment group and the placebo group showed weak evidence of effect (P = .052), although it demonstrates a dose-response relationship for IVIG (Fig. 3).[18] There was also a benefit in pemphigus activity score[19] and antibody titre demonstrated with IVIG.[18]

Plasmapheresis
Guillaume and colleagues[20] presented the results of a study of 40 participants investigating the efficacy of plasmapheresis in pemphigus. There was no difference in any outcome in this study, including disease control, cumulative steroid dose, or serum antibody titres.[20] Four individuals of the 22 composing the intervention cohort died of thromboembolism or infection and no deaths were reported in the control group. Although the difference between mortality rates was not calculated to be statistically significant (RR 7.43; 95% CI 0.43 to 129.55), it is, nevertheless, concerning. It is unclear if the mortality in this study was related to disease or protocol-related factors.[20] Since that time, no further RCTs evaluating the efficacy of this modality in pemphigus have been reported.

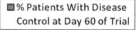

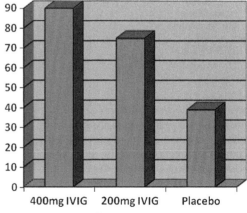

Fig. 3. Percentage of patients who had not achieved escape from protocol at day 60 of trial in 3 different treatment groups. (*From* Amagai M, Ikeda S, Shimizu H, et al. A randomized double blind trial of intravenous immunoglobulin for Pemphigus. J Am Acad Dermatol 2009;60:595–603; with permission.)

Topical Therapies

Topical epidermal growth factor

Tabrizi and colleagues present one study examining the effect of topical epidermal growth factor on healing time of cutaneous lesions in PV and PF when compared with a control cream (topical silver sulfadiazine [SSD]). Reanalysis of this data with survival analysis techniques demonstrated a benefit of topical epidermal growth factor in time to lesion healing compared with control[1] (hazard ratio 2.35, 95% CI 1.62 –3.41).[21] The long-term safety profile of this intervention is not well studied.

Topical pimecrolimus

A recent randomized, double-blind, left-right placebo-controlled study by Iraji and colleagues[22] assessed the effect of adjuvant topical 1% pimecrolimus cream in 11 patients treated with systemic glucocorticoids and azathioprine. Topical 1% pimecrolimus cream decreased the diameter of cutaneous lesions in patients with PV by a mean of 19% at day 30. Comparison with a placebo cream applied to a symmetric lesion on the same patient revealed a significant difference ($P<.0001$).[22]

Traditional Chinese Medicine

Traditional Chinese medicine was evaluated in 1 RCT of 40 participants.[23] In this study, the cumulative glucocorticoid dose was reported as superior in the traditional Chinese medicine group to the control; however, raw data was not reported.[23] No difference in serum antibody titre was observed for traditional Chinese medicine compared with glucocorticoids alone.[23] Overall, this study was poorly reported and, hence, the true efficacy of the intervention was difficult to assess.

PRACTICAL MANAGEMENT OF PEMPHIGUS: WHAT WE DO BASED ON THE EVIDENCE

Following a confirmed diagnosis of pemphigus, it is the authors' practice, based on the evidence presented earlier, to prescribe 1 mg/kg/d of oral prednisone while checking patients' thiopurine methyl transferase (TPMT) activity and other baseline safety investigations (such as full blood count, hepatic and renal function tests, bone density) before azathioprine. The prednisone dose is stable until patients reach the consolidation phase.[24] Azathioprine is commenced based on the TPMT activity levels and is chosen initially based on its low cost unless there are contraindications to its use. Safety bloods and blood pressure are monitored. After the consolidation phase, the steroids are gradually reduced by 10 mg every week until they reach 40 mg/d. After this, the authors use the taper developed by Victoria Werth as used in the dapsone trial previously quoted.[16] The azathioprine dose is maintained, unless adverse effects arise, until the steroids are tapered to zero. If there are problems with azathioprine, then mycophenolate mofetil at 2 g/d is substituted as the next drug of choice. If both of these approaches do not work or the pemphigus relapses, IVIG is commenced at 400 mg/d for 3 consecutive days per month for 3 to 6 months; and once stable, the prednisone is tapered. Rarely rituximab may be used for recalcitrant disease. Methotrexate may also be used as an adjunctive treatment in the place of azathioprine or mycophenolate. For PF, dapsone is also considered as a first-line agent.

SUMMARY OF FINDINGS

The optimal therapeutic strategy for pemphigus vulgaris and pemphigus foliaceus is not known. With multiple treatment modalities and regimens available, treatment choice is complex. In addition to the evidence of the efficacy discussed in this review, the adverse effect profile, cost, and patient comorbidities are also important considerations. Of the randomized controlled trials that have been conducted, many are limited by small sample sizes. Systemic glucocorticoids are central to the effective management of pemphigus, although evidence is not clear as to the optimal dose or regimen. Adjuvant immunosuppressants or modulatory agents have evidence supporting a steroid-sparing role; although, no direct benefits have been observed for remission or disease control. Topical preparations seem to decrease the time required for healing of erosions. The development of consensus definitions and disease activity scores[3,24,25] should assist with smaller studies being combined in meta-analyses when larger studies are difficult to perform. These efforts will bear fruit in the coming years with much more evidence available to combine into powerful meta-analyses. Overall, further trials will contribute additional information to help clarify the optimal treatments for pemphigus. Any management strategy for individual patients should include consideration of potential benefits and adverse events unique to the individual patient.

REFERENCES

1. Martin L, Agero AL, Werth V, et al. Interventions for pemphigus vulgaris and pemphigus foliaceus [review]. Cochrane Database Syst Rev 2009;1: CD006263.

2. Li W, Wei ML, Li JY, et al. Evidence-based treatment for a patient with oral pemphigus. Chinese Journal of Evidence-Based Medicine 2005;5(9):715–7.

3. Martin LK, Murrell DF. Treatment of pemphigus: the need for more evidence. Arch Dermatol 2008;144: 100–1.

4. Murrell DF, Dick S, Ahmed AR, et al. Consensus statement on definitions of disease, end points and therapeutic response for pemphigus. J Am Acad Dermatol 2008;58(6):1043–6.

5. Ratnam K, Phay K, Tan C. Pemphigus therapy with oral prednisolone regimens: a five year study. Int J Dermatol 1990;29:363–7.

6. Chams-Davatchi C, Esmaili N, Daneshpazhooh M, et al. Randomized controlled open label trial of four treatment regimens for pemphigus vulgaris. J Am Acad Dermatol 2007;57:622–8.

7. Rose E, Wever S, Zillikens D, et al. Intravenous dexamethasone-cyclophosphamide pulse therapy in comparison with oral methylprednisolone-azathioprine therapy in patients with pemphigus vulgaris: results of a multicenter prospectively randomized study. J Dtsch Dermatol Ges 2005;3:200–6.

8. Beissert S, Werfel T, Frieling U, et al. A comparison of oral methylprednisolone plus azathioprine or mycophenolate mofetil for the treatment of pemphigus. Arch Dermatol 2006;142:1447–54.

9. Daniel BS, Murrell DF. The actual management of pemphigus. G Ital Dermatol Venereol 2010;145: 689–702.

10. Sethy P, Khandpur S, Sharma V. Randomized open comparative trial of dexamethasone-cyclophosphamide pulse and daily oral cyclophosphamide versus cyclophosphamide pulse and daily oral prednisolone in pemphigus vulgaris. Indian J Dermatol Venereol Leprol 2009;75(5):476–82.

11. Mentink L, Mackenzie M, Toth G, et al. Randomized control trial of adjuvant oral dexamethasone pulse therapy in pemphigus vulgaris. Arch Dermatol 2007;143:570–6.

12. Beissert S, Mimouni D, Kanwar A, et al. Treating pemphigus vulgaris with prednisone and mycophenolate mofetil: a multicenter, randomized, placebo-controlled trial. J Invest Dermatol 2010;130:2041–8.

13. Harman K, Albert S, Black M. Guidelines for the management of pemphigus vulgaris. Br J Dermatol 2003;149:926–37.

14. Chrysomallis F, Ioannides D, Teknetzis A, et al. Treatment of oral pemphigus vulgaris. Int J Dermatol 1994;33:803–7.

15. Ioannides D, Chrysomallis F, Bystryn J. Ineffectiveness of cyclosporine as an adjuvant to corticosteroids in the treatment of pemphigus. Arch Dermatol 2000; 136:868–72.

16. Werth V, Fivenson D, Pandya A, et al. Multicenter randomized placebo controlled trial of dapsone as a glucocorticoid sparing agent in maintenance phase pemphigus vulgaris. Arch Dermatol 2008; 144:25–34.

17. El-Darouti M, Marzouk S, Abdel Hay R, et al. The use of sulfasalazine and pentoxifylline (low cost antitumour necrosis factor drugs) as adjuvant therapy for the treatment of pemphigus vulgaris: a comparative study. Br J Dermatol 2009;161:313–9.

18. Amagai M, Ikeda S, Shimizu H, et al. A randomized double blind trial of intravenous immunoglobulin for pemphigus. J Am Acad Dermatol 2009;60: 595–603.

19. Herbst A, Bystryn JC. Patterns of remission in pemphigus vulgaris. J Am Acad Dermatol 2000;42: 422–7.

20. Guillaume J, Roujeau J, Morel P, et al. Controlled study of plasma exchange in pemphigus. Arch Dermatol 1988;124:1659–63.

21. Tabrizi M, Chams-Davatchi C, Esmaeeli N, et al. Accelerating effects of epidermal growth factor on skin lesions of pemphigus vulgaris: a double blind, randomized controlled trial. J Eur Acad Dermatol Venereol 2007;21:79–84.

22. Iraji F, Asilian A, Siadat A. Pimecrolimus 1% cream in the treatment of cutaneous lesions of pemphigus vulgaris: a double-blind placebo controlled clinical trial. J Drugs Dermatol 2010;9:684–6.

23. Luo X, Zhu L, Tao L, et al. The clinical and laboratory research for Chinese traditional medicine in the treatment of pemphigus. J Clin Dermatol 2003;32:38–41.

24. Pfutze M, Niedermeier A, Hertl M, et al. Introducing a novel autoimmune bullous skin disorder intensity score (ABSIS) in pemphigus. Eur J Dermatol 2007; 17:4–11.

25. Rosenbach M, Murrell DF, Bystryn JC, et al. Reliability and convergent validity of two outcome instruments for pemphigus. J Invest Dermatol 2009;129: 2404–10.

26. U.S. Preventive Services Task Force. U.S. Preventive Services Task Force Ratings: grade definitions. 3rd edition. Guide to Clinical Preventive Services; 2000–2003. Available at: http://www.uspreventiveservice staskforce.org/3rduspstf/ratings.htm. Accessed December 29, 2010.

27. U.S. Preventive Services Task Force. Guide to clinical preventive services: report of the U.S. Preventive Services Task Force. Philadelphia: DIANE Publishing; 1989. p. 24.

Current Management Strategies in Paraneoplastic Pemphigus (Paraneoplastic Autoimmune Multiorgan Syndrome)

John W. Frew, MBBS, MMed (Clin Epi)[a,b],
Dédée F. Murrell, MA, BMBCh, FAAD, MD, FACD[c,*]

KEYWORDS
• Paraneoplastic pemphigus
• Paraneoplastic autoimmune multiorgan syndrome
• Management

Paraneoplastic pemphigus (PNP) or paraneoplastic autoimmune multiorgan syndrome (PAMS) is a life-threatening autoimmune blistering disease commonly associated with lymphoproliferative neoplasms.[1] It is characterized by painful mucosal erosions with a polymorphous skin eruption (not always defined by bullae) in association with an occult or verified neoplasm.[1–4] Mortality due to the disease has been reported to be as high as 90%.[4] Response to therapy is highly variable, with an incomplete knowledge of the pathogenesis of the disease making targeted therapies a challenge.[4–6] Our article in the previous issue of this journal entitled 'Paraneoplastic Pemphigus (Paraneoplastic Autoimmune Multiorgan Syndrome): Clinical Presentations and Pathogenesis' discusses the varied clinical presentations and pathologic characteristics pertaining to this condition.[7] This article focuses on current management strategies in PNP/PAMS, and reported instances of their treatment successes and failures.

However, due to the rarity of the condition and the high rates of treatment failure, no randomized control trials exist to guide the evidence-based treatment of this condition; all evidence to date on the efficacy of therapeutic modalities has been gained from individual case reports, small case series, and expert recommendations.

INITIAL MANAGEMENT IN SUSPECTED PNP/PAMS

The varied clinical presentations of PNP/PAMS supports the need for patients who present with an aggressive mucous membrane and/or cutaneous eruption, with overlapping features of pemphigus vulgaris, erosive lichen planus, or erythema multiforme, to be assessed for the possibility of PNP/PAMS prior to the institution of empirical immunosuppressive therapy. Empirical immunosuppression in the setting of an undiagnosed neoplasm may be highly detrimental to

[a] St George Hospital, Gray Street, Kogarah, Sydney, NSW 2217, Australia
[b] Faculty of Medicine, University of Sydney, Sydney, NSW 2006, Australia
[c] Department of Dermatology, St George Hospital, University of New South Wales, Gray Street, Kogarah, Sydney, NSW 2217, Australia
* Corresponding author.
E-mail address: d.murrell@unsw.edu.au

Dermatol Clin 29 (2011) 607–612
doi:10.1016/j.det.2011.06.016
0733-8635/11/$ – see front matter © 2011 Elsevier Inc. All rights reserved.

the patient's clinical condition, particularly as one hypothesis regarding the pathogenesis of PNP/PAMS involves direct production of autoantibodies by tumor cells.[6] Similarly, in individuals presenting with a known history of neoplastic disease, caution should be exercised in empirical immunosuppression prior to definitive diagnosis, and a reduced threshold for bladder IF testing should be considered.

In the acute inpatient setting, stabilization of the patient is paramount while identification of the suspected neoplasm, or assessment of the progression of a known neoplasm, occurs. Previous empirical immunosuppression may already have been initiated before the identification of a neoplasm, and this should be taken into account when assessing the need for monitoring and other supportive therapy, as sepsis may cause rapid and life-threatening deterioration. This deterioration is another reason why suspected cases of pemphigus are best managed in a specialist center familiar with autoimmune bullous diseases, of which there are a few in most countries.

MANAGEMENT STRATEGIES IN PNP/PAMS

Management strategies in PNP/PAMS can be divided into a series of 6 steps, which should begin when PNP/PAMS is suspected as a diagnosis:

1. Stabilization of the patient
2. Investigation for the presence of malignancy
3. Establishment of a definitive diagnosis of PNP/PAMS
4. Removal of the underlying neoplasm where feasible
5. Medical treatment of the underlying neoplasm
6. Treatment of the disease itself (individualized for the patient) through either:
   a. Immunosuppression
   b. Immunomodulation
   c. Removal of pathogenic autoantibodies.

The most definitive management of PNP in cases involving localized nonmetastatic neoplasm involves the elimination/removal of the causative neoplasm,[2,6] although in many cases the high and rapid progression to mortality in PNP/PAMS results in the acute management and stabilization of the patient to be of greater immediate priority than definitive surgical or oncologic therapy.[3] In cases of PNP/PAMS that have been associated with thymoma or Castleman tumor, surgical excision of the tumor has been shown to radically improve the cutaneous manifestations of the illness, although a few reports have shown persistent disease despite the elimination of the underlying neoplasm.[6]

As opposed to other forms of pemphigus, for which high-dose corticosteroids and immunosuppressive agents have a moderate success rate in reducing the severity of the disease, many cases of PNP/PAMS have been reported to be resistant to all forms of therapy as traditionally used in other autoimmune bullous diseases.[2,6] This high level of resistance to therapy supports several of the mechanisms as presented by Vezzoli and colleagues,[6] who suggest that the tumor cells either directly produce the autoantibodies as seen in PNP/PAMS (also seen in malignant acanthosis nigricans), or are indirectly involved in their production or activation.[6] Other contributing factors to the relatively large number of reports of resistant cases may be publication bias, as well as the knowledge that the success of treatment in PNP/PAMS is dependent on many complex and interacting factors, including the length of survival of the patient, the progression of underlying malignancy, and other cormorbidities such as concurrent infection secondary to immunosuppression from previously unsuccessful therapies. Many patients who may be successfully treated with particular therapies may not survive long enough to see the outcome, secondary to their underlying malignancy or sepsis. This aspect reiterates the importance of further investigation into the underlying pathophysiology of PNP/PAMS in order to correlate the mechanisms underlying the disease process with successful treatment modalities.

CORTICOSTEROIDS

Corticosteroids are usually considered a first-line therapy for PNP/PAMS[3,6]; however, in the majority of cases the disease progresses or fails to remit despite the use of pulsed and high-dose steroid regimens.[2,6] While the majority of case reports demonstrate a positive effect of corticosteroids on the cutaneous manifestation of the illness, there is typically little improvement in the stomatitis, which many investigators report to be poorly responsive to a variety of therapies.[2,3,6] Vezolli and colleagues[6] specifically comment that one of the clinical hallmarks of PNP is the resistance of the mucosal lesions to most therapeutic strategies. Case reports do exist as to the efficacy of steroids alone in PNP, usually in non-Hodgkin's lymphoma with relatively mild mucosal involvement.[2,6,8] This indication may be of a more benign form of PNP, which would be more responsive to steroids as a monotherapy.[2,6] High-dose corticosteroids are still recommended as the first line of treatment because they have some degree of efficacy, particularly for cutaneous lesions.[3]

Systemic corticosteroids are also used alongside other chemotherapy agents including azathioprine, cyclosporine, and mycophenolate mofetil, although response rates vary dramatically depending on the underlying neoplasm and combination of agents used.[3,6] Similarly to corticosteroids alone, although improvement is commonly seen in the cutaneous lesions of PNP, the mucous membrane involvement is particularly resistant to treatment.

CYCLOPHOSPHAMIDE

High-dose cyclophosphamide is a potentially effective treatment for PNP, with significant responses being reported with high doses of cyclophosphamide in combination with steroids.[9–11] Becker and colleagues[10] reported a case of PNP in the setting of Waldenstrom macroglobulinemia treated with dexamethasone (100 mg intravenously at 3-weekly intervals) and cyclophosphamide (500 mg intravenously days 1–3 every 3 weeks) with complete response of desquamation and erosions as well as oral and genital lesions between 4 and 6 weeks. Hertzberg and colleagues[9] presented cases of two patients non-Hodgkin lymphoma (one follicular and one large-cell) who developed PNP/PAMS with manifestations including buccal ulceration, hemorrhagic crusted lips, conjunctivitis, and papulosquamous cutaneous eruptions with sparse bullae. Both patients were successfully treated with 100 mg prednisone and 150 mg cyclophosphamide daily (reduced to 100 mg cyclophosphamide daily in the second instance), achieving successful resolution within 4 weeks from the onset of treatment. However, both eventually succumbed to their underlying neoplasm within the following months.[9] Nousari and colleagues[11] have also reported the effectiveness and safety of ablative intravenous cyclophosphamide (200 mg/kg daily over 4 days) in a patient with chronic lymphocytic leukemia-associated PNP.

MYCOPHENOLATE MOFETIL

A case report by Williams and colleagues[12] documented the successful treatment of mucocutaneous lesions in PNP/PAMS with underlying B-lymphocyte chronic lymphocytic leukemia (CLL), with mycophenolate mofetil in association with azathioprine and prednisone. Initially given as 1 g/d alongside 80 mg/d prednisone and 100 mg/d azathioprine, as the prednisone was tapered the mycophenolate mofetil was increased to 2 g/d and eventually was used as a monotherapy as the other drugs were withdrawn. This medication was the only one in this individual that controlled the oral and genital lesions, as prednisone,

azathioprine, and cyclosporine were unsuccessful in controlling the mucosal lesions.[12]

AZATHIOPRINE

As mentioned previously, both Hertzberg and Williams have described the use of azathioprine alongside corticosteroids and other immunosuppressive medications to control PNP/PAMS.[9,12] Krunic and colleagues[13] also reported the case of a patient with PNP/PAMS with underlying retroperitoneal liposarcoma who was treated with tumor resection, prednisone (0.75–1.0 mg/kg), and azathioprine (100 mg/d). After 2 weeks, the lichen planus–like cutaneous lesions and mucous membrane ulcerations had significantly improved, and complete resolution was seen within 6 weeks.[13] Another patient with underlying B-cell CLL was treated with prednisone, 40 mg and azathioprine, 100 mg daily, and experienced complete resolution of violaceous papular eruptions and marked alleviation of ulcerative stomatitis with only residual ulceration of the tongue 2 years after initial diagnosis of PNP/PAMS.[14]

CYCLOSPORINE

Cyclosporine in combination with glucocorticoids has been trialed in a handful of case reports; although it has benefits in improving cutaneous lesions, again its effect in resolving mucous membrane lesions is varied.[15,16] Miltenyi and colleagues[17] published a recent case report outlining the use of cyclosporine alongside steroids and thalidomide in a young female with Castleman disease, which was unable to be completely excised. Her initial presentation with gingival hyperplasia and buccal ulcerations were responsive to 25 mg methylprednisone, 200 mg thalidomide, and 150 mg cyclosporin A. The 18 months following the partial excision of the tumor saw continued control of the disease.[17] By contrast, the combination of oral cyclosporine 5 mg/kg daily and prednisone 35 mg daily has been reported to heal erosions of the mucous membranes substantially, but not completely, within a 2-month period in a patient with chronic lymphocytic leukemia.[15] Gergely and colleagues[18] reported success in resolving mucous membrane lesions in B-cell lymphoma–associated PNP/PAMS with doses up to 7 mg/kg/d of cyclosporine A; however, they also warned against the risk of B-cell proliferation with the use of cyclosporine A in B-cell malignancies.

INTRAVENOUS IMMUNOGLOBULIN

Intravenous immunoglobulin (IVIG) has been proposed for several years as holding promise for the treatment of PNP/PAMS, due to its direct effects on B-cell antibodies that are believed to be involved in the pathogenesis of this disease.[19–21] Nanda and colleagues[21] reported a favorable outcome in a patient with PNP/PAMS with underlying B-lymphocyte CLL and hepatitis C, with reduction in the severity of cutaneous lesions along with the use of corticosteroids. Regarding Castleman tumors preexcision and postexcision, Zhu and Zhang[19] reported on the facility of IVIG to reduce circulating autoantibodies intraoperatively and postoperatively.

PLASMAPHERESIS

Plasmapheresis, along with IVIG, has also been raised as a possible therapeutic candidate in this patient population.[2] Izaki and colleagues[22] reported the case of a patient with underlying CLL with severe mucous membrane involvement resistant to pulsed corticosteroid therapy. A modest improvement was noted with the initiation of twice-weekly plasmapheresis, and a decrease in the range of autoantibody titers from 1:640–1280 to 1:20–40 was also seen. Unfortunately, before the patient's condition could improve further, he succumbed to sepsis.[13] Vezzoli and colleagues[6] recommend the concurrent administration of a potent B-cell suppressor, such as cyclophosphamide with plasmapheresis, to prevent a rebound phenomenon of autoantibody production on withdrawal of plasmapheresis.

TOPICAL TACROLIMUS

A recent article by Vecchietti and colleagues[23] outlines their use of tacrolimus mouthwash in a patient with non-Hodgkin lymphoma whose cutaneous erosions responded well to systemic treatment with R-CHOP, but had persistent erosive stomatitis. This condition subsequently resolved with 2 weeks' use of tacrolimus mouthwash 3 times daily.

RITUXIMAB

The use of rituximab in PNP/PAMS has been an exciting new modality that shows promise for the effective treatment of PNP/PAMS.[6] A variety of case reports have shown its efficacy, particularly in follicular non-Hodgkin lymphoma whereby its mode of action is believed to be both on the B-cell autoantibodies underlying the pathophysiological mechanisms of PNP/PAMS and on the underlying malignancy itself. A variety of different rituximab regimens have been used in the literature, including use as a monotherapy in dosages of 375 mg/m^2 in weekly doses for 4 weeks[24]

followed by 8 weekly maintenance infusions, as well as weekly infusions for 4 weeks alongside corticosteroids[25] and other immunosuppressive agents such as cyclosporine A.[26] Schmidt and colleagues[27] recently reviewed 13 patients with PNP associated with CD20-positive B-cell malignancies treated with rituximab, and found that 2 patients had progression of disease despite therapy. Schadlow and other investigators anecdotally report that patients with advanced PNP/PAMS and advanced malignancy do not respond as well to rituximab therapy as do those patients earlier in the course of their disease. The reasons behind these observations are not yet clear.[6,27,28]

ALEMTUZUMAB

One case report by Hohwy and colleagues[29] reported remission of both PNP/PAMS and B-lymphocyte CLL through treatment with alemtuzumab, a CD52 monoclonal antibody that acts against both T and B lymphocytes, sparing hemopoietic stem cells. This treatment was given in a patient with a 4-year history of CLL refractory to treatment with a variety of other therapies including corticosteroids, topical tacrolimus for stomatitis, cyclosporine, and IVIG. Alemtuzumab was administered 30 mg intravenously 3 times a week for 12 weeks. Cutaneous and mucosal lesions remitted during the first 2 to 4 weeks of therapy. Twelve months post therapy the patient still remained in remission on maintenance therapy of 500 mg mycophenolate mofetil and 5 mg prednisone.[29]

SUMMARY

The initial identification of potential cases of PNP/PAMS and early assessment, diagnosis, and control of the underlying neoplasm are the essential components to maximizing beneficial outcomes for patients with PNP/PAMS. In controlling the disease process and reducing the impact of the illness, several therapeutic modalities have been explored with variable rates of success. Through the anecdotal evidence supplied in a variety of case reports examining treatments in PNP/PAMS, it is made clear that much still needs to be learnt regarding the underlying pathophysiology of PNP/PAMS to identify targeted mechanisms and to disrupt the progression of this frequently fatal illness. The relative success seen by biological therapies such as rituximab and alemtuzumab lend credence to the suggestion, as given by Vezzoli and colleagues,[6] that as individual patients have unique pathologic contributions of T and B lymphocytes to the degree of their illness, this may explain the variability in therapies that target only T or B lymphocytes specifically. Speculation may occur as to the connection between the clinical manifestation of PNP/PAMS mimicking other well-known T- or B-lymphocyte–mediated conditions[4] and their underlying pathophysiology and response to therapies, although at the moment these remain only speculations. Overall, the treatment of PNP/PAMS is far from straightforward, and individual patients have widely variable responses to therapy depending on their underlying malignancy, progression of disease at the time of treatment, and preexisting comorbidities.

REFERENCES

1. Zimmerman J, Bahmer F, Rose C, et al. Clinical and immunopathological spectrum of paraneoplastic pemphigus. J Dtsch Dermatol Ges 2010;8:598–605 [in English, German].

2. Robinson ND, Hashimoto T, Amagai M, et al. The new pemphigus variants. J Am Acad Dermatol 1999;40:649–71.

3. Sehgal VN, Srivastava G. Paraneoplastic pemphigus/ paraneoplastic autoimmune multiorgan syndrome. Int J Dermatol 2009;48:162–9.

4. Nguyen VT, Ndoye A, Bassler KD, et al. Classification, clinical manifestations and immunopathological mechanisms of the epithelial variant of paraneoplastic autoimmune multiorgan syndrome. Arch Dermatol 2001;137:193–206.

5. Joly P, Richard C, Gilbert D, et al. Sensitivity and specificity of clinical, histologic, and immunologic features in the diagnosis of paraneoplastic pemphigus. J Am Acad Dermatol 2000;43:619–26.

6. Vezzoli P, Berti E, Marzano AV. Rationale and efficacy for the use of rituximab in paraneoplastic pemphigus. Expert Rev Clin Immunol 2008;4(3):351–64.

7. Frew JW, Murrell DF. Paraneoplastic pemphigus (paraneoplastic autoimmune multiorgan syndrome): clinical presentations and pathogenesis. Dermatol Clin 2011;29(3):419–25.

8. Martínez De Pablo MI, Iranzo P, Mascaró JM, et al. Paraneoplastic pemphigus associated with non-Hodgkin B-cell lymphoma and good response to prednisone. Acta Derm Venereol 2005;85(3):233–5.

9. Herzberg MS, Schiffer M, Sullivan J, et al. Paraneoplastic pemphigus in two patients with B-cell non-Hodgkin's lymphoma: significant responses to cyclophosphamide and prednisolone. Am J Hematol 2000;63:105–6.

10. Becker LR, Bastian BC, Wesselmann U, et al. Paraneoplastic pemphigus treated with dexamethasone/ cyclophosphamide pulse therapy. Eur J Dermatol 1998;8:551–3.

11. Nousari HC, Brodsky RA, Jones RJ, et al. Immunoablative high-dose cyclophosphamide without stem cell rescue in paraneoplastic pemphigus: report of a case and review of this new therapy for severe autoimmune disease. J Am Acad Dermatol 1999; 40:750–4.

12. Williams J, Marks J, Billingsley E. Use of mycophenolate mofetil in the treatment of paraneoplastic pemphigus. Br J Dermatol 2000;142(3):506–8.

13. Krunic AL, Kokai D, Bacetic B, et al. Retroperitoneal round-cell liposarcoma associated with paraneoplastic pemphigus presenting as lichen planus pemphigoides-like eruption. Int J Dermatol 1997; 36:526–9.

14. Camisa C, Helm TN, Liu YC, et al. Paraneoplastic pemphigus: a report of three cases including one long-term survivor. J Am Acad Dermatol 1992;27: 547–53.

15. Perniciaro C, Kuechle MK, Colon-Otero G, et al. Paraneoplastic pemphigus: a case of prolonged survival. Mayo Clin Proc 1994;69:851–5.

16. Lee JS, Pei-Lin Ng P, Tao M, et al. Paraneoplastic pemphigus resembling linear IgA bullous dermatosis. Int J Dermatol 2006;45(9):1093–5.

17. Miltenyi Z, Toth J, Gonda A, et al. Successful immunomodulatory therapy in Castleman disease with paraneoplastic pemphigus vulgaris. Pathol Oncol Res 2009;15:375–81.

18. Gergely L, Váróczy L, Vadász G, et al. Successful treatment of B cell chronic lymphocytic leukemia-associated severe paraneoplastic pemphigus with cyclosporin A. Acta Haematol 2003;109(4):202–5.

19. Zhu X, Zhang B. Paraneoplastic pemphigus. J Dermatol 2007;34:503–11.

20. Van Rossum M, Verhaegen N, Jonkman M, et al. Follicular non-Hodgkin's lymphoma with refractory paraneoplastic pemphigus: case report with review of novel treatment modalities. Leuk Lymphoma 2004;45(11):2327–32.

21. Nanda M, Nanda A, Al-Sabah H, et al. Paraneoplastic pemphigus in association with B-cell lymphocytic leukemia and hepatitis C: favorable response to intravenous immunoglobulins and prednisolone. Int J Dermatol 2007;46(7):767–9.

22. Izaki S, Yoshizawa Y, Kitamura K, et al. Paraneoplastic pemphigus: potential therapeutic effect of plasmapheresis. Br J Dermatol 1996;134(5):987–9.

23. Vecchietti G, Kerl K, Hugli A, et al. Topical Tacrolimus (FK506) for relapsing erosive stomatitis in paraneoplastic pemphigus. Br J Dermatol 2003;148: 833–4.

24. Borradori L, Lombardi T, Samson J, et al. Anti CD20 monoclonal antibody (Rituximab) for refractory erosive stomatitis secondary to CD20+ follicular lymphoma associated paraneoplastic pemphigus. Arch Dermatol 2001;137:269–72.

25. Heizmann M, Itin P, Wernli M, et al. Successful treatment of paraneoplastic pemphigus in follicular NHL with rituximab: report of case and review of

treatment for paraneoplastic pemphigus in NHL and CLL. Am J Hematol 2001;66:142–4.

26. Barnadas M, Roe E, Brunet S, et al. Therapy of paraneoplastic pemphigus with rituximab: a case report and review of the literature. J Eur Acad Dermatol Venereol 2006;20:69–74.

27. Schmidt E, Goebler M, Zillikens D. Rituximab in severe pemphigus. Ann N Y Acad Sci 2009;1173:683–91.

28. Schadlow M, Anhalt G, Sinha A. Using rituximab (CD20 antibody) in a patient with paraneoplastic pemphigus. J Drugs Dermatol 2003;2:564–7.

29. Hohwy T, Bang K, Steiniche T, et al. Alemtuzumab induced remission of both severe paraneoplastic pemphigus and leukaemic bone marrow infiltration in a case of treatment resistant B-cell chronic lymphocytic leukaemia. Eur J Haematol 2004;73:206–9.

Evidence-Based Management of Bullous Pemphigoid

Benjamin S. Daniel, BA, BCom, MBBS, MMed (Clin Epi)[a,b],
Luca Borradori, MD[c], Russell P. Hall III, MD[d],
Dédée F. Murrell, MA, BMBCh, FAAD, MD, FACD[e,*]

KEYWORDS

- Bullous pemhigoid • Autoimmune bullous disease
- Topical corticosteroids • Systemic corticosteroids

Bullous pemphigoid (BP) is the most common auto-immune bullous disease, preferentially affecting the elderly.[1,2] It is characterized by generalized pruritus with subsequent subepidermal bullous formation as well as the detection of autoantibodies against the BP180 (BPAG2, type XVIII collagen) and BP230 (BPAg1-e) antigens. Multiple treatments have been used, though evidence supporting their use is deficient because of a paucity of adequate clinical trials. This shortcoming is partly due to the low prevalence and heterogeneous nature of the disease, and differing study designs with small numbers of patients.

Elderly patients are more likely to have multiple comorbidities and be susceptible to changes in medications than other populations. As a result, adverse effects and potential drug interactions should be considered when treating BP. It is therefore important to provide a review of the evidence supporting the various treatments for BP, so that clinicians can select the best and most efficient medication for their patients. Each treatment regimen must be individualized according to the severity of disease, comorbidities, and patients' expectations. Furthermore, the physician's personal

experience and drug availability also affect the final choice. Clinical manifestations, epidemiology, and pathogenesis have been reviewed in the previous issue of *Dermatologic Clinics*. This article focuses on the adaptation of the evidence-based trials in BP to a practical system of managing BP. The authors consider the treatment approach under 3 headings: (1) the context, (2) the treatments, and (3) the morbidity and mortality.

THE CONTEXT OF THE TREATMENT

The average age of presentation in BP is usually between 75 and 85 years,[3–6] with many comorbidities, and hence there is a need to be cautious with treatments.[7] BP patients are often either in nursing homes or are already dependent on relatives for care. Three independent case-control studies have shown that there is a high risk of prior neurologic problem 5 to 10 years before the onset of BP.[8–10] Hence, when treating patients with BP, consideration should be given to 3 important factors that may increase the morbidity and/or mortality of the treatment: (1) patient age, (2) underlying diagnosis such as diabetes mellitus,

Funding: This work was in part supported by grants from the Swiss National Foundation for Scientific Research (31003A-121966 and 31003A-09811, to L.B.) and the European Community's FP7 (Coordination Theme 1-HEALTH-F2-2008-200515, to L.B.).

[a] Department of Dermatology, St George Hospital, Gray Street, Kogarah, Sydney, NSW 2217, Australia
[b] Faculty of Medicine, University of New South Wales, Sydney, NSW 2052, Australia
[c] Department of Dermatology, Inselspital and University of Bern, 3010 Bern, Switzerland
[d] Department of Dermatology, Duke University Medical Center, Durham, NC 27710, USA
[e] Department of Dermatology, St George Hospital, University of New South Wales, Gray Street, Kogarah, Sydney, NSW 2217, Australia
* Corresponding author.
E-mail address: d.murrell@unsw.edu.au

Dermatol Clin 29 (2011) 613–620
doi:10.1016/j.det.2011.06.003
0733-8635/11/$ – see front matter © 2011 Elsevier Inc. All rights reserved.

hypertension, or cardiovascular disease, and (3) the multitude of side effects associated with the use of high doses of systemic corticosteroids. The drugs given to this population need to be tempered with the understanding that they could interfere with other medical problems and will require the assistance of third parties to administer it in most cases. The first consideration is to do no more good than harm to this vulnerable group of patients, no matter how effective a particular treatment may appear in trials perhaps involving healthier patients.

THE EVIDENCE FOR THE TREATMENTS

The treatments under discussion include corticosteroids (oral and topical) and steroid-sparing agents. The latter include, among others, azathioprine, mycophenolate mofetil (MMF), tetracyclines with or without nicotinamide, dapsone, cyclophosphamide, intravenous immunoglobulin (IVIG), plasmapheresis, and rituximab. These agents and their overall important treatment questions are discussed.

THE SAFETY OF THE TREATMENTS

As each type of treatment is discussed, the drawbacks of each type of treatment are mentioned, this being particularly important in the context of the elderly population with BP.

QUESTIONS THAT REMAIN TO BE ANSWERED

There are 3 main questions remaining to be answered in BP management:

1. What is the optimal dose and route of administration of corticosteroids for newly diagnosed BP?
2. What population of BP patients should be treated with oral versus topical corticosteroids versus steroid-sparing drugs?
3. Are steroid-sparing drugs safe and effective?

The goal of treatment in BP is to arrest disease progression, reduce itch, and rapidly stimulate healing of blisters. Quick and efficient therapy is important, as extensive disease with delayed healing is also prone to infection and may require antibiotic coverage and, in severe cases, hospitalization. Patients may present at various stages of clinical severity, due to a delay in diagnosis (particularly in types presenting with diffuse pruritus only, urticarial or eczematous BP before the blistering develops).

A recent Cochrane review of the 7 randomized controlled trials (RCTs) concluded the following: (1) very potent topical steroids are effective and safe treatments for BP; (2) their use in extensive disease may be limited by side effects and practical factors; (3) starting doses of prednisolone greater than 0.75 mg/kg/d do not seem to give

additional benefit in disease control and they may reduce the incidence and severity of adverse reactions; (4) the effectiveness of the addition of plasma exchange or azathioprine to corticosteroids has not been established; and (5) combination treatment with tetracycline and nicotinamide may be useful, but this needs further validation.[10] A summary of these trials is given in **Table 1**.

For question (1), the optimal starting dose for oral prednisone/prednisolone should be no higher than 0.75 mg/kg/d, as there was no significant difference in resolution of blistering between days 21 and 50 using this dose in comparison with 1.25 mg/kg/d.[11] The formulation of steroid does not seem to matter, because Dreno's[12] study comparing methylprednisolone versus prednisolone found no significant difference.

The type of steroid, dosage, and duration of therapy varies among clinicians. A survey of German dermatologists[13] found that 53% of the hospitals prescribed less than 1 mg/kg/d as the initial dose whereas the remainder (47%) used the higher dose of 1 to 2 mg/kg/d. About one-third of hospitals aim to maintain patients on less than 7.5 mg/d prednisone (or equivalent), whereas others prefer tapering until prednisone can be stopped. The effectiveness of prednisone is related to the number of blisters before initiation of treatment, and it has been suggested that they should not be discontinued if response is not observed within a certain timeframe.[14] Duration of treatment or an increased dose may be required for extensive disease to respond. However, systemic corticosteroids are responsible for multiple adverse effects, and can be detrimental and potentially fatal in the elderly.[15]

Although systemic steroids have conventionally been used as the mainstay of treatment, their long-term use increases the risk of steroid-associated side effects (**Box 1**)[16] and should therefore be minimized or tapered once clinical improvement is detected. The use of topical corticosteroids has been evaluated as a possible way to avoid systemic corticosteroids in some patients with BP.

A landmark study of bullous diseases by a French group randomized BP patients to topical versus oral steroids,[17] and found that topical clobetasol propionate (40 g/d) was associated with improved overall survival (P = .02) and fewer severe adverse effects (P = .006) than oral prednisone in patients with extensive BP (defined as presence of more than 10 new blisters per day on 3 consecutive days). In severe BP, survival in the oral prednisone group at 1 year was 58% and in the topical steroid group was 76%, and severe complications were more common in the oral (54%) than in the topical (29%) treatment groups. There was no difference in disease control detected between the two treatments or in the survival and severe side effects of the moderate BP groups with either topical or systemic treatment. This finding would suggest that severe BP patients would be better managed on topical corticosteroids. To apply this evidence internationally, one needs to compare these mortality rates in France with those published from abroad. In the United States, where oral corticosteroids are favored for BP management, Colbert and colleagues[18] showed a 1-year survival of 89% for BP, significantly higher than the 76% in France for topical treatment and 58% for oral prednisone. Korman's group[19] found a 1-year survival of 76%. Roujeau and colleagues,[20] on the other hand, found a 1-year survival of 58%. Langan and colleagues[21] in the United Kingdom found a 1-year mortality of 19%. The French group attributes the differences to their inclusion of every BP case in France, including the moribund, whereas they believe the United States studies, which are based at tertiary centers, have a bias toward patients who are well enough to travel to these centers and are treatable in an outpatient setting.[22]

A further prospective multicenter randomized study in France of 312 BP patients with moderate or extensive BP was conducted with a 1-year follow-up. This RCT compared the efficacy and safety of 40 g clobetasol propionate per day reduced over 12 months versus 10 to 30 g clobetasol propionate per day (adapted to the weight and disease extent) reduced over 4 months.[4] No difference in the rate of BP control or event-free survival occurred between the two treatment groups. There was a strong beneficial effect of the mild regimen versus the moderate regime, with reduction of mortality rate and serious side effects. The mild regimen resulted in a 70% lower cumulative dose of topical corticosteroids (1314 g vs 5760 g).

There are practical limitations on the implementation of this routine. These limits include the need to apply the cream on almost the entire body, and that the assistance of either a relative or a nurse is often required. In some patients the severity of the disease may require more aggressive therapy with systemic corticosteroids initially, with topical corticosteroids being used as steroid-sparing agents. Furthermore, the possibility of systemic side effects should not be forgotten. Hence, careful management of patients is still required, for example, for diabetes, electrolyte imbalance, and adrenal axis suppression. There are higher costs than for oral corticosteroids, but fewer major side effects and mortality compared with oral corticosteroids. Topical steroids have lower costs than IVIG and new immunosuppressive drugs, such as MMF. As the French health system pays for

nurses to administer the topical steroids, which improves compliance, in the patients' homes/ nursing homes up to twice daily after discharge, the treatment becomes affordable for BP patients in France. Some health systems do not subsidize the cost of highly potent topical steroids. A cost-benefit analysis comparing this with the complications derived from systemic treatment would be of value but has not been performed. For Australia, the difficulty is that only one class I topical steroid is available, and only on private script at $30 per 15-g tube with no discounts, with private insurance (held by a third of the population) not covering much of the cost toward drugs. Furthermore, most people are managed as outpatients, and there is no easy provision of visiting nurses even for once a day, let alone on weekends.

Therefore, the evidence from these studies demonstrates that a mild regimen of topical corticosteroids is superior to systemic steroids, with fewer adverse effects.[23] Patients in countries where the cost of the potent topical steroids is not prohibitory for the patient and where help is available to apply these creams once or twice daily are ideally suited to the topical steroid regimen. The experience in Switzerland is that in approximately half of the patients, topical treatment is practically not feasible because of either lack of regular assistance or the patient being bedridden.

The use of several different drugs has been proposed as adjuvant therapy as a means to reduce the cumulative steroid dose.[24] Despite the beneficial intention, iatrogenic complications such as immunosuppression, susceptibility to infections, and renal or hepatic injury are relatively common. Doses and duration of therapy need to be individualized, depending on severity of disease, comorbidities, and general health. Regular hematologic and biochemistry monitoring during therapy is warranted. Although guidelines and systematic reviews have been published, good evidence supporting adjuvant treatments is lacking.[25,26]

The studies on the steroid-sparing drugs are now presented and discussed to address question (3) above.

Azathioprine

Beissert and colleagues[27] performed an RCT comparing oral methylprednisolone (0.5 mg/kg/d) plus azathioprine (2 mg/kg/d) with methylprednisolone (0.5 mg/kg/d) plus MMF (1000 mg twice a day). Complete resolution was observed in 35 of 38 (92%) of patients in the azathioprine group and in 35 of 35 (100%) of those in the MMF group with a median of 24 and 42 days, respectively. These differences were not statistically significant.

Table 1
Summary of randomised controlled trials of treatments in bullous pemphigoid

Study	Year	Treatment Arms	No. of Patients	Follow-Up	Main Finding
Beissert et al[27]	2007	Azathioprine + methylprednisolone	38		No difference between the 2 treatment arms in achieving disease remission
		Mycophenolate mofetil + methylprednisolone	35		
Burton et al[29]	1978	Prednisone 30–80 mg/kg/d + azathioprine	12		No difference in the percentage of patients with disease control at 3-year follow-up
		Prednisone 30–80 mg/kg/d	13	3 y	Corticosteroid-sparing effect was significant in the combination group ($P<.01$)
Dreno et al[12]	1993	Prednisolone (average) 1.16 mg/kg/d	29		Both methylprednisolone and prednisolone result in a reduction in the number of blisters. There was no statistically significant difference between the 2 treatments
		Methylprednisolone (average) 1.17 mg/kg/d	28		
Fivenson et al[34]	1994	Combination of nicotinamide 500 mg total dissolved solids + tetracycline 500 mg 4 times a day	14	10 mo	No statistical difference between the 2 groups in complete response
		Prednisone (40–80 mg)	6		
Guillaume et al[30]	1993	prednisone 1 mg/kg/d	31	6 mo	No statistical significance between the treatment groups. No additional effect in those treated with azathioprine or plasma exchange
		Prednisone 1 mg/kg/d + azathioprine	36		
		Prednisone 1 mg/kg/d + plasma exchange	31		
Joly et al[17]	2002	Moderate disease	—	3 wk	In the moderate disease, both topical and oral steroids were equally effective in achieving disease control
		Topical 0.05% clobetasol propionate twice a day	77		
		Prednisone 0.5 mg/kg/d	76		
		Extensive disease	—	3 wk	In the extensive group, topical steroids resulted in a greater disease control compared with oral steroids
		Topical steroids	93		
		Prednisone 1 mg/kg/d	95		

(continued on next page)

Table 1
(continued)

Study	Year	Treatment Arms	No. of Patients	Follow-Up	Main Finding
Joly et al[4]	2009	Topical clobetasol propionate 10–30 g/d	159	3 wk	No significant difference between the 2 treatment regimes. Cumulative dose of topical steroids was statistically reduced in the mild regime
		Topical clobetasol propionate 40 g/d	153		
Liu et al[59]	2006	Jingui Shenqi pill + prednisone	15	4 wk	No significant difference between the 2 groups when assessing partial or complete healing
		Prednisone alone	15		
Morel and Guillaume[11]	1984	Prednisolone 0.75 mg/kg/d	26		No significant difference in the percentage of patients who were clear of skin lesions at days 21 and 51
		Prednisolone 1.25 mg/kg/d	24	—	
Roujeau et al[37]	1984	Prednisolone 0.3 mg/kg/d	17	1 mo	Disease control was achieved with a lower dose of prednisone in the plasma exchange group
		Plasma exchange + prednisolone 0.3 mg/kg/d	24		

There was no significant difference between the time of remission and disease recurrence. Severe or life-threatening events occurred in 9 of 38 (24%) of those in the azathioprine group compared with 6 of 35 (17%) in the MMF group. It should be noted that doses of azathioprine were not adapted to thiopurine methyltransferase activity in the latter study.

Although there have been reports of improvement in disease severity with the use of azathioprine,[28] evidence from RCTs is lacking. A study comparing azathioprine plus prednisolone with prednisolone alone found no difference in outcomes. There was, however, a reduction in the maintenance dose of prednisolone in the combination group.[29] Another study randomized 100 patients with active BP to 1 of 3 groups: prednisolone therapy alone, azathioprine (100–150 mg/d) plus prednisolone, or plasma exchange plus prednisolone. All patients were commenced on prednisolone 1 mg/kg divided into 2 daily doses. Those in group 3 had 4 plasma exchanges within the first 2 weeks. There was no significant difference in disease control between the 3 groups at 6 months. Therefore, there is no additional benefit in using azathioprine or plasma exchange instead of prednisolone alone.[30]

Tetracycline and Nicotinamide

BP has also been treated with tetracycline and nicotinamide, with success.[31] In 1986, 4 patients treated with tetracycline or erythromycin and niacinamide (initially 500 mg 3–4 times a day) showed significant improvement.[32] Subsequent case reports also support the beneficial use of this approach. Seven patients treated with tetracycline (2 g/d) and nicotinamide (2 g/d) had

Box 1
Common adverse effects associated with systemic corticosteroids

Diabetes

Hypertension

Osteoporosis

Cataracts and glaucoma

Peptic ulcer disease

Infections and sepsis

Myopathy and myalgia

Mood swings

Data from Daniel BS, Murrell DF. The actual management of pemphigus. G Ital Dermatol Venereol 2010;145(5):689–702.

improvement within 2 weeks, and all patients had disease clearance at 2-year follow-up, though 2 of 7 (29%) patients reported occasional blisters.[33] A trial comparing the combination of tetracycline (500 mg 4 times a day) plus nicotinamide (500 mg 3 times a day) with prednisone failed to a show statistically significant difference between the two groups.[34] There were 5 complete responders and 5 partial responders in the combination group (n = 12), compared with 1 complete response and 5 partial responses in the prednisone monotherapy group (n = 6). A larger RCT may demonstrate statistical significance. Adverse effects reported include gastrointestinal symptoms, acute tubular necrosis (ATN), and tinnitus. The patient who developed ATN had an elevated serum creatinine at baseline and was taking nonsteroidal anti-inflammatory medications. The renal function improved within 2 weeks of cessation of tetracycline and nicotinamide.[26,34]

Methotrexate

Methotrexate is an immunosuppressive agent that inhibits the metabolism of folic acid. To date there are no published RCTs comparing methotrexate with another treatment in BP. Despite this, however, methotrexate has been used successfully in BP.[35] A retrospective analysis of 98 patients treated with either methotrexate alone or methotrexate plus prednisone found the 2-year remission rate was higher in the monotherapy group as compared with the combination regimen (43% vs 35%, respectively).[23] A search of the literature[36] found clinical improvement in 42 of 45 (93%) cases. Abnormal liver function tests, gastrointestinal symptoms, infection, and anemia are known side effects of methotrexate.

Plasma Exchange

One RCT showed that the addition of plasma exchange to steroids had a significant reduction in the mean cumulative dose of systemic steroids.[37] Another study, however, concluded that plasma exchange was not an effective adjuvant in the treatment of BP.[30] It is unlikely that future trials will definitely address the role of plasma exchange in this area.

Other Treatments

Cyclosporine,[38] dapsone,[39] and topical tacrolimus[40] have been reported to have some benefit. In line with previous uncontrolled series, the authors have personally (L.B.) used chlorambucil for years, with good results.[41,42] Large controlled trials are required to confirm the efficacy of these agents.

Although IVIG may be beneficial as an adjuvant to other therapies, its true effect has not been analyzed in an RCT and its use is limited by its cost.[43,44]

Most of the studies of steroid-sparing agents were underpowered in determining the correct answer. The effectiveness of the addition of plasma exchange or azathioprine to corticosteroids has not been established,[5] and combination treatment with tetracycline and nicotinamide may be useful, but this needs further validation.[10]

Rituximab has been used recently for many autoimmune diseases, and there is literature supporting its utility in patients with pemphigus vulgaris. Scattered case reports suggest it may be of value in BP. An open-label study using rituximab in the treatment of 8 patients with BP, all of whom required ongoing systemic corticosteroid therapy of 17.5 mg/d or more of prednisone, has been conducted. Six of the 8 patients were controlled with less than 5 mg of prednisone at 12 months after starting therapy.[45] Further studies with an RCT are needed to confirm this finding.

SUMMARY

- Some investigators have suggested that the disease usually resolves after 5 years, but prospective studies addressing the long-term course of BP are lacking. In fact, a significant proportion of BP patients will die within 3 years after diagnosis. In a prospective nationwide study in Switzerland, the authors found a 3-year probability of death of 38.8%.[46] Furthermore, a recent prospective study of 114 BP patients found that up to 45% of the evaluable individuals experienced a relapse, which in most cases occurred within 6 months after cessation of therapy.[47]
- In this context, therapies are aimed at ameliorating skin lesions and itch, inducing remission, and reducing both morbidity and mortality. Oral steroids need to be used judiciously in BP, as the elderly are more prone to adverse effects and drug interactions. Although the aim of adjuvant therapy is to reduce the cumulative steroid dose and hence steroid-associated effects,[48,49] they also contribute to morbidity and mortality through their harmful profiles. Hospitalization may facilitate monitoring and avoid complications, though some research indicates an increased mortality with prolonged hospitalization.

From the RCTs available, the evidence supports the use of potent topical corticosteroids in acute BP, wherever feasible. Systemic corticosteroids are effective in managing BP although the evidence supporting adjuvant use is lacking. The same applies for the use of tetracyclines in combination with nicotinamide which, however, may be tried in mild disease without major concern. In specific situations, it may be necessary to try and take advantage of other molecules such topical tacrolimus (for example, in the case of severe local side effects of corticosteroids[40,50,51]), IVIG (useful, eg, in immunocompromised patients),[52] anti-CD20 monoclonal antibody (rituximab [Mabthera]),[53–55] anti-IgE monoclonal antibody (omalizumab, [Xolair]),[56] or even immunoadsorption/immunoapheresis.[57,58] Due to the poor methodological quality and underpowered studies, the evidence supporting many of the therapies in BP is lacking. The development of scoring systems to grade BP will assist with the clinical trial evidence.[37]

REFERENCES

1. Bernard P, Vaillant L, Labeille B, et al. Incidence and distribution of subepidermal autoimmune bullous skin diseases in three French regions. Bullous Diseases French Study Group. Arch Dermatol 1995;131(1):48–52.
2. Zillikens D, Wever S, Roth A, et al. Incidence of autoimmune subepidermal blistering dermatoses in a region of central Germany. Arch Dermatol 1995;131(8):957–8.
3. Jung M, Kippes W, Messer G, et al. Increased risk of bullous pemphigoid in male and very old patients: a population-based study on incidence. J Am Acad Dermatol 1999;41(2 Pt 1):266–8.
4. Joly P, Roujeau JC, Benichou J, et al. A comparison of two regimens of topical corticosteroids in the treatment of patients with bullous pemphigoid: a multicenter randomized study. J Invest Dermatol 2009;129(7):1681–7.
5. Korman N. Bullous pemphigoid. J Am Acad Dermatol 1987;16(5 Pt 1):907–24.
6. Marazza G, Pham HC, Scharer L, et al. Incidence of bullous pemphigoid and pemphigus in Switzerland: a 2-year prospective study. Br J Dermatol 2009; 161(4):861–8.
7. Risser J, Lewis K, Weinstock MA. Mortality of bullous skin disorders from 1979 through 2002 in the United States. Arch Dermatol 2009;145(9):1005–8.
8. Taghipour K, Chi CC, Vincent A, et al. The association of bullous pemphigoid with cerebrovascular disease and dementia: a case-control study. Arch Dermatol 2010;146(11):1251–4.
9. Langan SM, Groves RW, West J. The relationship between neurological disease and bullous pemphigoid: a population-based case-control study. J Invest Dermatol 2011;131(3):631–6.
10. Bastuji-Garin S, Joly P, Lemordant P, et al. Risk factors for bullous pemphigoid in the elderly: a prospective case-control study. J Invest Dermatol 2011;131(3):637–43.
11. Morel P, Guillaume JC. Treatment of bullous pemphigoid with prednisolone only: 0.75 mg/kg/day versus 1.25 mg/kg/day. A multicenter randomized study. Ann Dermatol Venereol 1984;111(10):925–8 [in French].
12. Dreno B, Sassolas B, Lacour P, et al. Methylprednisolone versus prednisolone methylsulfobenzoate in pemphigoid: a comparative multicenter study. Ann Dermatol Venereol 1993;120(8):518–21.
13. Hofmann SC, Kautz O, Hertl M, et al. Results of a survey of German dermatologists on the therapeutic approaches to pemphigus and bullous pemphigoid. J Dtsch Dermatol Ges 2009;7(3):227–33.
14. Chosidow O, Saada V, Diquet B, et al. Correlation between the pretreatment number of blisters and the time to control bullous pemphigoid with prednisone 1 mg/kg/day. Br J Dermatol 1992;127(2):185–6.
15. Thomas TP. The complications of systemic corticosteroid therapy in the elderly. A retrospective study. Gerontology 1984;30(1):60–5.
16. Daniel BS, Murrell DF. The actual management of pemphigus. G Ital Dermatol Venereol 2010;145(5): 689–702.
17. Joly P, Roujeau JC, Benichou J, et al. A comparison of oral and topical corticosteroids in patients with bullous pemphigoid. N Engl J Med 2002;346(5):321–7.
18. Colbert RL, Allen DM, Eastwood D, et al. Mortality rate of bullous pemphigoid in a US medical center. J Invest Dermatol 2004;122(5):1091–5.
19. Parker SR, Dyson S, Brisman S, et al. Mortality of bullous pemphigoid: an evaluation of 223 patients and comparison with the mortality in the general population in the United States. J Am Acad Dermatol 2008;59(4):582–8.
20. Roujeau JC, Lok C, Bastuji-Garin S, et al. High risk of death in elderly patients with extensive bullous pemphigoid. Arch Dermatol 1998;134(4):465–9.
21. Langan SM, Smeeth L, Hubbard R, et al. Bullous pemphigoid and pemphigus vulgaris–incidence and mortality in the UK: population based cohort study. BMJ 2008;337:a180.
22. Joly P, Benichou J, Saiag P, et al. Response to: mortality rate of bullous pemphigoid in a US medical center. J Invest Dermatol 2005;124(3):664–5.
23. Kjellman P, Eriksson H, Berg P. A retrospective analysis of patients with bullous pemphigoid treated with methotrexate. Arch Dermatol 2008;144(5):612–6.
24. Khumalo NP, Murrell DF, Wojnarowska F, et al. A systematic review of treatments for bullous pemphigoid. Arch Dermatol 2002;138(3):385–9.
25. Wojnarowska F, Kirtschig G, Highet AS, et al. Guidelines for the management of bullous pemphigoid. Br J Dermatol 2002;147(2):214–21.
26. Kirtschig G, Middleton P, Bennett C, et al. Interventions for bullous pemphigoid. Cochrane Database Syst Rev 2010;10:CD002292.
27. Beissert S, Werfel T, Frieling U, et al. A comparison of oral methylprednisolone plus azathioprine

or mycophenolate mofetil for the treatment of bullous pemphigoid. Arch Dermatol 2007;143(12):1536–42.

28. Greaves MW, Burton JL, Marks J, et al. Azathioprine in treatment of bullous pemphigoid. Br Med J 1971; 1(5741):144–5.

29. Burton JL, Harman RR, Peachey RD, et al. Azathioprine plus prednisone in treatment of pemphigoid. Br Med J 1978;2(6146):1190–1.

30. Guillaume JC, Vaillant L, Bernard P, et al. Controlled trial of azathioprine and plasma exchange in addition to prednisolone in the treatment of bullous pemphigoid. Arch Dermatol 1993;129(1):49–53.

31. Shiohara J, Yoshida K, Hasegawa J, et al. Tetracycline and niacinamide control bullous pemphigoid but not pemphigus foliaceus when these conditions coexist. J Dermatol 2010;37(7):657–61.

32. Berk MA, Lorincz AL. The treatment of bullous pemphigoid with tetracycline and niacinamide. A preliminary report. Arch Dermatol 1986;122(6):670–4.

33. Kolbach DN, Remme JJ, Bos WH, et al. Bullous pemphigoid successfully controlled by tetracycline and nicotinamide. Br J Dermatol 1995;133(1):88–90.

34. Fivenson DP, Breneman DL, Rosen GB, et al. Nicotinamide and tetracycline therapy of bullous pemphigoid. Arch Dermatol 1994;130(6):753–8.

35. Bara C, Maillard H, Briand N, et al. Methotrexate for bullous pemphigoid: preliminary study. Arch Dermatol 2003;139(11):1506–7.

36. Gurcan HM, Ahmed AR. Analysis of current data on the use of methotrexate in the treatment of pemphigus and pemphigoid. Br J Dermatol 2009;161(4):723–31.

37. Roujeau JC, Guillaume JC, Morel P, et al. Plasma exchange in bullous pemphigoid. Lancet 1984; 2(8401):486–8.

38. Thivolet J, Barthelemy H, Rigot-Muller G, et al. Effects of cyclosporin on bullous pemphigoid and pemphigus. Lancet 1985;1(8424):334–5.

39. Venning VA, Millard PR, Wojnarowska F. Dapsone as first line therapy for bullous pemphigoid. Br J Dermatol 1989;120(1):83–92.

40. Chu J, Bradley M, Marinkovich MP. Topical tacrolimus is a useful adjunctive therapy for bullous pemphigoid. Arch Dermatol 2003;139(6):813–5.

41. Chave TA, Mortimer NJ, Shah DS, et al. Chlorambucil as a steroid-sparing agent in bullous pemphigoid. Br J Dermatol 2004;151(5):1107–8.

42. Milligan A, Hutchinson PE. The use of chlorambucil in the treatment of bullous pemphigoid. J Am Acad Dermatol 1990;22(5 Pt 1):796–801.

43. Czernik A, Bystryn JC. Improvement of intravenous immunoglobulin therapy for bullous pemphigoid by adding immunosuppressive agents: marked improvement in depletion of circulating autoantibodies. Arch Dermatol 2008;144(5):658–61.

44. Harman KE, Black MM. High-dose intravenous immune globulin for the treatment of autoimmune blistering diseases: an evaluation of its use in 14 cases. Br J Dermatol 1999;140(5):865–74.

45. Edhegard K, Ronaghy A, Streilein RD, et al. Low serum BAFF response and increased IgD B-cell recovery predict clinical flares in bullous pemphigoid (BP) patients treated with rituximab. J Invest Dermatol 2011;131:s10.

46. Cortes, B Marazza G, Naldi L, et al. Mortality of bullous pemphigoid in Switzerland: a prospective study. Br J Dermatol, May 17, 2011 [online].

47. Bernard P, Reguiai Z, Tancrede-Bohin E, et al. Risk factors for relapse in patients with bullous pemphigoid in clinical remission: a multicenter, prospective, cohort study. Arch Dermatol 2009;145(5):537–42.

48. Downham TF 2nd, Chapel TA. Bullous pemphigoid: therapy in patients with and without diabetes mellitus. Arch Dermatol 1978;114(11):1639–42.

49. Paul MA, Jorizzo JL, Fleischer AB Jr, et al. Low-dose methotrexate treatment in elderly patients with bullous pemphigoid. J Am Acad Dermatol 1994;31(4):620–5.

50. Ko MJ, Chu CY. Topical tacrolimus therapy for localized bullous pemphigoid. Br J Dermatol 2003; 149(5):1079–81.

51. Chuh AA. The application of topical tacrolimus in vesicular pemphigoid. Br J Dermatol 2004;150(3):622–3.

52. Gurcan HM, Jeph S, Ahmed AR. Intravenous immunoglobulin therapy in autoimmune mucocutaneous blistering diseases: a review of the evidence for its efficacy and safety. Am J Clin Dermatol 2010; 11(5):315–26.

53. Szabolcs P, Reese M, Yancey KB, et al. Combination treatment of bullous pemphigoid with anti-CD20 and anti-CD25 antibodies in a patient with chronic graft-versus-host disease. Bone Marrow Transplant 2002; 30(5):327–9.

54. Schmidt E, Seitz CS, Benoit S, et al. Rituximab in autoimmune bullous diseases: mixed responses and adverse effects. Br J Dermatol 2007;156(2):352–6.

55. Reguiai Z, Tchen T, Perceau G, et al. Efficacy of rituximab in a case of refractory bullous pemphigoid. Ann Dermatol Venereol 2009;136(5):431–4 [in French].

56. Fairley JA, Baum CL, Brandt DS, et al. Pathogenicity of IgE in autoimmunity: successful treatment of bullous pemphigoid with omalizumab. J Allergy Clin Immunol 2009;123(3):704–5.

57. Schmidt E, Zillikens D. Immunoadsorption in dermatology. Arch Dermatol Res 2010;302(4):241–53.

58. Marker M, Derfler K, Monshi B, et al. Successful immunoapheresis of bullous autoimmune diseases: pemphigus vulgaris and pemphigoid gestationis. J Dtsch Dermatol Ges 2011;9(1):27–31.

59. Liu BG, Li ZY, Du M. [Effects of jingui shenqi pill combined prednisone on expression of glucocorticoid receptor and its clinical effect in treating bullous pemphigoid patients]. Zhongguo Zhong Xi Yi Jie He Za Zhi 2006;26(10):881–4 [in Chinese].

Pemphigoid Gestationis: Current Management

Lizbeth R.A. Intong, MD, DPDS[a,b],
Dédée F. Murrell, MA, BMBCh, FAAD, MD, FACD[c],*

KEYWORDS

• Pemphigoid gestationis • Management • Treatment

Pemphigoid gestationis (PG) is a rare autoimmune bullous disease and has been reported as occurring in 1 in 20,000 to 50,000 pregnant women.[1,2] Due to pregnancy being an exclusion criteria in most clinical trials and the extensive list of medications contraindicated during pregnancy, it is no surprise that there is a scarcity of literature when it comes to management of this condition. Breastfeeding also imposes limitations on recommended treatments. Most reports are small case series and retrospective reviews. It has been accepted that potent topical corticosteroids are helpful in milder cases, whereas more extensive disease requires systemic corticosteroids, which are considered the mainstay of therapy.[1–8] There have been reports of the success of immunosuppressive treatment in recalcitrant, chronic, relapsing cases.[1–5,8]

There is recent evidence that suggests that early-onset PG and blister formation is associated with adverse pregnancy outcomes in the form of decreased gestational age at delivery, perterm birth, and low-birth-weight babies.[9,10] This finding suggests that in these more severe cases, early institution of treatment, mainly systemic corticosteroids, is essential to prevent these adverse outcomes.

This article focuses on the use of topical and systemic corticosteroids, as well as immunosuppressives, in the management of PG.

MANAGEMENT OF PEMPHIGOID GESTATIONIS

This section discusses the various treatments reported for PG. **Table 1** summarizes the treatment options, while **Table 2** shows the different pregnancy categories assigned to various medications by the United States Food and Drug Administration (US FDA). **Table 3** shows the classification recommended for use by the Therapeutic Goods Authority (TGA) in Australia. The Australian categorization system is not hierarchical and differs from that of the US FDA. The subcategorization of the B category is based on animal data, as human data are lacking or inadequate. Furthermore, a B category does not imply greater safety than a C category. Some medications in the same drug class (ie, topical and systemic corticosteroids) are assigned different categories, as the risk of birth defects may be dependent on the dose, route of administration, and dosing regimen.

General Measures

One of the main aims of therapy is to provide symptomatic relief for discomfort and pruritus, as well as to address psychological anxiety. Systemic therapy should only be initiated when the symptom severity outweighs the risks to the fetus.[2,3] Following a confirmed diagnosis of PG, before starting immunosuppressants baseline

[a] Department of Dermatology, James Laws House, St George Hospital, Gray Street, Kogarah, Sydney, NSW 2217, Australia
[b] Faculty of Medicine, University of New South Wales, Sydney, NSW 2052, Australia
[c] Department of Dermatology, St George Hospital, University of New South Wales, Gray Street, Kogarah, Sydney, NSW 2217, Australia
* Corresponding author.
E-mail address: d.murrell@unsw.edu.au

Dermatol Clin 29 (2011) 621–628
doi:10.1016/j.det.2011.06.013
0733-8635/11/$ – see front matter © 2011 Elsevier Inc. All rights reserved

Table 1
Summary of treatment for pemphigoid gestationis

Medication/Treatment	Pregnancy Category[a]	Type of Study/Author(s)	Dose	Use (Prepartum or Postpartum)
Topical corticosteroids	C A[b]	Multiple reports Mainstay of treatment	Potent CS applied twice a day (ie, clobetasol propionate 0.05% or betamethasone dipropionate 0.05%)	Both
Systemic corticosteroids	C A[b]	Multiple reports Mainstay of treatment	PSN 1 mg/kg/d or equivalent dose	Both
Tetracyclines and nicotinamide	D	Case reports Amato et al,[15] 2002; Loo et al,[16] 2001	Doxycycline 200 mg/d + nicotinamide 500 mg/d Minocycline 100 mg/d + nicotinamide 1000 mg/d	Postpartum
Cyclophosphamide	D	Case report Castle et al,[17] 1996	0.75 g/m² slow IV infusion	Postpartum
Cyclosporin	C	Case report Hern et al,[18] 1998	100 mg/d + PSN 10–20 mg/d IVIG 0.4 g/kg/d × 5 d	Postpartum
Azathioprine	D	Case reports Kreuter et al,[19] 2004 Sereno et al,[20] 2005 Cianchini et al,[21] 2007 Amato et al,[22] 2003	50–100 mg/d (+ IVIG 0.5 g/kg/d × 2 d + PSN 15 mg) 150 mg/g ineffective followed by IVIG 0.4 g/kg/d × 6 cycles 150 mg/d (+ dapsone 125 mg/d + PSN 100 mg/d + IVIG 0.5 g/kg/d × 3 d) ineffective followed by rituximab 375 mg/m² weekly for 4 wk 100 mg/d (+ PSN 40–150 mg/d + dapsone 50 mg/d + 5 plasmaphereses)	Postpartum
Dapsone	C B2[b]	Case reports Cianchini et al,[21] 2007 Amato et al,[22] 2003	Dapsone 125 mg/d (+ PSN 100 mg/d + azathioprine 150 mg/d + IVIG 0.5 g/kg/d × 3 d) ineffective followed by rituximab 375 mg/m² weekly for 4 wk 50 mg/d (+ PSN 40–150 mg/d + azathioprine 100 mg/d + 5 plasmaphereses)	Postpartum

Drug	CS category	Source	Regimen	Prepartum/Postpartum
IVIG	C	Case reports Doiron and Pratt,[23] 2010 Hern et al,[18] 1998 Kreuter et al,[19] 2004 Sereno et al,[20] 2005	40 g IV × 3 d monthly during pregnancy	Both
			0.4 g/kg/d × 5 d (+ cyclosporin 100 mg/d + PSN 10–20 mg/d)	Prepartum
			0.5 g/kg/d × 2 d (+ PSN 15 mg imuran 50–100 mg/d)	Postpartum
			IVIG 0.4 g/kg/d × 6 cycles	Postpartum
Rituximab	C	Case report Cianchini et al,[21] 2007	Rituximab 375 mg/m² weekly for 4 wk	Postpartum
Plasmapheresis	Unclassified	Case reports Amato et al,[22] 2003 Van de Wiel et al,[24] 1980 Marker et al,[25] 2011	5 plasmaphereses + (PSN 40–150 mg/d + azathioprine 100 mg/d + dapsone 50 mg/d)	Both
				Postpartum
			3 plasma exchanges during 26 wk, 5 during delivery, and 2 postpartum	Both
			15 immunoapheresis sessions (14 pre- and 1 postpartum) in addition to methylprednisolone 60 mg/d tapered	Both
Goserelin	X Dᵇ	Case report Garvey et al,[26] 1992	6-Month course of goserelin (in addition to PSN 20–80 mg/d)	Postpartum

Abbreviations: CS, corticosteroid; IV, intravenous; IVIG, intravenous immunoglobulin; PSN, prednisolone.
[a] Labeling of medications in pregnancy and lactation vary in different countries.
[b] Category in Australia.

Table 2
Definitions of pregnancy categories of medications in the United States

Pregnancy Category	Details	Examples
A	Adequate and well-controlled studies have failed to demonstrate a risk to the fetus in the first trimester of pregnancy (and there is no evidence of risk in later trimesters)	
B	Animal reproduction studies have failed to demonstrate a risk to the fetus and there are no adequate and well-controlled studies in pregnant women	
C	Animal reproduction studies have shown an adverse effect on the fetus and there are no adequate and well-controlled studies in humans, but potential benefits may warrant use of the drug in pregnant women despite potential risks	Cyclosporin, rituximab, dapsone, IVIG Topical CS (betamethasone, mometasone, triamcinolone, hydrocortisone) Systemic CS (prednisone, prednisolone, methylprednisolone)
D	There is positive evidence of human fetal risk based on adverse reaction data from investigational or marketing experience or studies in humans, but potential benefits may warrant use of the drug in pregnant women despite potential risks	Azathioprine, cyclophosphamide, doxycycline, minocycline
X	Studies in animals or humans have demonstrated fetal abnormalities and/or there is positive evidence of human fetal risk based on adverse reaction data from investigational or marketing experience, and the risk involved in use of the drug in pregnant women clearly outweighs potential benefits	Goserelin, systemic isotretinoin, thalidomide, methotrexate

Data from The US FDA pregnancy and lactation labeling system is undergoing revisions at this time. Available at: http://www.fda.gov/Drugs/DevelopmentApprovalProcess/DevelopmentResources/Labeling/ucm093307.htm. Accessed May 1, 2011.

blood tests (full blood count, liver and renal function tests) should be ordered, including specific enzyme levels related to specific drugs (ie, glucose-6-phosphate-dehydrogenase [G6PD] for dapsone and thiopurine methyltransferase for azathioprine). Fortnightly to monthly monitoring blood tests are also ordered while on treatment. This condition is generally pruritic, and if required, in addition to systemic corticosteroids, category A antihistamines such as chlorpheniramine or dexchlorpheniramine are suitable choices. Cool compresses may be applied to the skin to relieve pruritus. Intact large blisters may be drained with a sterile, large-bore needle, but care must be taken to avoid unroofing the blisters. Nonstick vaseline gauze or silicone dressings may be applied to the blisters. Secondary bacterial infection is treated with an appropriate antibiotic.

Corticosteroids

In milder and localized forms of PG, potent topical corticosteroids (CS) such as betamethasone dipropionate may be used to control the disease. A large systematic review on the safety of topical CS did not find any significant associations with congenital abnormality, preterm delivery, or still-birth. The study suggested, however, that there was a link between very potent topical CS and low birth weight.[11,12] It has been recently suggested in a study of 39 women with PG in a comparison with 22 normal controls that onset of PG in the first and second trimester and presence of blisters may lead to adverse pregnancy outcomes, including decreased gestational age, preterm birth, and low-birth-weight babies. In the same study, the use of systemic CS, on the other hand, did not have any adverse effects on

Table 3
Definitions of pregnancy categories of medications in Australia

Pregnancy Category	Details	Examples
A	Drugs which have been taken by a large number of pregnant women and women of childbearing age without any proven increase in the frequency of malformations or other direct or indirect harmful effects on the fetus having been observed	Topical CS (betamethasone, triamcinolone) Systemic CS (prednisone, prednisolone, methylprednisolone, dexamethasone, triamcinolone)
B1	Drugs which have been taken by only a limited number of pregnant women and women of childbearing age, without an increase in the frequency of malformation or other direct or indirect harmful effects on the human fetus having been observed Studies in animals have not shown evidence of an increased occurrence of fetal damage	Mupirocin, calcipotriol
B2	Drugs which have been taken by only a limited number of pregnant women and women of childbearing age, without an increase in the frequency of malformation or other direct or indirect harmful effects on the human fetus having been observed Studies in animals are inadequate or may be lacking, but available data show no evidence of an increased occurrence of fetal damage	Dapsone
B3	Drugs which have been taken by only a limited number of pregnant women and women of childbearing age, without an increase in the frequency of malformation or other direct or indirect harmful effects on the human fetus having been observed Studies in animals have shown evidence of an increased occurrence of fetal damage, the significance of which is considered uncertain in humans	Topical CS (mometasone), Inhaled CS (triamcinolone), pimecrolimus
C	Drugs which, owing to their pharmacologic effects, have caused or may be suspected of causing, harmful effects on the human fetus or neonate without causing malformations. These effects may be reversible. Accompanying texts should be consulted for further details	Cyclosporine, rituximab Topical CS (methylprednisolone aceponate)
D	Drugs which have caused, are suspected to have caused, or may be expected to cause an increased incidence of human fetal malformations or irreversible damage. These drugs may also have adverse pharmacologic effects. Accompanying texts should be consulted for further details	Azathioprine, cyclophosphamide, goserelin, doxycycline, minocycline, methotrexate, mycophenolate mofetil
X	Drugs which have such a high risk of causing permanent damage to the fetus that they should not be used in pregnancy or when there is a possibility of pregnancy	Systemic isotretinoin, acitretin, thalidomide

Data from http://www.tga.gov.au/hp/medicines-pregnancy.htm. Accessed May 1, 2011.

pregnancy outcomes, and its use was justified.[3] The preferred systemic steroid is prednisolone, as unlike its prodrug prednisone, it bypasses metabolism in the liver, and therefore is safer in pregnancy.[13] Prednisolone is usually started at a dose of 0.5 to 1 mg/kg/d and may be increased or tapered slowly, depending on the response.

This drug is generally safe during pregnancy, but one must keep in mind that long-term use of CS results in adverse effects such as hypertension, Cushing syndrome, osteopenia/osteoporosis, and abnormalities in glucose metabolism. In cases of severe, persistent PG requiring long-term CS, a bone mineral density scan is taken, and calcium and vitamin D supplements are commenced. There is a report of a young Asian woman with PG who developed gestational diabetes after just a week of high-dose prednisolone.[14]

Doxycycline/Minocycline and Nicotinamide

There have been two small case series reporting the success of combination treatment with doxycycline 200 mg/d and nicotinamide 500 mg/d, or minomycin 100 mg/d and nicotinamide 1000 mg/d for a period of 6 months in postpartum patients with persistent PG, that is, persistent bullae months to years after giving birth.[15,16] However, tetracyclines are listed as category D in pregnancy, due to potential harm to the bone formation in the fetus as well as permanent discoloration of the teeth and enamel hypoplasia. No long-term follow-up of these sequelae were given in these reports from the United Kingdom and Italy.[15,16]

Cyclophosphamide

A patient with severe and persistent PG in the postpartum period who also had antiphospholipid antibody syndrome had an excellent clinical response to pulsed-dose intravenous cyclophosphamide. The patient was started on oral prednisone 20 mg/d, which was increased to 120 mg/d. She delivered a baby at 32 weeks of gestation by emergency cesarean section. Despite high doses of prednisone, blistering continued, and azathioprine was added to her treatment at 8 months postpartum. This treatment was discontinued after 4 weeks because of significant elevation of her liver enzymes. At 9 months postpartum, in consultation with her rheumatologist, cyclophosphamide at 0.75 g/m^2 was commenced. She received 2 doses in an 8-week period, followed by another dose 5 months later, resulting in complete remission off therapy up to 18 months after birth.[17]

Cyclosporine

Cyclosporine at a dose of 100 mg/d has been used in conjunction with low-dose prednisolone and intravenous immunoglobulin (IVIG) at a dose of 0.4 g/kg/d for 5 days in a case of severe PG. This therapy was started 7 months postpartum as blistering continued. The patient was a young 17-year-old female Kuwaiti who was noted to have PG at 20 weeks of gestation. She received up to 80 mg prednisolone, but unfortunately she had a fetal death in utero at 30 weeks' gestation. Of interest, this patient continued to have blistering for up to 1.5 years postpartum, and was thought to have an overlap with bullous pemphigoid due to the cyclical, persistent blistering without hormonal mediation.[18]

Azathioprine

Azathioprine has been used as an adjunct to systemic corticosteroids in cases of severe, persistent PG in the postpartum period, with breastfeeding being avoided, usually at doses of 50 to 150 mg/d, with varying success.[4,5,19–22]

Dapsone

Dapsone has been another popular adjuvant to systemic corticosteroids in severe, persistent PG. Doses reported range from 50 to 150 mg/d. There have been varying degrees of response to this drug. It is important to order a blood test for G6PD before starting this medication, to reduce the risk of a severe dapsone hypersensitivity reaction.[4,5,21,22]

Intravenous Immunoglobulin

IVIG has been demonstrated to be safe during pregnancy, and there have been several reports on its use both during pregnancy and in the postpartum period. IVIG is often added to an existing regimen of corticosteroids and other immunosuppressives, and doses range from 0.4 to 0.5 g/kg/d for 2 to 5 days in monthly cycles.[18–20,23]

Rituximab

There has been a recent report of the success of rituximab in a case of severe, persistent PG failing treatment with a combination treatment of dapsone, high-dose prednisone, and azathioprine. After receiving 4 weekly infusions of rituximab at 375 mg/m^2, the patient went into remission for about 6 months. Four more rituximab infusions were again administered at 2-month intervals to treat a flare, with complete remission. Rituximab was well tolerated, and no side effects were noted.[21]

Plasmapheresis

Plasmapheresis has been reported in a woman with severe, persistent PG up to 2 years postpartum. Plasmapheresis was used in conjunction with high-dose prednisone, azathioprine, and dapsone, without much success.[22] An earlier article reported the success of plasma exchanges in a 40-year-old woman in the 20th week of her fifth pregnancy. She received several plasma exchanges (plasmapheresis) during 26 weeks, delivery, and postpartum, with rapid resolution of pruritus and skin lesions.[24]

There have been reports of the success of adjuvant immunoapheresis (IA), which is a specific type of plasmapheresis, in the treatment of severe PG. The most recent one is that of a 30-year-old woman with severe PG not adequately controlled by high-dose methylprednisolone. She received 15 IA sessions (14 prepartum and 1 postpartum) in addition to methylprednisolone, with excellent response.[25]

Goserelin

There has been a case reported of a 46-year-old woman in the United Kingdom with a 17-year history severe PG requiring high-dose oral prednisolone for up to 10 years after her last pregnancy, who went into complete remission after chemical oophorectomy with goserelin, a luteinizing hormone-releasing hormone (LHRH) analogue.[26]

Others

A retrospective review of 87 patients with PG in the United Kingdom also cited the use of pyridoxine and sulfapyridine as an adjunct to corticosteroids.[4]

SUMMARY

Corticosteroids are the mainstay of treatment in PG, as they are relatively safe during pregnancy and in the postpartum period. There are some reports of success with the use of IVIG, immunoapheresis, and plasma exchange during pregnancy and in the postpartum period. Most other small reports demonstrate the efficacy of anti-inflammatory antibiotics, immunosuppressives, and an LHRH analogue in the postpartum period, in conjunction with corticosteroids, for severe, persistent cases.

REFERENCES

1. Shornick JK. Herpes gestationis. J Am Acad Dermatol 1987;17:539–56.
2. Ingen-Housz-Oro S. Pemphigoid gestationis: a review. Ann Dermatol Venereol 2011;138:209–13 [in French].
3. Semkova K, Black M. Pemphigoid gestationis: current insights into pathogenesis and treatment. Eur J Obstet Gynecol Reprod Biol 2009;145:138–44.
4. Jenkins RE, Hern S, Black MM. Clinical features and management of 87 patients with pemphigoid gestationis. Clin Exp Dermatol 1999;24:255–9.
5. Castro LA, Lundell RB, Krause PK, et al. Clinical experience in pemphigoid gestationis: report of 10 cases. J Am Acad Dermatol 2006;55:823–8.
6. Bedocs PM, Kumar V, Mahon MJ. Pemphigoid gestationis: a rare case and review. Arch Gynecol Obstet 2009;279:235–8.
7. Lu PD, Ralston J, Kamino H, et al. Pemphigoid gestationis. Dermatol Online J 2010;16:10.
8. Ambros-Rudolph CM, Müllegger RR, Vaughan-Jones SA, et al. The specific dermatoses of pregnancy revisited and reclassified: results of a retrospective two-center study on 505 pregnant patients. J Am Acad Dermatol 2006;54:395–404.
9. Chi CC, Wang SH, Charles-Holmes R, et al. Pemphigoid gestationis: early onset and blister formation are associated with adverse pregnancy outcomes. Br J Dermatol 2009;160:1222–8.
10. Shornick JK, Black MM. Fetal risks in herpes gestationis. J Am Acad Dermatol 1992;26:63–8.
11. Chi CC, Mayon-White RT, Wojnarowska FT. Safety of topical corticosteroids in pregnancy: a population-based cohort study. J Invest Dermatol 2011;131:884–91.
12. Chi CC, Wang SH, Kirtschig G, et al. Systematic review of the safety of topical corticosteroids in pregnancy. J Am Acad Dermatol 2010;62:694–705.
13. Little BB. Immunosuppressant therapy during gestation. Semin Perinatol 1997;21:143–8.
14. Heazell AEP, Sinha A, Bhatti NR. A case of gestational diabetes arising following treatment with glucocorticoids for pemphigoid gestationis. J Matern Fetal Neonatal Med 2005;18:353–5.
15. Amato L, Coronella G, Berti S, et al. Successful treatment with doxycycline and nicotinamide of two cases of persistent pemphigoid gestationis. J Dermatolog Treat 2002;13:143–6.
16. Loo WJ, Dean D, Wojnarowska F. A severe persistent case of recurrent pemphigoid gestationis successfully treated with minocycline and nicotinamide. Clin Exp Dermatol 2001;26:726–7.
17. Castle SP, Mather-Mondrey M, Bennion S, et al. Chronic herpes gestationis and antiphospholipid antibody syndrome successfully treated with cyclophosphamide. J Am Acad Dermatol 1996;34:333–6.

18. Hern S, Harman K, Bhogal BS, et al. A severe persistent case of pemphigoid gestationis treated with intravenous immunoglobulins and cyclosporine. Clin Exp Dermatol 1998;23:185–8.

19. Kreuter A, Harati A, Breuckmann F, et al. Intravenous immune globulin in the treatment of persistent pemphigoid gestationis. J Am Acad Dermatol 2004;51: 1027–8.

20. Sereno C, Filipe P, Marques-Gomes, et al. Refractory herpes gestationis responsive to intravenous immunoglobulin: a case report. J Am Acad Dermatol 2005;52(3 Suppl 1):116 [abstract: P1604].

21. Cianchini G, Masini C, Lupi F, et al. Severe persistent pemphigoid gestationis: long-term remission with rituximab. Br J Dermatol 2007;157:388–9.

22. Amato L, Mei S, Gallerani I, et al. A case of herpes gestationis: persistent disease or conversion to bullous pemphigoid. J Am Acad Dermatol 2003;49: 302–7.

23. Doiron P, Pratt M. Antepartum intravenous immunoglobulin therapy in refractory pemphigoid gestationis: case report and literature review. J Cutan Med Surg 2010;14:189–92.

24. Van de Wiel A, Hart CH, Flinterman J, et al. Plasma exchange in herpes gestationis. Br Med J 1980;281: 1041–2.

25. Marker M, Derfler K, Monshi B, et al. Successful immunoapheresis of bullous autoimmune disease: pemphigus vulgaris and pemphigoid gestationis. J Dtsch Dermatol Ges 2011;9:27–31.

26. Garvey MP, Handfield-Jones SE, Black MM. Pemphigoid gestationis-response to chemical oophorectomy with goserelin. Clin Exp Dermatol 1992;17: 443–5.

Management of Linear IgA Disease

Sue Yin Ng, MBBS, BSc, MRCP (UK),
Vanessa V. Venning, BMBCh, DM, FRCP*

KEYWORDS

- Linear IgA disease • Management • Immunoglobulin A
- Autoimmunity

DEFINITION

Linear immunoglobulin A (IgA) disease is an acquired autoimmune blistering disease of the skin and mucous membranes that runs a chronic course over 3 to 6 years before remitting. It typically presents with papulovesicles and blisters configured in an arcuate pattern on an urticated base with 2 peaks in age of onset, although it can occur at any age. The first peak is in young prepubescent children, called chronic bullous disease of childhood, and the second peak affects patients older than 60 years of age.

The disease is characterized by subepidermal blistering and linear deposition of IgA along the dermoepidermal basement membrane zone. The clinical presentation, diagnosis, and pathogenesis have been covered in a recent issue of *Dermatologic Clinics* (Venning, 2011).[1] In this article, the management of linear IgA in adults is considered, the management of children will be dealt with in the article by Mintz & Morel elsewhere in this issue.

TREATMENT

Linear IgA can be induced by drugs, including vancomycin; captopril; cephalosporins; nonsteroidal antiinflammatory drugs, such as diclofenac; as well as a wide range of other drugs reported in the literature.[2–5] When drug-induced disease is considered, withdrawal of the suspect drug is essential.

The treatment of linear IgA disease should be tailored to the extent of involvement and the severity of the disease, with consideration being given to preexisting comorbidities that may influence treatment choice. Potent topical steroids in the form of clobetasol propionate can be an effective monotherapy for patients with mild disease.[2,6] There have been case reports of successful control of this disease with antiinflammatory antibiotics, such as tetracyclines, and macrolide antibiotics alone or in combination with nicotinamide and topical steroids.[2,6–9]

The majority of patients with cutaneous disease respond effectively to dapsone as a first-line therapy in dosages of 50 to 200 mg/d. This response is usually rapid, with a clinical response occurring within the first few days of starting therapy.[6,10] Mucous membrane involvement is typically more resistant to single-agent treatment with dapsone.

Before commencing patients on dapsone, a glucose-6-phosphate dehydrogenase (G6PD) level should be obtained because a deficiency in this enzyme can lead to severe hemolysis. A reduction of 1 to 2 g/dL of hemoglobin is frequently observed in patients with normal G6PD levels and is usually well tolerated as long as the reduction is gradual and there are no significant comorbidities of anemia or ischemic heart disease.

Other well-established side effects associated with dapsone therapy are dose-related methemoglobinemia; bone marrow suppression, including agranulocytosis; and a motor peripheral neuropathy. Other less-common side effects include hepatitis, pneumonitis, nephritis, erythema multiforme, and dapsone hypersensitivity.

Sulfonamides, including sulfapyridine or sulfamethoxypyridazine (dosages range from 250 mg to 2 g/d), are alternatives to dapsone and can be used either as an alternative or in combination with dapsone.[6,11] Both drugs have a similar

Department of Dermatology, Churchill Hospital, Old Road, Oxford OX3 7LJ, UK
* Corresponding author.
E-mail address: vanessa.venning@orh.nhs.uk

Dermatol Clin 29 (2011) 629–630
doi:10.1016/j.det.2011.06.014
0733-8635/11/$ – see front matter © 2011 Elsevier Inc. All rights reserved.

side-effect profile to dapsone, but dapsone intolerance does not preclude their use.

For patients resistant or achieving only partial response to dapsone therapy, systemic corticosteroids/prednisolone in combination with dapsone can be trialed in dosages of up to 40 mg daily to achieve optimal control.[6]

In patients who are resistant to the aforementioned therapies, azathioprine or cyclosporine has had favorable reports of achieving disease control.[12–14] There have been isolated case reports of treatment with mycophenolate mofetil,[15] nicotinamide/niacinamide,[8,13,14] colchicines,[14,16] intravenous immunoglobulins,[17] and immunosorption.[18]

It is postulated that patients who are more resistant to treatment have both IgG and IgA deposits on the basement membrane zone, which indicates multiple target antigens and possible prolonged antigenic stimulation.[2]

Because this disease can spontaneously remit, there should be repeated attempts at tapering treatment once control has been achieved to ascertain whether remission has occurred.

REFERENCES

1. Venning VA. Linear IgA disease: clinical presentation, diagnosis, and pathogenesis. Dermatol Clin 2011;29(3):453–8.

2. Herron M, Zone J. Dermatitis herpetiformis and Linear IgA bullous dermatosis. In: Bolognia J, Jorizzo J, Rapini R, editors. Dermatology. 1st edition. Boston (MA): Mosby Elsevier Ltd; 2003. p. 479–87.

3. Rao C, Russell P. Linear IgA Dermatosis and chronic bullous disease of childhood. In: Wolff K, Goldsmith L, Katz S, et al, editors. Fitzpatrick's dermatology in general medicine. 7th edition. New York: McGraw Hill Medical; 2008. p. 485–90.

4. Baden L, Apovian C, Imber M, et al. Vancomycin induced linear IgA bullous dermatosis. Arch Dermatol 1988;124:1186–8.

5. Kuechle M, Stegemeir E, Maynard B, et al. Drug induced linear IgA bullous dermatosis: report of six cases and review of the literature. J Am Acad Dermatol 1994;30:187–92.

6. Korman N. Linear IgA bullous dermatosis. In: Heymann W, Berth-Jones J, et al, editors. Treatment of skin disease. Comprehensive therapeutic strategies. 2nd edition. Boston (MA): Mosby Elsevier Ltd; 2006. p. 358–60.

7. Cooper S, Powell J, Wognarowska F. Linear IgA disease: successful treatment with erythromycin. Clin Exp Dermatol 2002;27:677–9.

8. Chaffins M, Collison D, Fivenson D. Treatment of pemphigus and linear IgA dermatosis with nicotinamide and tetracycline: review of 13 cases. J Am Acad Dermatol 1993;28:998–1000.

9. Powell J, Kirtchig G, Allen J, et al. Mixed immunobullous disease of childhood: a good response to antimicrobials. Br J Dermatol 2001;144:769–74.

10. Wojnarowska F. Linear IgA dapsone responsive bullous dermatosis. J R Soc Med 1980;73:371–3.

11. McFadden J, Leonard J, Powles A, et al. Sulphamethoxypyridazine for dermatitis herpetiformis, linear IgA disease and cicatricial pemphigoid. Br J Dermatol 1989;121:759–62.

12. Young H, Coulson I. Linear IgA disease: successful treatment with cyclosporine. Br J Dermatol 2000; 143:204–5.

13. Wojnarowska F. Linear IgA disease of adults. In: Wojnarowska F, Briggaman R, editors. Management of blistering diseases. New York: Raven Press; 1990. p. 105–18.

14. Venning VA, Wojnarowska FT. Immunobullous diseases. In: Burns DA, Cox NH, Griffiths CE, editors. Rook's textbook of dermatology. 8th edition. Oxford (UK): Wiley-Blackwell Publishing Ltd; 2010. p. 45–51.

15. Glaser R, Sticherlin M. Successful treatment of linear IgA bullous dermatosis with mycophenolate mofetil. Acta Derm Venereol 2002;82:308–9.

16. Arum H. Linear IgA bullous dermatosis: successful treatment with colchicines. Arch Dermatol 1984; 120:160–1.

17. Ishii N, Hashimoto T, Zillikens D, et al. High dose intravenous immunoglobulin (IVIG) therapy in autoimmune skin blistering diseases. Clin Rev Allergy Immunol 2010;38:186–95.

18. Kasperkiewicz M, Meier M, Zillikens D. Linear IgA disease: successful application of immunoadsorption and review of the literature. Dermatology 2010; 220:259–63.

Management of Dermatitis Herpetiformis

Adela Rambi G. Cardones, MD, Russell P. Hall III, MD*

KEYWORDS

- Dermatitis herpetiformis • Management
- Gluten-sensitive enteropathy • Pruritus

Dermatitis herpetiformis (DH) is a severely pruritic cutaneous disease characterized by markedly pruritic, symmetrically distributed papulovesicles that usually affect the extensor surfaces: the scalp (especially the posterior hairline), elbows, knees, back, and buttocks.[1,2] Histology of skin lesions in DH is characterized by a subepidermal blister with a predominantly neutrophilic infiltrate in the dermal papillary tips,[3] although a mixed or even predominantly lymphocytic dermal infiltrate may also be found.[4,5] Direct immunofluorescence reveals granular deposition of immunoglobulin A (IgA) at the dermal-epidermal junction in both involved and uninvolved skin as well as the oral mucosa.[6–10] Patients with DH have an associated gluten-sensitive enteropathy (GSE),[11] and dietary control is sufficient in abrogating the cutaneous symptoms of DH.[12,13] The condition is chronic, but it waxes and wanes with no clear triggering factors. This disease tends to be chronic, although approximately 10% to 12% of these patients can go into spontaneous remission.[14,15]

Epidermal transglutaminase (eTG) or transglutaminase 3 has been identified as the target autoantigen in DH.[16,17] Serum eTG IgA compared with tissue transglutaminase IgA and IgG was more sensitive in detecting GSE.[18] These serologic studies, however, should not be used to confirm the diagnosis of DH because the presence of IgA anti-eTG has a sensitivity for diagnosis of DH of only 70%. Furthermore, dietary intake seems to correlate with eTG IgA; that is, avoidance of gluten resulted in the gradual decrease of antibody levels.

TREATMENT

The 2 major options for the treatment of DH are medical treatment with dapsone or a sulfone drug and dietary treatment by the strict restriction of gluten intake.[19] Medical therapy with dapsone results in a rapid clinical improvement of skin findings, but it can be associated with side effects. Furthermore, it does not improve the gastrointestinal pathology in patients with DH.[20,21] On the other hand, dietary restriction of gluten has been proven to attenuate both the cutaneous and gastrointestinal signs and symptoms of DH.[13] However, this can be difficult because strict adherence is often required and the improvement of cutaneous symptoms may take weeks if not months.

Gluten-free Diet

Both the skin and the gastrointestinal manifestations of DH are gluten sensitive.[12,13] Leonard and coworkers[22] rechallenged 12 patients whose DH had previously been controlled on a gluten-free diet, and both the rash and the gastrointestinal changes recurred in response to the reintroduction of gluten. As many as 80% of patients with DH are able to stop or reduce their dose of dapsone on a strict gluten-free diet.[23] Those who are able to reduce but not completely eliminate gluten from their diet may see some benefit[15] but not enough to completely control their cutaneous symptoms.[20,24] Patients with DH treated with a gluten-free diet need at least 5 months before they are able to reduce their dapsone dose and

Department of Dermatology, Duke University Medical Center, Durham, NC 27710, USA
* Corresponding author. Room 4044, Purple Zone, Duke South, 200 Trent Drive, Durham, NC 27710.
E-mail address: hall0009@mc.duke.edu

Dermatol Clin 29 (2011) 631–635
doi:10.1016/j.det.2011.06.015
0733-8635/11/$ – see front matter © 2011 Elsevier Inc. All rights reserved.

anywhere from 8 to 48 months before they can stop dapsone treatment altogether.[12,13,23] In some patients, gluten restriction need not be lifelong because long-term remission can occur in as many as 10% to 12% of patients.[14,15] Bardella and colleagues[25] reported that 7 out of 38 patients who reverted to a normal, gluten-containing diet after an average of 8 years of gluten restriction continued to experience remission of their skin and gut disease after a mean follow-up of 12 years. Fry and coworkers[20] observed that macroscopic and microscopic small intestinal abnormalities among patients with DH on a gluten-free diet decreased significantly when compared with those who were on a normal diet, including a decrease in intraepithelial lymphocytic infiltration.[20] In this same study, they found that the improvement of cutaneous symptoms and gastrointestinal abnormality was directly related to the degree of strictness of the gluten-free diet. The incidence of lymphoma and other malignancies in patients with DH and GSE, although low, has been reported to increase when compared with the normal population.[26,27] Recent studies, however, have not found a similar increased risk of malignancy.[28] The reason for this discrepancy is not clear. It has been suggested that adherence to a gluten-free diet may play a role in moderating the risk of developing a malignancy, but a controlled study has not been done.[26,29] Van Der Meer and colleagues[30] have reported that an elemental diet can lead to the control of the eruption of DH. Kandunce and coworkers[31] have also shown that an elemental diet is effective at achieving control of DH often within 2 to 4 weeks.[31] Of interest, this effect seems to be independent of gluten ingestion. These studies suggest that other dietary proteins may also be important in the pathogenesis of dermatitis herpetiformis. IgA deposition in the skin appears to improve, albeit over a course of several years, on a gluten-free diet.[20,32,33] Fry and coworkers[32] noted that only 4 out of 23 patients with DH on a gluten-free diet had complete clearance of IgA deposition in their skin and only after several years. They further described that there was no difference in the quantity of IgA, as assessed by the amount of fluorescence, whether patients were controlled with a gluten-free diet alone, gluten-free diet and dapsone, dapsone alone, or in those in clinical remission. Frodin and coworkers[33] followed 32 patients with DH on either a gluten-free or gluten-reduced diet for 15 to 43 months and, although there was a decrease in the intensity of IgA deposition in the skin of these patients, none had a complete disappearance of cutaneous IgA deposition in spite of a good clinical response. In patients with DH controlled on a gluten-free diet and with clearance of cutaneous IgA deposition, gluten challenge results in the reappearance of cutaneous IgA deposits within 1 month.[22] A more direct immunologic effect of a gluten-free diet is reflected in serum interleukin (IL)-8 levels among patients with DH. Serum IL-8 is elevated in patients with DH, and a gluten-free diet normalizes or reduces the amount of circulating IL-8 in these patients.[34] Patients with DH on a gluten-free diet had a decreased mRNA expression of IL-8 compared with those on a normal diet, suggesting that the elevated circulating IL-8 in patients with DH is produced in the intestinal mucosa as a response to gluten.[34]

Adherence to a gluten-free diet is effective in the majority of patients with DH at controlling the cutaneous manifestations of DH with a resultant decrease or elimination of the need for dapsone therapy. Even patients with DH with a normal initial small-bowel biopsy experience improvement of their rash when placed on a gluten-free diet.[35] In addition, a gluten-free diet may prevent or lessen the possibility of an increased risk of lymphoma and other malignancies in patients with DH. Adherence to a gluten-free diet, however, is difficult and requires significant knowledge and strong compliance by patients and their families. Fry and coworkers[20] noted that only 23 of 42 patients who thought that they were on a gluten-free diet were actually adhering to a strict gluten-free diet when evaluated by a dietitian. Consultation with a registered dietitian with expertise in gluten-free diets is often extremely valuable in improving patients' compliance with the diet. In addition, several patient groups are extremely useful for patients learning more about the diet (Celiac Sprue Association, csaceliacs.org).

Dapsone

The cutaneous signs and symptoms of DH can often be quickly and adequately controlled by 100 to 200 mg of dapsone with minimal side effects, although there is considerable variability in response.[19] Some patients require as little as 25 mg by mouth daily, whereas others may need up to 400 mg daily. Treatment can be initiated at a dosage of 100 mg daily unless patients have other significant risk factors, such as cardiovascular, pulmonary, or hematologic disease, and those who would likely not tolerate the hemolytic anemia and methemoglobinemia that may result from dapsone therapy. A complete review of the pharmacology and adverse effects of dapsone is beyond the scope of this review and readers are referred to several recent reviews for further information.[36,37] Most patients with DH will respond to dapsone within 24 to 36 hours of initiating the medication, and withdrawal of dapsone results in recurrence of signs and symptoms within 24 to 48 hours. Treatment with dapsone, however, does not alter gastrointestinal mucosal changes.[20,21] Furthermore, sulfone treatment does not appear to affect deposition of complement in the skin of patients with DH even when their cutaneous lesions were controlled.[38] This finding suggests that the therapeutic effect of dapsone is exerted at the effector cells of the cutaneous pathology; that is, there is neutrophilic infiltration of the skin and not at the initiation of the immunologic response, which is thought to occur when gut mucosa is exposed to gluten. Indeed, dapsone has been demonstrated to interfere with neutrophil chemotaxis[39] and the adhesion to antibodies[40] as well as with the release of IL-8 from keratinocytes.[41]

Careful monitoring of the side effects of dapsone is required. Aside from a careful history and physical examination to evaluate the cardiovascular, pulmonary, gastrointestinal, neurologic, and renal status of patients, a baseline complete blood count with differential, renal function test, liver function test, urinalysis, and G6PD level are recommended. Although a complete review of the pharmacology of dapsone is beyond the scope of the review, it is critical that the physician prescribing this drug be aware of the most severe adverse events. All patients will develop a dose-dependent hemolytic anemia with a resultant decrease in hemoglobin. In addition, some degree of methemoglobinemia will develop in all patients on dapsone, also in a dose-dependent manner. Concomitant administration of cimetidine, 400 mg by mouth 3 times a day, reduces dapsone-induced methemoglobinemia without affecting the clinical response in patients with DH.[42] Idiosyncratic side effects, including agranulocytosis, and hepatic function abnormalities may also occur. These side effects may be severe, and appropriate monitoring for side effects is essential. Because many of these side effects can be noted early and are reversible, monitoring of complete blood counts should be performed weekly for 1 month, every other week for 1 month, and then at 3- to 4-month intervals. Monitoring of liver and renal function should be performed periodically or as dictated by symptoms. Because many of these side effects are dose related, patients should be told not to adjust dapsone dosage without consulting their physician. Dapsone is also associated with a distal motor neuropathy. This event is relatively rare, but it is reversible and also requires monitoring by clinical examination and nerve-conduction studies as needed. Although dapsone is an extremely effective drug for the control of DH, the potential for toxicity is great and close follow-up is needed. Physicians who prescribe dapsone should be familiar with the pharmacology and adverse effects of the drug.[36,37] In addition, because of the unfamiliarity of some physicians with the use of dapsone, it is recommended that patients carry cards describing their use of dapsone and the associated adverse effects, including methemoglobinemia and a low-grade hemolytic anemia.

Sulfapyridine and Sulfasalazine

Sulfapyridine is an alternative medical treatment for DH, although less effective than dapsone, and patients are usually controlled with 1 to 2 g by mouth daily. This medication, however, is not readily available in the United States. Sulfasalazine, which is more readily available, is metabolized into 5-amino-salicylic acid (5-ASA) and sulfapyridine. Patients have been reported to respond to 2 to 4 g/d of sulfasalazine.[43,44] Once sulfasalazine is metabolized in the gut, most of the sulfapyridine is absorbed and excreted in the urine, whereas most of the 5-ASA remains in the gut and is thought to exert a local antiinflammatory effect that makes it useful in the treatment of inflammatory bowel disease.[45] It is not yet known if sulfasalazine exerts any effect on the gastrointestinal pathology in DH, but in one report of a patient with DH and ulcerative colitis, both the cutaneous and gastrointestinal symptoms improved on treatment with sulfasalazine.[46]

SUMMARY

The major treatment strategies for DH are gluten restriction or medical treatment with sulfones. Control of the cutaneous manifestations, but not the gastrointestinal changes, is rapid with dapsone. In addition to control of the cutaneous signs and symptoms of DH, dietary gluten restriction also induces improvement of gastrointestinal morphology and is possibly protective against the development of lymphoma.

REFERENCES

1. Duhring LA. Landmark article, Aug 30, 1884: dermatitis herpetiformis. By Louis A. Duhring. JAMA 1983; 250(2):212–6.
2. Katz SI. Dermatitis herpetiformis. Clinical, histologic, therapeutic and laboratory clues. Int J Dermatol 1978;17(7):529–35.
3. Rose C, Brocker EB, Zillikens D. Clinical, histological and immunpathological findings in 32 patients with dermatitis herpetiformis Duhring. J Dtsch Dermatol Ges 2010;8(4):265–70, 265–71.

4. Alonso-Llamazares J, Gibson LE, Rogers RS 3rd. Clinical, pathologic, and immunopathologic features of dermatitis herpetiformis: review of the Mayo Clinic experience. Int J Dermatol 2007;46(9):910–9.

5. Warren SJ, Cockerell CJ. Characterization of a subgroup of patients with dermatitis herpetiformis with nonclassical histologic features. Am J Dermatopathol 2002;24(4):305–8.

6. Seah PP, Fry L, Stewart JS, et al. Immunoglobulins in the skin in dermatitis herpetiformis and coeliac disease. Lancet 1972;1(7751):611–4.

7. Haffenden G, Wojnarowska F, Fry L. Comparison of immunoglobulin and complement deposition in multiple biopsies from the uninvolved skin in dermatitis herpetiformis. Br J Dermatol 1979;101(1):39–45.

8. Nisengard RJ, Chorzelski T, Maciejowska E, et al. Dermatitis herpetiformis: IgA deposits in gingiva, buccal mucosa, and skin. Oral Surg Oral Med Oral Pathol 1982;54(1):22–5.

9. van der Meer JB. Granular deposits of immunoglobulins in the skin of patients with dermatitis herpetiformis. An immunofluorescent study. Br J Dermatol 1969;81(7):493–503.

10. Chorzelski TP, Beutner EH, Jablonska S, et al. Immunofluorescence studies in the diagnosis of dermatitis herpetiformis and its differentiation from bullous pemphigoid. J Invest Dermatol 1971;56(5):373–80.

11. Marks J, Shuster S, Watson AJ. Small-bowel changes in dermatitis herpetiformis. Lancet 1966; 2(7476):1280–2.

12. Fry L, McMinn RM, Cowan JD, et al. Gluten-free diet and reintroduction of gluten in dermatitis herpetiformis. Arch Dermatol 1969;100(2):129–35.

13. Fry L, McMinn RM, Cowan JD, et al. Effect of gluten-free diet on dermatological, intestinal, and haematological manifestations of dermatitis herpetiformis. Lancet 1968;1(7542):557–61.

14. Paek SY, Steinberg SM, Katz SI. Remission in dermatitis herpetiformis: a cohort study. Arch Dermatol 2011;147(3):301–5.

15. Garioch JJ, Lewis HM, Sargent SA, et al. 25 years' experience of a gluten-free diet in the treatment of dermatitis herpetiformis. Br J Dermatol 1994;131(4):541–5.

16. Sardy M, Karpati S, Merkl B, et al. Epidermal transglutaminase (TGase 3) is the autoantigen of dermatitis herpetiformis. J Exp Med 2002;195(6):747–57.

17. Donaldson MR, Zone JJ, Schmidt LA, et al. Epidermal transglutaminase deposits in perilesional and uninvolved skin in patients with dermatitis herpetiformis. J Invest Dermatol 2007;127(5):1268–71.

18. Jaskowski TD, Hamblin T, Wilson AR, et al. IgA anti-epidermal transglutaminase antibodies in dermatitis herpetiformis and pediatric celiac disease. J Invest Dermatol 2009;129(11):2728–30.

19. Katz SI, Hall RP 3rd, Lawley TJ, et al. Dermatitis herpetiformis: the skin and the gut. Ann Intern Med 1980;93(6):857–74.

20. Fry L, Leonard JN, Swain F, et al. Long term follow-up of dermatitis herpetiformis with and without dietary gluten withdrawal. Br J Dermatol 1982;107(6):631–40.

21. Reunala T, Kosnai I, Karpati S, et al. Dermatitis herpetiformis: jejunal findings and skin response to gluten free diet. Arch Dis Child 1984;59(6):517–22.

22. Leonard J, Haffenden G, Tucker W, et al. Gluten challenge in dermatitis herpetiformis. N Engl J Med 1983;308(14):816–9.

23. Fry L, Seah PP, Riches DJ, et al. Clearance of skin lesions in dermatitis herpetiformis after gluten withdrawal. Lancet 1973;1(7798):288–91.

24. Ljunghall K, Tjernlund U. Dermatitis herpetiformis: effect of gluten-restricted and gluten-free diet on dapsone requirement and on IgA and C3 deposits in uninvolved skin. Acta Derm Venereol 1983;63(2):129–36.

25. Bardella MT, Fredella C, Trovato C, et al. Long-term remission in patients with dermatitis herpetiformis on a normal diet. Br J Dermatol 2003;149(5):968–71.

26. Hervonen K, Vornanen M, Kautiainen H, et al. Lymphoma in patients with dermatitis herpetiformis and their first-degree relatives. Br J Dermatol 2005; 152(1):82–6.

27. Askling J, Linet M, Gridley G, et al. Cancer incidence in a population-based cohort of individuals hospitalized with celiac disease or dermatitis herpetiformis. Gastroenterology 2002;123(5):1428–35.

28. Lewis NR, Logan RF, Hubbard RB, et al. No increase in risk of fracture, malignancy or mortality in dermatitis herpetiformis: a cohort study. Aliment Pharmacol Ther 2008;27(11):1140–7.

29. Lewis HM, Renaula TL, Garioch JJ, et al. Protective effect of gluten-free diet against development of lymphoma in dermatitis herpetiformis. Br J Dermatol 1996;135(3):363–7.

30. van der Meer JB, Zeedijk N, Poen H, et al. Rapid improvement of dermatitis herpetiformis after elemental diet. Arch Dermatol Res 1981;271(4):455–9.

31. Kadunce DP, McMurry MP, Avots-Avotins A, et al. The effect of an elemental diet with and without gluten on disease activity in dermatitis herpetiformis. J Invest Dermatol 1991;97(2):175–82.

32. Fry L, Haffenden G, Wojnarowska F, et al. IgA and C3 complement in the uninvolved skin in dermatitis herpetiformis after gluten withdrawal. Br J Dermatol 1978;99(1):31–7.

33. Frodin T, Gotthard R, Hed J, et al. Gluten-free diet for dermatitis herpetiformis: the long-term effect on cutaneous, immunological and jejunal manifestations. Acta Derm Venereol 1981;61(5):405–11.

34. Hall RP 3rd, Benbenisty KM, Mickle C, et al. Serum IL-8 in patients with dermatitis herpetiformis is produced in response to dietary gluten. J Invest Dermatol 2007;127(9):2158–65.

35. Buckley DA, McDermott R, O'Donoghue D, et al. Should all patients with dermatitis herpetiformis follow a gluten-free diet? J Eur Acad Dermatol Venereol 1997;9(3):222–5.

36. Zhu YI, Stiller MJ. Dapsone and sulfones in dermatology: overview and update. J Am Acad Dermatol 2001;45(3):420–34.

37. Hall RP III, Mickle CP. Dapsone. In: Wolverton SE, editor. Comprehensive dermatologic drug therapy. Philadelphia: Saunders; 2001. p. 239–57.

38. Katz SI, Hertz KC, Crawford PS, et al. Effect of sulfones on complement deposition in dermatitis herpetiformis and on complement-mediated guinea-pig reactions. J Invest Dermatol 1976;67(6):688–90.

39. Wozel G, Blasum C, Winter C, et al. Dapsone hydroxylamine inhibits the LTB4-induced chemotaxis of polymorphonuclear leukocytes into human skin: results of a pilot study. Inflamm Res 1997; 46(10):420–2.

40. Thuong-Nguyen V, Kadunce DP, Hendrix JD, et al. Inhibition of neutrophil adherence to antibody by dapsone: a possible therapeutic mechanism of dapsone in the treatment of IgA dermatoses. J Invest Dermatol 1993;100(4):349–55.

41. Schmidt E, Reimer S, Kruse N, et al. The IL-8 release from cultured human keratinocytes, mediated by antibodies to bullous pemphigoid autoantigen 180, is inhibited by dapsone. Clin Exp Immunol 2001; 124(1):157–62.

42. Coleman MD, Rhodes LE, Scott AK, et al. The use of cimetidine to reduce dapsone-dependent methemoglobinemia in dermatitis-herpetiformis patients. Br J Clin Pharmacol 1992;34(3):244–9.

43. Goldstein BG, Smith JG Jr. Sulfasalazine in dermatitis herpetiformis. J Am Acad Dermatol 1990;22(4):697.

44. Willsteed E, Lee M, Wong LC, et al. Sulfasalazine and dermatitis herpetiformis. Australas J Dermatol 2005;46(2):101–3.

45. Klotz U. Clinical pharmacokinetics of sulphasalazine, its metabolites and other prodrugs of 5-aminosalicylic acid. Clin Pharmacokinet 1985;10(4):285–302.

46. Lambert D, Collet E, Foucher JL, et al. Dermatitis herpetiformis associated with ulcerative colitis. Clin Exp Dermatol 1991;16(6):458–9.

Therapeutic Approaches to Patients with Mucous Membrane Pemphigoid

A. Shadi Kourosh, MD*, Kim B. Yancey, MD

KEYWORDS

- Immunosuppressives • Mucosal sites • Interdisciplinary
- Glucocorticosteroids

This article summarizes the treatment of mucous membrane pemphigoid (MMP), a treatment-resistant disease for which the goal of therapy is control of symptoms and preservation of function. The arsenal of therapeutics is roughly the same as that for bullous pemphigoid with additional emphasis on site-directed therapy as the guiding principle of management.

Vigilant review of symptoms, examination of mucous membranes and skin to determine all sites of involvement, and prompt referral to subspecialists (ie, ophthalmologists, otolaryngologists and so forth) to assist in evaluation and management of affected sites, can make the difference between independent functioning and disability for patients with MMP, especially those with ocular and laryngeal involvement. The involvement of certain mucosal sites (ie, ocular, genital, nasopharyngeal, esophageal, and laryngeal mucosal sites) is considered high risk and warrants more aggressive intervention. As in the treatment of any autoimmune disease, effective treatment must be reconciled with efforts to minimize the adverse effects of exposure to systemic glucocorticosteroids and/or other immunosuppressives.

APPROACH TO PATIENTS WITH LOW-RISK DISEASE

Low-risk disease (eg, involvement of only the oral mucosa and/or skin sites with less tendency and/or clinical significance of scarring) is managed first with topical corticosteroids of moderate to high potency. Available forms include mouthwash (dexamethasone swish-and-spit) and topical corticosteroid gels or ointments. To facilitate adsorption, gels and ointments can be used under occlusion with oral, insertable, vinyl, prosthetic devices (ie, dental trays).[1,2] Avoidance of toothpastes containing sodium lauryl sulfate and mouthwashes containing alcohol may further aid in the control of symptoms. Treatment may be escalated with intralesional glucocorticosteroid injections and systemic therapies, such as dapsone, low morning doses of prednisone, or the prednisone in combination with azathioprine or mycophenolate mofetil (**Table 1**).[3–6]

APPROACH TO PATIENTS WITH HIGH-RISK DISEASE

For patients with high-risk disease (eg, with involvement of ocular, genital, nasopharyngeal, esophageal, and/or laryngeal mucosal sites) systemic glucocorticosteroids (ie, prednisone at doses of 1 mg/kg/d) in combination with glucocorticosteroid-sparing agents have been the mainstay of treatment (**Table 1**). Although the lack of large-scale, randomized, controlled studies of therapeutic regimens has been limiting in guiding evidence-based practices for clinicians in this arena, the First International Consensus Conference on MMP supports initial treatment with prednisone (1 mg/kg/d) in combination with an agent that disrupts the purine

Disclosures: None.
Conflicts of Interest: None.
Department of Dermatology, University of Texas Southwestern Medical Center in Dallas, 5323 Harry Hines Boulevard, Dallas, TX 75390, USA
* Corresponding author.
E-mail address: askderm@gmail.com

Dermatol Clin 29 (2011) 637–641
doi:10.1016/j.det.2011.06.022
0733-8635/11/$ – see front matter © 2011 Elsevier Inc. All rights reserved.

Table 1
Complications and treatment by mucosal site

Site	Possible Complications	Site-Specific Therapy

Mouth	• Adhesions between tongue and floor of mouth and around uvula and tonsils
	• Dental complications:
	  ○ Gingival loss
	  ○ Caries
	  ○ Periodontal ligament damage
	  ○ Loss of bone mass
	  ○ Loss of teeth
		Mild:
		• Initial treatment with topical glucocorticosteroids
		  ○ Moderate to high potency (class I–III steroids) gels or ointments bid/qid
		  ○ Mouthwash (dexamethasone 100 g/mL, 5 mL per rinse) used in a swish-and-spit regimen for 5 min bid/tid
		  ○ Under occlusion (ie, beneath prosthetic vinyl dental trays)
		  ○ Avoidance of toothpastes containing sodium lauryl sulfate
		  ○ Avoidance of mouthwashes containing alcohol
		  ○ Topical agents for pain (eg, lidocaine or benzocaine [beware potential complications])
		• Topical calcineurin inhibitor (eg, tacrolimus)
		• Intralesional glucocorticosteroids
		Moderate:
		• Dapsone (25–200 mg/d)
		• Low morning doses of prednisone (0.5 mg/kg or 20–40 mg/d with or without azathioprine [2.0–2.5 mg/kg/d], mycophenolate mofetil [1.0 to 2.5 g/d], or cyclophosphamide [1.0 to 2.0 mg/kg/d])
		Severe:
		• Higher dose of prednisone (1 mg/kg or 60 mg/d with or without azathioprine [2.0–2.5 mg/kg/d], mycophenolate mofetil [1.0–2.5 g/d], or cyclophosphamide [1.0–2.0 mg/kg/d])
		Alternatives/Miscellaneous:
		• Thalidomide, tetracycline/niacinamide, IVIG, plasmapheresis, rituximab
		• Surgery for scarring, tissue loss

Eye	• Painful, erosive, conjunctivitis
	• Conjunctival scarring
	• Shortened fornices
	• Loss of goblet cells
	• Decrease in tear mucus content, unstable tear film
	• Symblepharon
	• Ankyloblepharon
	• Ectropion
	• Trichiasis
	• Corneal irritation
	• Superficial punctate keratinopathy
	• Corneal neovascularization
	• Corneal ulcers
	• Scarring, occlusion, secondary infection of the tear ducts
	• Blindness
		• Epilation of eyelashes for trichiasis
		• Topical glucocorticosteroids per decision of ophthalmologist
		Mild to Moderate:
		• Dapsone (25–200 mg/d)
		• Low morning doses of prednisone (0.5 mg/kg or 20–40 mg/d with or without azathioprine [2.0–2.5 mg/kg/d], mycophenolate mofetil [1.0–2.5 g/d], or cyclophosphamide [1.0–2.0 mg/kg/d])
		Severe:
		• Higher dose of prednisone (1 mg/kg or 60 mg/d with or without azathioprine [2.0–2.5 mg/kg/d], mycophenolate mofetil [1.0–2.5 g/d], or cyclophosphamide [1.0–2.0 mg/kg/d])
		• IVIG (2 g/kg of body weight) over 2–3 days every 2–6 weeks for 4–6 months
		• Biologic agents:
		  ○ Anti-TNF agents (eg, etanercept, infliximab)
		  ○ Anti-CD 20 (rituximab)
		Alternatives/Miscellaneous:
		• Subconjunctival mitomycin
		• Surgical interventions per ophthalmology

Nose	• Scarring • Tissue loss	Mild: • Irrigation with isotonic saline or tap water 2 or 3 times a day • Nasal emollients • Topical corticosteroids (eg, nasal sprays, inhalers) Mild, Moderate, and/or Severe: • The same as outlined for ocular treatments

Larynx	• Chronic erosions, edema, scarring leading to:
	  ○ Supraglottic stenosis
	  ○ Airway compromise
		Mild, Moderate, and/or Severe:
		• The same as outlined for ocular treatments
		• Tracheostomy for airway compromise

Esophagus	• Esophageal dysfunction and reflux, causing:
	  ○ Exacerbation of laryngeal disease
	  ○ Bronchospasm
	• Stricture formation
	• Weight loss
	• Aspiration
		Mild, Moderate, and/or Severe:
		• The same as outlined for ocular treatments
		• Esophageal dilation

Anogenital region	• Urethral stricture • Vaginal and/or anal stenosis • Secondary infection	• Topical corticosteroids • Topical calcineurin inhibitor (tacrolimus) Mild, Moderate, and/or Severe: • The same as outlined for ocular treatments • Surgical interventions per urology/gynecology
Skin	• Scarring	• Topical corticosteroids • Topical calcineurin inhibitors Mild, Moderate, and/or Severe: • The same as outlined for ocular treatments

pathway (eg, azathioprine [2.0–2.5 mg/kg/d] or mycophenolate mofetil [1.0–2.5 g/d]). After this regimen brings MMP under control, prednisone is tapered gradually over approximately 6 months and the patient is maintained on the alternate agent alone for an additional 6 to 12 months.[7–12]

For patients with severe eye involvement, 2 small, randomized, controlled trials have supported combined regimens of prednisone (1 mg/kg/d initially, tapered over 6 months) and cyclophosphamide (2 mg/kg/d) over prednisone alone, in halting the advancement of severe ocular disease and producing long-term remission. To avoid the possible adverse effects of cyclophosphamide (eg, alopecia, anemia, leucopenia, male sterility, hemorrhagic cystitis, and DNA damage with potential for malignancy),[13] dapsone may be tried initially for patients with moderate disease. However, treatment should be escalated (to prednisone plus cyclophosphamide) if dapsone does not achieve control in a short time (eg, approximately 1 month) so that mucosal inflammation and scarring sequelae may be curbed in a timely manner.[6,7,11,13,14] Subconjunctival mitomycin may also assist in reducing mucosal fibrosis,[15–17] although this intervention has not been widely used.

In cases of refractory disease, intravenous immunoglobulin (IVIG) has served as a safe and effective therapy in selected patients.[14,18] Biologics, in particular the inhibitors of tumor necrosis factor alpha (eg, etanercept, infliximab) and the anti-CD20 monoclonal antibody rituximab, are emerging as more commonly used drugs.[19,20]

In managing high-risk patients, it is important to consider that those on long-term prednisone and other immunosuppressive treatments may require prophylaxis for *Candida* and or *Pneumocystis* infections as well as therapies for prevention of osteoporosis (eg, calcium, vitamin D, and/or bisphosphonates). All patients with MMP require long-term follow-up because of the likelihood of relapse of this chronic disease, as well as interdisciplinary management with specialists who have expertise about particularly threatening sites of involvement.

SUMMARY

The therapeutic approach to MMP is site specific, with the goal of preserving function for patients with chronic and treatment-resistant disease. Control of disease must be balanced with minimizing the sequelae of long-term exposure to systemic glucocorticosteroids and/or other immunosuppressives. Timely interventions and multidisciplinary management are essential in preventing disability.

REFERENCES

1. Lozada-Nur F, Huang MZ, Zhou GA. Open preliminary clinical trial of clobetasol propionate ointment in adhesive paste for treatment of chronic oral vesiculoerosive diseases. Oral Surg Oral Med Oral Pathol 1991;71:283–7.
2. Lozada-Nur F, Miranda C, Maliksi R. Double-blind clinical trial of 0.05% clobetasol propionate (corrected from proprionate) ointment in orabase and 0.05% fluocinonide ointment in orabase in the treatment of patients with oral vesiculoerosive diseases. Oral Surg Oral Med Oral Pathol 1994;77:598–604.
3. Poskitt L, Wojnarowska F. Treatment of cicatricial pemphigoid with tetracycline and nicotinamide. Clin Exp Dermatol 1995;20:258–9.
4. Reiche L, Wojnarowska F, Mallon E. Combination therapy with nicotinamide and tetracyclines for cicatricial pemphigoid: further support for its efficacy. Clin Exp Dermatol 1998;23:254–7.
5. Lozada F. Prednisone and azathioprine in the treatment of patients with vesiculoerosive oral diseases. Oral Surg Oral Med Oral Pathol 1981;52:257–63.
6. Rogers RS 3rd, Seehafer JR, Perry HO. Treatment of cicatricial (benign mucous membrane) pemphigoid with dapsone. J Am Acad Dermatol 1982;6:215–23.
7. Tauber J, Sainz De La Maza M, Foster CS. Systemic chemotherapy for ocular cicatricial pemphigoid. Cornea 1991;10:185–95.
8. Brody HJ, Pirozzi DJ. Benign mucous membrane pemphigoid. Response to therapy with cyclophosphamide. Arch Dermatol 1977;113:1598–9.
9. Mondino BJ, Brown SI. Immunosuppressive therapy in ocular cicatricial pemphigoid. Am J Ophthalmol 1983;96:453–9.
10. Elder MJ, Lightman S, Dart JK. Role of cyclophosphamide and high dose steroid in ocular cicatricial pemphigoid. Br J Ophthalmol 1995;79:264–6.
11. Chan LS, Ahmed AR, Anhalt GJ, et al. The first international consensus on mucous membrane pemphigoid: definition, diagnostic criteria, pathogenic factors, medical treatment, and prognostic indicators. Arch Dermatol 2002;138:370–9.
12. Lazarova Z, Yancey KB. Cicatricial pemphigoid: immunopathogenesis and treatment. Dermatol Ther 2002;15:382–8.
13. Kirtschig G, Murrell DF, Wojnarowska F, et al. Interventions for mucous membrane pemphigoid and epidermolysis bullosa acquisita. Cochrane Database Syst Rev 2009;2. DOI:10.1002/14651858.CD004056.
14. Foster CS, Ahmed AR. Intravenous immunoglobulin therapy for ocular cicatricial pemphigoid: a preliminary study. Ophthalmology 1999;106:2136–43.
15. Yamamoto T, Varani J, Soong HK, et al. Effects of 5-fluorouracil and mitomycin C on cultured rabbit subconjunctival fibroblasts. Ophthalmology 1990;97:1204–10.

16. Donnenfeld ED, Perry HD, Wallerstein A, et al. Subconjunctival mitomycin C for the treatment of ocular cicatricial pemphigoid. Ophthalmology 1999;106: 72–8 [discussion: 79].

17. Secchi AG, Tognon MS. Intraoperative mitomycin C in the treatment of cicatricial obliterations of conjunctival fornices. Am J Ophthalmol 1996;122:728–30.

18. Letko E, Bhol K, Foster SC, et al. Influence of intravenous immunoglobulin therapy on serum levels of anti-beta 4 antibodies in ocular cicatricial pemphigoid.

A correlation with disease activity. A preliminary study. Curr Eye Res 2000;21:646–54.

19. Dupuy A, Viguier M, Bedane C, et al. Treatment of refractory pemphigus vulgaris with rituximab (anti-CD 20 monoclonal antibody). Arch Dermatol 2004; 140:91–6.

20. Sacher C, Rubbert A, Konig C, et al. Treatment of recalcitrant cicatricial pemphigoid with the tumor necrosis factor alpha antagonist etanercept. J Am Acad Dermatol 2002;46:113–5.

Management of Epidermolysis Bullosa Acquisita

Lizbeth R.A. Intong, MD, DPDS[a,b],
Dédée F. Murrell, MA, BMBCh, FAAD, MD, FACD[c],*

KEYWORDS

- Epidermolysis bullosa acquisita • Management • Treatment

Epidermolysis bullosa acquisita (EBA) is a rare, chronic, autoimmune, blistering disease primarily due to circulating IgG autoantibodies to the various domains of type VII collagen, the major component of anchoring fibrils.[1] Clinical features are similar to those seen in inherited forms of dystrophic epidermolysis bullosa, as well as other autoimmune bullous diseases such as the pemphigoid group. They include blistering in areas prone to trauma, resulting in scarring and milia formation, nail dystrophy, and varying degrees of mucosal involvement.[2–7]

MANAGEMENT OF EBA
General Measures and Supportive Treatment

Owing to the similarity of this disease to inherited dystrophic epidermolysis bullosa, avoidance of trauma and wearing protective padding is recommended to reduce blistering. Sterile rupturing of bullae to release pressure from fluid and the use of nonstick dressings (ie, silicone or petroleum jelly gauze) is recommended for covering erosions. During procedures when the patient is unconscious, such as esophageal dilatations, care needs to be taken to not put too much pressure on blood pressure cuffs and nonstick tape should be used to minimize blistering. Appropriate oral antibiotics may be given in the setting of secondary bacterial infection.[8]

Management of Mucosal Involvement

Mucosal involvement, especially of the ocular, oral, nasopharyngeal, esophageal, and genital mucosa, is often found in patients with EBA. The presence of mucosal involvement is a one of the main causes of disease morbidity.[4]

In addition to the immunosuppressive treatment required to suppress the disease, patients may need specific treatment directed at involved mucosal sites.

Eye involvement is EBA may range from a mild conjunctivitis to symblepharon, trichiasis, and even cicatrizing conjunctivitis with scarring and blindness if left untreated.[4–6,9,10] It is, therefore, imperative that EBA patients with ocular involvement be comanaged with an ophthalmologist to determine the response to the treatment modalities being given and to prescribe appropriate eye drops. Procedures such as repeated endoscopic esophageal dilatations are required under steroid cover if patients have esophageal strictures. There has been a case report of an adult male patient with EBA with recalcitrant disease for more than 13 years requiring repeated endoscopic dilatations due to esophageal strictures. He was covered with oral corticosteroids to reduce new blister formation that occurs after these procedures.[11]

Ankyloglossia and microstomia are additional mucosal complications of EBA that require comanagement with a dentist who specializes in

[a] Department of Dermatology, James Laws House, St George Hospital, Gray Street, Kogarah, Sydney, NSW 2217, Australia
[b] Faculty of Medicine, University of New South Wales, Sydney, NSW 2052, Australia
[c] Department of Dermatology, St George Hospital, University of New South Wales, Gray Street, Kogarah, Sydney, NSW 2217, Australia
* Corresponding author.
E-mail address: d.murrell@unsw.edu.au

Dermatol Clin 29 (2011) 643–647
doi:10.1016/j.det.2011.06.020
0733-8635/11/$ – see front matter © 2011 Elsevier Inc. All rights reserved.

complex cases. Sometimes, teeth have to be removed as the mouth becomes smaller and the treatments given for osteopenia or osteoporosis can have negative effects on the jaw or teeth.

Medications Used in the Treatment of EBA

There have been no randomized controlled trials to assess the management of EBA because it is such a rare disease and includes various subtypes.[12] The mainstay of treatment has been primarily systemic corticosteroids; however, the long-term immunosuppression required results in increased morbidity and mortality due to the known side effects of the drugs.[3,13] EBA patients do not necessarily respond well to corticosteroids when compared with other autoimmune blistering diseases (AIBD), particularly patients that have mechanobullous EBA rather than inflammatory EBA. Various immunosuppressants have been used, with varying success.[12–15] An algorithm has been suggested in a recent paper by a Japanese group. They suggest that mild EBA should be treated first with oral steroids 0.5 to 1.0 mg/kg/d with additional colchicine 50 to 100 mg/day and dapsone 100 to 300 mg/day, if required. Moderate EBA should be treated with a higher dose of oral steroids at 1.0 to 1.5 mg/kg/day with additional colchicine 100 to 200 mg/day. Finally, intractable

EBA should be treated with the same treatment given to patients with moderate EBA, with the addition of one or a combination of steroid pulses, cyclosporine 3 to 6 mg/kg/day, plasmapheresis, intravenous immunoglobulin (IVIG), or rituximab.[3] The median time to remission on combination treatment has been reported to range from 10 months in patients with classic EBA to 18 months in patients with bullous-pemphigoid–like EBA.[16] The Cochrane Review of interventions for EBA found only 11 nonrandomized trials of treatments for EBA. The majority were on the use of prednisone in combination with colchicine, additional topical steroids, dapsone, azathioprine, sulfapyridine, and cyclosporine. There were also studies on the use of IVIG, as well as 8-methoxypsoralen, before leukapheresis that showed some improvement in the first few months but with recurrence. The investigators concluded that it is not possible to draw definite conclusions about the best treatments for EBA.[12]

A review of articles on the treatment for EBA follows and a suggested algorithm is shown in **Table 1**. It is clear, though, that monotherapy is often unsuccessful, and that a multimodality approach is often necessary. It is also prudent to weigh the benefits of these medications over their risks and the potential side effects of long-term immunosuppression.

Table 1
Suggested treatment algorithm for EBA

Mild EBA[a]	Moderate EBA[b]	Severe EBA[c]
Oral steroids 0.5–1.0 mg/kg/d +	Oral steroids 1.0–1.5 mg/kg/d +	Oral steroids 1.0–1.5 mg/kg/d +
Colchicine 0.5–1 mg/d ±	Colchicine 1–3 mg/d ±	Colchicine 1–3 mg/d ±
Dapsone 1–2 mg/kg/d	Dapsone 1–2 mg/kg/d	Dapsone 1–2 mg/kg/d ±
		IV steroid pulses ±
		Cyclosporine 3–6 mg/kg/d or Mycophenolate mofetil 1–2 mg/kg/d ±
		Plasmapheresis or photopheresis ±
		IVIG 1–2 g/kg over 3–5 d for 1 mo ±
		Rituximab 375 mg/m² /wk for 4 wk

[a] Less than 5% body surface area without mucous membrane involvement; inflammatory type.
[b] From 5% to 15% body surface area and/or two or fewer mucous membranes involvement, not including ocular involvement.
[c] Greater than 5% body surface area and/or greater than two mucous membranes involved or ocular involvement.
Data from Ishii N, Hamada T, Dainichi T, et al. Epidermolysis bullosa acquisita: what's new? J Dermatol 2010;37:220–30.

Corticosteroids

Corticosteroids are still the mainstay in the treatment of EBA, with doses commonly ranging from 0.5 to 1.5 mg/kg/day.[3,12-14] A study using high-dose methylprednisolone (>8 mg/day) for at least 1 month was shown to induce remission in 2 months, in contrast to remission in 12 months in those given low dose methylprednisolone (≤8 mg/day).[16] The length of remission is unclear. Corticosteroids are often used in combination with dapsone in cases of childhood EBA, which has a different autoantibody profile, often to the triple helical collagen domain[17] Superpotent topical corticosteroids in the form of clobetasol propionate cream have been used in a patient with EBA and chronic hepatitis C. A total of 40 g of cream was applied daily for 2 months with remission lasting for 8 years, with no increases in blood sugar and blood pressure.[18]

Antiinflammatory Agents: Dapsone, Colchicine, Sulfapyridine, or Sulfasalazine

This group of drugs exerts their antiinflammatory effects via their antineutrophil action and are ideal owing to fewer side effects.[9] Dapsone at doses of 25 to 100 mg/day or 1 to 2 mg/kg/day has been used successfully in combination with topical and systemic corticosteroids in both adults and children with EBA.[12,14,18]

Colchicine has been used to treat EBA at doses of 0.5 to 2 mg/day as a monotherapy or in combination with other immunosuppressants. Response was seen as early as 2 weeks in some patients. Sulfapyridine, sulfasalazine, and mesalazine have also been given with some benefit in some EBA patients, with clinical response within a few weeks for some patients. In addition, it was possible to wean them off other immunosuppressive treatments.[3,12,14,19,20]

The authors have personal experience of an EBA patient with ulcerative colitis who has been in complete remission of his EBA on low-dose sulfasalazine for many years. Long-term control with this medication is unclear, and it is often used in conjunction with other immunosuppressives such as prednisone or cyclophosphamide.[12,14]

Immunosuppressive Agents: Cyclosporine, Mycophenolate, Mofetil, and Others

These medications are often used as immunosuppressive adjuvants to systemic corticosteroids, colchicine, and dapsone. Dose ranges for cyclosporine have been reported at 4 to 9 mg/kg with remission in recalcitrant case of EBA.[14,21,22]

Mycophenolate mofetil (MMF) has been administered at 1 to 2 mg/kg/day in case of adult and pediatric EBA, with varying responses.[14,23] There have reports of azathioprine, cyclophosphamide, and gold, as additional adjuvants in small studies.[12,14]

IVIG

IVIG is used as an off-label treatment for AIBD including EBA.[24] It is generally given at doses of 2 g/kg over 3 to 5 days, and reports of its use in fewer than 20 patients have suggested success in treating recalcitrant EBA. It is either administered as a monotherapy with doses of 1 to 2 g/kg or in combination with systemic corticosteroids.[14,24,25]

There is a small study suggesting that 7-month cycles of low-dose, 40 mg/kg/day for 5 days can help induce long-term remission, as seen in a patient with recalcitrant EBA of 7 years duration.[26] Another paper reports high-dose IVIG at 1 g/kg over 3 days given at monthly intervals achieved remission in 18 months.[27] IVIG has also been administered subcutaneously at a dose of 0.9 g/kg/month in divided doses over 5 days, as an immunomodulation therapy in a patient with severe EBA.[28]

Rituximab

Rituximab, a CD-20 monoclonal antibody has become increasingly popular in refractory mucocutaneous autoimmune disease such as pemphigus vulgaris, and has been trialed in a small group of EBA patients. There are seven patients reported in literature, with five patients showing improvement, one without improvement, and another dying of septicemia.[14]

The standard dose of 375 mg/m^2 of body surface area given at weekly intervals for 4 weeks was used in patients with recalcitrant EBA, and mostly in combination with other immunosuppressives such as MMF and systemic corticosteroids.[29-35] Rituximab has also been used successfully in combination with immunoadsorption, and various papers suggest that the depletion of memory B-cells parallels the decline in titers of circulating antibasement membrane zone antibodies.[32,33]

Other Biologic Agents

One paper examined the use of daclizumab, a humanized monoclonal antibody to the α–subunit of the high-affinity interleukin-2 receptor also known as CD25 or Tac. Three patients received between 6 and 12 intravenous infusions of daclizumab, given at 1 mg/kg at 2 to 4 week intervals. One patient with inflammatory disease had a favorable response without complications. The two remaining patients with dermolytic disease did not respond.[36] Reports have suggested the potential use of tumor necrosis factor (TNF-α) inhibitors, such as infliximab, in the treatment of EBA.[3]

Plasmapheresis and Extracorporeal Photochemotherapy (Photopheresis)

Plasmapheresis has been suggested as an adjunct to conventional treatments in recalcitrant EBA.[37] Adjuvant extracorporeal photochemotherapy (ECP), that is, ECP with administration of 8-methoxypsoralen before plasmapheresis, has been shown to induce partial-to-complete remission after three to six cycles of ECP in a small number of recalcitrant cases of EBA.[12,14,38,39]

THE FUTURE

The development of consensus definitions for EBA, as have been achieved for pemphigus and pemphigoid, should aid in standardizing reporting of outcomes in case reports and case series of EBA, which will assist in comparing treatment outcomes.[40,41] The development of a validated disease extent score for EBA, as has been done with the Autoimmune Bullous Skin Disorder Intensity Score (ABSIS) and Pemphigus Disease Area Index (PDAI) for pemphigus, should greatly assist in meta-analysis of small studies in EBA.[42]

SUMMARY

EBA is a chronic, debilitating, heterogenous disease with a high morbidity. Treatment is often challenging and remission is quite difficult to achieve despite multiple treatment modalities. The primary treatment is systemic corticosteroids, but this often remains unsatisfactory. Owing to the prolonged and progressive course of the disease, various antiinflammatory drugs and immunosuppressant adjuvants are used to control disease flares.

REFERENCES

1. Caux F. Diagnosis and clinical features of epidermolysis bullosa acquisita. Dermatol Clin 2011;29: 485–91.
2. Woodley DT, Chang C, Saadat P, et al. Evidence that anti-type VII collagen antibodies are pathogenic and responsible for the clinical, histological, and immunological features of epidermolysis bullosa acquisita. J Invest Dermatol 2005;124:958–64.
3. Ishii N, Hamada T, Dainichi T, et al. Epidermolysis bullosa acquisita: what's new? J Dermatol 2010;37: 220–30.
4. Delgado L, Aoki V, Santi T, et al. Clinical and immunopathological evaluation of epidermolysis bullosa acquisita. Clin Exp Dermatol 2011;36:12–8.
5. Palestine RF, Kossard S, Dicken CH. Epidermolysis bullosa acquisita: a heterogenous disease. J Am Acad Dermatol 1981;5:43–53.
6. Gammon WR, Briggaman RA, Woodley DT, et al. Epidermolysis bullosa acquisita—a pemphigoid-like disease. J Am Acad Dermatol 1984;11:820–32.
7. Lehman JS, Camilleri MJ, Gibson LE. Epidermolysis bullosa acquisita: concise review and practical considerations. Int J Dermatol 2009;48:227–36.
8. Parker SR, MacKelfresh J. Autoimmune blistering diseases in the elderly. Clin Dermatol 2011;29: 69–79.
9. Elchalal S, Kavosh ER, Chu DS. Ocular manifestations of blistering diseases. Immunol Allergy Clin N Am 2008;28:119–36.
10. Letko E, Bhol K, Anzaar F, et al. Chronic cicatrizing conjunctivitis in a patient with epidermolysis bullosa acquisita. Arch Ophthalmol 2006;124:1615–8.
11. Shipman AR, Agero AL, Cook I, et al. Epidermolysis bullosa acquisita requiring multiple oesophageal dilatations. Clin Exp Dermatol 2008;33:787–9.
12. Kirtschig G, Murrell DF, Wojnarowska F, et al. Interventions for mucous membrane pemphigoid and epidermolysis bullosa acquisita. Cochrane Database Syst Rev 2009;1:CD004056.
13. Le Roux-Villet C, Prost-Squarcioni C. Epidermolysis bullosa acquisita: literature review. Ann Dermatol Venereol 2011;138:228–46 [in French].
14. Gürcan HK, Ahmed AR. Current concepts in the treatment of epidermolysis bullosa acquisita. Expert Opin Pharmacother 2011;12:1259–68.
15. Engineer L, Ahmed AR. Emerging treatment for epidermolysis bullosa acquisita. J Am Acad Dermatol 2001;44:818–28.
16. Kim JH, Kim YH, Kim SC. Epidermolysis bullosa acquisita: a retrospective clinical analysis of 30 cases. Acta Derm Venereol 2011;91:307–12.
17. Arpey CJ, Elewski BE, Moritz DK, et al. Childhood epidermolysis bullosa acquisita. J Am Acad Dermatol 1991;24:706–14.
18. Abecassis S, Joly P, Genereau T, et al. Superpotent topical steroid therapy for epidermolysis bullosa acquisita. Dermatology 2004;209:164–6.
19. Tanaka N, Dainichi T, Ohyama B, et al. A case of epidermolysis bullosa acquisita with clinical features of Brunsting-Perry pemphigoid showing an excellent response to colchicine. J Am Acad Dermatol 2009; 61:715–9.
20. Cunningham BB, Kirchmann TT, Woodley D. Colchicine for epidermolysis bullosa acquisita. J Am Acad Dermatol 1996;34:781–4.
21. Connolly SM, Sander HM. Treatment of epidermolysis bullosa acquisita with cyclosporine. J Am Acad Dermatol 1987;16:890.
22. Crow LL, Finkle JP, Gammon WR, et al. Clearing of epidermolysis bullosa acquisita with cyclosporine. J Am Acad Dermatol 1988;19:937–42.

23. Tran MM, Anhalt GJ, Barrett T, et al. Childhood IgA-mediated epidermolysis bullosa acquisita responding to mycophenolate mofetil as a corticosteroid-sparing agent. J Am Acad Dermatol 2006;54: 734–44.

24. Smith DI, Swamy PM, Heffernan MP. Off-label uses of biologics in dermatology: interferon and intravenous immunoglobulin (part 1 of 2). J Am Acad Dermatol 2007;56:e1–54.

25. Mosquiera CB, Furlani LA, Xavier AFP, et al. Intravenous immunoglobulin for treatment of severe acquired bullous epidermolysis refractory to conventional immunosuppressive therapy. An Bras Dermatol 2010;85:521–4.

26. Kofler H, Wambacher-Gasser B, Topar G, et al. Intravenous immunoglobulin treatment in therapy-resistant epidermolysis bullosa acquisita. J Am Acad Dermatol 1996;34:331–5.

27. Segura S, Iranzo P, Martinez-dePablo I, et al. High-dose intravenous immunoglobulins for the treatment of autoimmune mucocutaneous blistering diseases: evaluation of its use in 19 cases. J Am Acad Dermatol 2007;56:960–7.

28. Tayal U, Burton J, Chapel H. Subcutaneous immunoglobulin therapy for immunomodulation in a patient with severe epidermolysis bullosa acquisita. Clin Immunol 2008;129:518–9.

29. Crichlow SM, Mortimer NJ, Harman KE. A successful therapeutic trial of rituximab in the treatment of a patient with recalcitrant, high-titre epidermolysis bullosa acquisita. Br J Dermatol 2007;156:194–6.

30. Saha M, Cutler T, Bhogal B, et al. Refractory epidermolysis bullosa acquisita: successful treatment with rituximab. Clin Exp Dermatol 2009;34:e979–80.

31. Schmidt E, Benoit S, Bröcker EB, et al. Successful adjuvant treatment of recalcitrant epidermolysis bullosa acquisita with anti-CD20 antibody rituximab. Arch Dermatol 2006;142:147–50.

32. Niedermeier A, Eming R, Pfütze M, et al. Clinical response of severe mechanobullous epidermolysis bullosa acquisita to combined treatment with immunoadsorption and rituximab (anti-CD20 monoclonal antibodies). Arch Dermatol 2007;143:192–8.

33. Li Y, Foshee JB, Sontheimer RD. Sustained clinical response to rituximab in a case of life-threatening overlap subepidermal autoimmune blistering disease. J Am Acad Dermatol 2011;64:773–8.

34. Cavailhes A, Balme B, Gilbert D, et al. [Successful use of combined corticosteroids and rituximab in the treatment of recalcitrant epidermolysis bullosa acquisita]. Ann Dermatol Venereol 2009;136:795–9 [in French].

35. Graves JE, Nunley K, Heffernan MP. Off-label uses of biologics in dermatology: rituximab, omalizumab, infliximab, etanercept, adalimumab, efalizumab, and alefacept (part 2 of 2). J Am Acad Dermatol 2007;56:e55–79.

36. Egan CA, Brown M, White JD, et al. Treatment of epidermolysis bullosa acquisita with the humanized anti-Tac mAb daclizumab. Clin Immunol 2001;101: 146–51.

37. Furue M, Iwata M, Yoon HI, et al. Epidermolysis bullosa acquisita: clinical response to plasma exchange therapy and circulating anti-basement membrane zone antibody titer. J Am Acad Dermatol 1986;14: 873–8.

38. Miller JL, Stricklin GP, Fine JD, et al. Remission of severe epidermolysis bullosa acquisita induced by extracorporeal photochemotherapy. Br J Dermatol 1995;133:467–71.

39. Sanli H, Akay BN, Ayyildiz E, et al. Remission of severe autoimmune bullous disorders induced by long-term extracorporeal photochemotherapy. Transfus Apher Sci 2010;43:353–9.

40. Murrell DF, Dick S, Ahmed AR, et al. Consensus statement on definitions of disease, end points, and therapeutic response for pemphigus. J Am Acad Dermatol 2008;58:1043–6.

41. Martin LK, Murrell DF. Pemphigus: directions for the future. J Am Acad Dermatol 2011;64:909–10.

42. Rosenbach M, Murrell DF, Bystryn JC, et al. Reliability and convergent validity of two outcome instruments for pemphigus. J Invest Dermatol 2009;129:2404–10.

Bullous Systemic Lupus Erythematosus

Deshan F. Sebaratnam, MBBS (Hons)[a],
Dédée F. Murrell, MA, BMBCh, FAAD, MD, FACD[b],*

KEYWORDS

- Systemic lupus erythematosus
- Vesiculobullous skin disease • Type VII collagen

Systemic lupus erythematosus (SLE) is a multisystem autoimmune disease with 76% of patients reporting dermatologic involvement at some point during their clinical course, 5% of which have chronic vesicobullous disease.[1] The blisters may represent primary SLE lesions, typically demonstrating basement membrane zone (BMZ) vacuolization and a mononuclear cell infiltrate in the upper dermis with cleavage of the epidermis from the dermis, manifesting as bullae.[2] Alternatively, patients with SLE may have concomitant separate bullous dermatoses, with cases of SLE and dermatitis herpetiformis (DH),[3] bullous pemphigoid (BP),[4] pemphigus,[5] mucous membrane pemphigoid,[6,7] epidermolysis bullos acquisita (EBA),[8] and linear IgA disease[9,10] all reported in the literature. Another category of SLE patients forms a special subgroup based on the presence of distinctive clinical and histologic features and is described as having a specific manifestation of SLE—bullous SLE (BSLE).

PATHOGENESIS

BSLE is believed caused by circulating autoantibodies to type VII collagen. Type VII collagen is an important element of the anchoring fibrils that maintain adhesion at the epidermal-dermal junction by cross-linking the lamina densa and dermal matrix.[11] Antibodies of patients with BSLE recognize epitopes in the region of the amino-terminal noncollagenous (NC1) domain of collagen VII.[12,13] These epitopes are shared between BSLE and EBA, and further analysis with immunoblotting and enzyme linked immunoassay studies have shown that BSLE sera also react with the collagenous domain adjacent to the carboxyl-terminal non-collagenous (NC2) domain, as reactivity of a construct of this domain and NC2 abolished the reactivity.[13]

There are several mechanisms through which these pathogenic autoantibodies could result in the development of bullae. Interference between type VII collagen and its extracellular matrix ligands could block or weaken connection of the anchoring fibrils to the lamina densa and anchoring plaques resulting in ineffective lamina densa–dermal adhesion.[14] Autoantibodies bound to the collagenous region near the NC2 domain may interfere with the antiparallel dimer alignment of collagen VII disrupting adherence at the dermis.[15] In vitro studies have demonstrated that antibodies to type VII collagen have the potential to activate complement and generate complement-dependent peptides, which precipitate neutrophil-mediated proteolysis at the epidermal-dermal junction.[16,17] Furthermore the peribullous skin of BSLE patients has been shown to active complement and generate inflammatory mediators to a significantly greater degree than uninvolved skin from the same patients or SLE patients without bullous disease.

Autoimmunity to type VII collagen remains the central focus of the pathogenesis of BSLE; however, more recent studies have demonstrated that this may not be the exclusive target antigen. A study of BSLE patients also identified

Conflict of interest: none declared.
[a] Department of Dermatology, St George Hospital, Gray Street, Sydney, NSW 2217, Australia
[b] Department of Dermatology, St George Hospital, University of New South Wales, Gray Street, Kogarah, Sydney, NSW 2217, Australia
* Corresponding author.
E-mail address: d.murrell@unsw.edu.au

Dermatol Clin 29 (2011) 649–653
doi:10.1016/j.det.2011.06.002

autoantibodies to other elements of the basement membrane, including laminin-5, laminin-6, and BP antigen I.[18] Epitope spreading may account for this. The primary autoimmune insult against collagen VII could expose epitopes otherwise sequestered, leading to a secondary autoimmune response to the newly exposed targets, accounting for the increasing repertoire of autoantibodies observed in BSLE.

Although the exact mechanism of bullae formation in BSLE has yet to be elucidated, it is likely that the underlying pathogenesis revolves around immunoglobulin deposition causing dysadhesion of the lamina densa subregion of the basement membrane from the upper dermis.

CLINICAL FEATURES

The clinical presentation of BSLE is typically that of an acute, generalized vesicobullous eruption in patients who satisfy the American Rheumatism Association revised criteria for SLE.[19] Typically patients are black women in the second or third decade of life, although BSLE may manifest in patients of either gender or of any race or age.[16] Lesions may erupt anywhere, although there exists a predilection for the upper trunk, neck, and supraclavicular regions as well as axillary folds and the oral and vulvar mucosa. There is a tendency for areas of sun-exposed skin to be most often affected although several cases exist without any suggestion of photosensitivity. Bullae usually arise from erythematous macules and may be preceded by inflammatory plaques but can also arise from normal skin.[20] Bullae may be large and tense, like those of BP (**Fig. 1**), or small and grouped, like those of DH. The lesions evolve to erosions and typically heal without scarring although may progress to hypopigmented or, less commonly, hyperpigmented macules (**Fig. 2**). Pruritus is not usually present. The mechanical fragility and healing with scars and milia, which are characteristic of EBA, are not typically present in BSLE.[16] The clinical trajectory of BSLE lesions does not usually correlate with the systemic manifestations of a patient's SLE.[21] Furthermore, the primary lesions of SLE and discoid lupus are rarely observed in patients with BSLE.

HISTOPATHOLOGY

Histologic findings in BSLE are relatively consistent across cases and resemble lesions seen in DH. Bullae demonstrate separation of the epidermis from the dermis at the BMZ. The epidermal roof is typically intact and the blister cavity contains fibrin and abundant neutrophils. There is

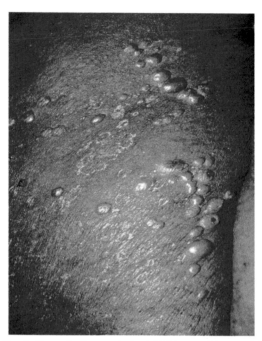

Fig. 1. Tense bullae typical of BLSE on a 21-year-old African American woman.

also a neutrophil-dominated inflammatory infiltrate of the upper dermis[16] and dermal edema. In some cases, the infiltrate is most pronounced in the dermal papillae, as seen in DH, and in other cases, it distributed evenly in a band beneath the BMZ, as seen in linear IgA disease.[22] Some monocytes and eosinophils are normally present within the infiltrate and in some cases there is histologic evidence of necrotizing vasculitis demonstrated by leukocytoclasis, extravasation of erythrocytes, and vessel necrosis.[21] Basal keratinocyte vacuolisation, BMZ thickening and epidermal atrophy

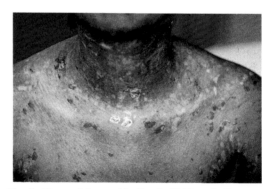

Fig. 2. The vesicles and bullae in BLSE typically progress to erosions, then heal without scarring or milia, although pigmentary changes (typically hypopigmentation) are common in patients with darker skin types.

characteristic of primary SLE lesions are generally absent in the lesions of BSLE.

DIRECT IMMUNOFLUORESCENCE

Immunoglobulin deposits in the upper dermis and the BMZ are a consistent finding in BSLE. Perilesional and unaffected skin demonstrate deposits of IgG, IgA, IgM, and complement at the BMZ under direct immunofluorescence (DIF). A review of immunohistochemistry in 30 cases of BSLE reported IgG was present in 93% of cases and IgM and IgA in approximately 70% of cases.[23] Complement was present in 77% of cases and has been reported more commonly observed in lesional skin than in clinically uninvolved skin.[16] Two major patterns of immunoglobulin deposition have been described with a granular pattern present in approximately 60% of cases and a linear pattern present in approximately 40%.[23] In some cases, thready or fibrillar deposits have been reported or a mixed pattern compromising a band of homogenous deposits punctuated by scattered granular deposits.[16] Irrespective of the pattern of immunoglobulin deposition, the clinical and histologic features of BSLE are consistent.

INDIRECT IMMUNOFLUORESCENCE

The results of indirect immunofluorescence (IIF) in BSLE patients correlate with findings on DIF. In those patients with granular immunoglobulin deposition on DIF, IIF is negative. In those patients with a linear pattern of immunoreactants on DIF, IIF on normal skin is usually negative but positive on sodium chloride split skin, most showing dermal binding.[24]

IMMUNOELECTRON MICROSCOPY

Immunoelectron microscopy studies demonstrate immunoglobulin deposition as a continuous band of granular reaction products in the upper dermis beneath the lamina densa. Occasionally, deposition is observed on the lamina densa and in the deeper dermis the region where anchoring fibrils are seen in the dermis.[16] The epidermal-dermal cleavage plane is usually the area of immunoglobulin deposition.[20]

IMMUNOBLOTTING AND ELISA

Immunoblotting has demonstrated reaction between antibodies in the sera of BSLE patients and 290-kDa and 145-kDa autoantigens extracted from normal human dermis.[25,26] These autoantigens have been identified as components of type VII collagen,[27] the target antigen in EBA. Fusion proteins of smaller components of the collagen VII NC-1 domain were created and tested by both immunoblotting and ELISA by one of the authors (DFM) and two epitope regions were identified within the type III fibronectin repeat region.[12] These epitope regions were the same ones recognized by the EBA sera in the study, at that time not explaining the clinical differences in phenotype of the two conditions. The epitopes were independently verified by Jones and colleagues[28] using 8-mer peptides from within these two epitope regions, confirming cross-reaction of BSLE sera and EBA sera with two peptide regions within each of the two previously defined epitope regions. Four epitope regions within the NC1 domain were also found by Woodley and colleagues in addition to reactivity against the collagenous domain adjacent to the NC2 domain.[13]

DIAGNOSIS

Camisa and Sharma first proposed diagnostic criteria for BSLE in 1983,[29] which were later revised after the administration of salt split-skin immunofluorescence.[30] The criteria essentially necessitated (1) a diagnosis of SLE by American Rheumatism Association criteria, (2) a vesiculobullous eruption, (3) subepidermal histopathology consistent with DH and leucocytoclastic vasculitis, (4) negative or positive IIF for BMZ autoantibodies, and (5) positive DIF at the BMZ.

Gammon and coworkers then divided patients into two types depending on the presence of antibodies to type VII collagen.[16] Those patients with antibodies to collagen VII identifiable by IIF or immunoelectron microscopy, usually with linear or mixed patterns of immunoglobulin deposition, were designated has having type I BSLE. Patients who did not demonstrate antibodies to type VII collagen were designated has having type II BSLE. Clinically it is not possible to distinguish between the two types of BSLE; rather, subtyping is performed through immunohistochemistry.

A third type of BSLE was proposed by Yell and colleagues[2] in 1995, who also suggested revised criteria for diagnosis. They highlighted that there existed BSLE patients with classical clinical and histologic features whose sera bound to epidermal rather than dermal epitopes and that these patients should be designated as having type III BSLE.

As understanding of the pathogenesis underling BSLE evolves, these criteria are likely to change accordingly. At present, however, a diagnosis of BSLE is still made according to the revised criteria put forward by Camisa and Sharma, with further subtyping performed according to the results of immunofluorescence, immunoblotting, and ELISA.

MANAGEMENT

The mainstay of treatment of BSLE is dapsone. The response to dapsone is rapid and often occurs at low doses (25–50 mg) with cessation of blister formation observed within 48 hours and clearance of the eruption occurring within a week.[21] (For full guidelines on the use of dapsone in BSLE, see the review article in by Piette and Werth elsewhere in this issue.) To minimize risk of hemolysis, it is recommended that the therapeutic dosage of dapsone should not exceed 1.5 mg/kg per day.[31] Rapid relapses may occur with withdrawal of dapsone with prompt remission observed when therapy is re-instituted. Discontinuance of treatment is normally possible within 12 months.[32]

In contrast, BSLE lesions are often recalcitrant to the high-dose systemic corticosteroids and immunomodulators used to treat the other manifestations of SLE. In settings where BSLE occurs simultaneously with a flare of SLE, however, it has been advocated that increasing the dosages of corticosteroids and other immunosuppressants can control both clinical problems and should, therefore, be used in this setting.[33] Success has been reported using prednisone and azathioprine[16] and methotrexate monotherapy.[34] A recent article outlined the efficacy of rituximab in a patient with disease refractory to first-line therapies.[35] Consideration of such modalities is warranted where control of visceral SLE symptoms in needed or when dapsone is contraindicated.

SUMMARY

BSLE is a rare bullous dermatosis in patients with SLE. It is characterized by clinical and histologic features resembling BP or DH and a heterogenous immunologic profile, usually characterized by autoimmunity to components of type VII collagen, much like EBA. Dapsone is the mainstay of treatment, with patients usually showing a prompt response to treatment and complete resolution normally achieved within 12 months. As understanding of the pathology of this dermatologic condition has evolved, so have the criteria and profiling of BSLE. The distinct clinical, histologic, and immunologic features of BSLE represent a unique bullous disease phenotype.

REFERENCES

1. Gammon WR, Briggaman RA. Bullous eruption of systemic lupus erythematosus. In: Wojnarowska F, Briggaman RA, editors. Management of blistering diseases. London: Chapman and Hall Ltd; 1990. p. 263–75.
2. Yell JA, Allen J, Wojnarowska G, et al. Bullous systemic lupus erythematosus: revised criteria for diagnosis. Br J Dematol 1995;132(6):921–8.
3. Thomas JR 3rd, Daniel Su WP. Concurrence of lupus erythematosus and dermatitis herpetiformis. A report of nine cases. Arch Dermatol 1974;119(9):740–5.
4. Bittencourt AL, Brito E, Sadigursky M, et al. [Systemic lupus erythematosus with bullous manifestations. Association with bullous pemphigoid and a rare presentation of systemic lupus erythematosus]. Acta Medica Portuguesa 1984;5(4–5):119–25 [in Portuguese].
5. Chorzelski T, Jablonska S, Blaszczyk M. Immunopathological investigation in the Senear-Usher syndrome (coexistence of pemphigus and lupus erythematosus). Br J Dermatol 1968;80(4):211–7.
6. Malik M, Gurcan HM, Ahmed AR. Coexistence of mucous membrane pemphigoid and connective-tissue disease. Clin Exp Dermatol 2010;35(2):156–9.
7. Stoll DM, King LE Jr. Association of bullous pemphigoid with systemic lupus erythematosus. Arch Dermatol 1984;120(3):362–6.
8. Dotson AD, Raimer SS, Pursley TV, et al. Systemic lupus erythematosus occurring in a patient with epidermolysis bullosa acquisita. Arch Dermatol 1981; 117(7):422–6.
9. Alba D, Alvarex-Doforno R, Casado M. [Linear bullous IgA dermatosis and systemic lupus erythematosus]. Medicina Clinica 1995;105(2):77–8 [in Spanish].
10. Lau M, Kaufmann-Grunzinger I, Raghunanth M. A case report of a patient with features of systemic lupus erythematosus and linear IgA disease. Br J Dermatol 1991;124(5):498–502.
11. Morris NP, Keene DR, Glanville RW, et al. The tissue form of type VII collagen is an antiparallel dimer. J Biol Chem 1997;261(12):5638–44.
12. Gammon WR, Murrell DF, Jenison MW, et al. Autoantibodies to type VII collagen recognise epitopes in a fibronectin-like region of the noncollagenous (NC1) domain. J Invest Dermatol 1993;100(5):618–22.
13. Chen M, Marinkovich P, Veis A. Interactions of the amino-terminal non-collagenous (NC1) domain of type VII collagen with extracellular matrix proteins. J Biol Chem 1997;272(23):14516–22.
14. Gammon WR. Autoimmunity to collagen VII: autoantibody-mediated pathomechanisms regulate clinico-pathological phenotypes of acquired epidermolysis bullosa and bullous SLE. J Cutan Path 1993; 20(2):109–14.
15. Chen M, Keene DR, Costa FK, et al. The carboxyl terminus of type VII collagen mediates antiparallel dimer formation and constitutes a new antigenic epitope for epidermolysis bullosa acquisita autoantibodies. J Biol Chem 2001;276(24):21649–55.
16. Gammon WR, Briggaman RA, Bullouse SL. A phenotypically distinctive but immunologically

heterogenous bullous disorder. J Invest Dermatol 1993;100(1):28S–34S.

17. Gammon WR, Briggaman RA, Inman AO III, et al. Evidence supporting a role for immune complex-mediated inflammation in the pathogenesis of bullous lesions of systemic lupus erythematosus. J Invest Dermatol 1983;81(4):320–5.

18. Chan LS, Lapiere JC, Chen M, et al. Bullous systemic lupus erythematosus with autoantibodies recognizing multiple skin basement membrane components, bullous pemphigoid antigen 1, laminin-5, laminin-6 and type VII collagen. Arch Dermatol 1999;135(5):569–73.

19. Tan EM, Cohen AS, Fries JF, et al. The 1982 revised criteria for the classification of systemic lupus erythematosus. Arthritis Rheum 1982;25(11):1271–7.

20. Vassileva S. Bullous systemic lupus erythematosus. Clin Dermatol 2004;22(2):129–38.

21. Hall RP, Lawley TJ, Smith HR, et al. Bullous eruption of systemic lupus erythematosus. Dramatic response to dapsone therapy. Ann Intern Med 1982;97(2):165–70.

22. Burrows NP, Bhogal BS, Black MM, et al. Bullous eruption of systemic lupus erythematosus: a clinicopathological study of four cases. Br J Dermatol 1993;128(3):332–8.

23. Fleming MG, Bergfield MF, Tomecki KJ. Bullous systemic lupus erythematosus. Int J Dermatol 1989;28(5):321–6.

24. Yell AJ, Wojnarowska F. Bullous skin disease in lupus erythematosus. Lupus 1997;6(2):112–21.

25. Barton DD, Fine JD, Gammon WR, et al. Bullous systemic lupus erythematosus: an unusual clinical course and detectable circulating autoantibodies to the epidermolysis bullosa antigen. J Am Acad Dermatol 1986;15(2):369–73.

26. Gammon WR, Woodley DT, Dole KC, et al. Evidence that anti-basement membrane zone antibodies in bullous eruption of systemic lupus erythematosus recognise epidermolysis bullosa acquisita autoantigen. J Invest Dermatol 1985;84(6):472–6.

27. Tatnall FM, Whitehead PC, Black MM, et al. Identification of the epidermolysis bullosa acquisita antigen by LH7.2 monoclonal antibody: use in diagnosis. Br J Dermatol 1989;120(4):533–9.

28. Jones DA, Hunt SW 3rd, Prisayanh PS, et al. Immunodominant autoepitopes of type VII collagen are short, paired peptide sequences within the fibronectin type III homology region of the noncollagenous (NC1) domain. J Invest Dermatol 1995;104(2):231–5.

29. Camisa C, Sharma HM. Vesiculobullous systemic lupus erythematosus. J Am Acad Dermatol 1983;9(6):924–33.

30. Camisa C, Grimwood RE. Indirect immunofluorescence in vesiculobullous eruption of systemic lupus erythematosus. J Invest Dermatol 1986;86(5):606.

31. Zhu YI, Stiller MJ. Dapsonse and sulfones in dermatology: overview and update. J Am Acad Dermatol 2001;45(3):420–34.

32. Yung A, Oakley A. Bullous systemic lupus erythematosus. Aust J Dermatol 2000;41(4):234–7.

33. Fernandez-Sanchez A, Charli-Joseph Y, Saeb-Lima M, et al. Are corticosteroids and immunosuppressors an efficacious treatment for bullous lupus erythematosus with systemic manifestations? Eur J Dermatol 2010;20(6):823–4.

34. Malcangi G, Brandozzi G, Giangiacomi M, et al. Bullous SLE: response to methotrexate and relationship with disease activity. Lupus 2003;12(1):63–6.

35. Alsanafi S, Kovarik C, Mermelstein A. Rituximab in the treatment of bullous systemic lupus erythematosus. J Clin Rheum 2011;17(3):142–4.

The International Pemphigus and Pemphigoid Foundation

Dédée F. Murrell, MA, BMBCh, FAAD, MD, FACD[a],
Victoria P. Werth, MD[b,c], Janet Segall, BA[d],
Will Zrnchik, MBA[d], Molly Stuart, JD[d],
David Sirois, MD, PhD[e,*]

KEYWORDS

- International Pemphigus Pemphigoid Foundation
- Pemphigus • Pemphigoid • Pemphigus vulgaris

HISTORY

The International Pemphigus Pemphigoid Foundation (IPPF) was founded by Janet Segall in California in 1994. Janet suffers from pemphigus vulgaris and wanted to help other patients to find the right doctors to treat them. Dédée Murrell encountered her sitting at a small table within the exhibit area at an American Academy of Dermatology meeting in San Francisco and told her that she would introduce her to the late Dr Jean-Claude Bystryn, the expert in pemphigus at New York University, who would be keen to help her. And he was. From that moment, the IPPF blossomed. Grant Anhalt was recruited as the first Medical Advisory Board (MAB) president and David Sirois, oral medicine expert from New York University, became the overall president of the then-called International Pemphigus Pemphigoid Foundation. Other MAB members recruited were Razzaque Ahmed from Boston; Luis Diaz from the University of North Carolina at Chapel Hill; Sergei Grando from University of California, Irvine; Russell Hall from Duke University; Bob Jordan from Texas; Neil Korman from Cincinatti; Amit Pandya from the University of Texas Southwestern Medical Center; John Stanley and Victoria Werth from the University of Pennsylvania; and Dédée Murrell from Sydney, Australia. Gradually more international experts have been included in the MAB, including Masa Amagai, Takashi Hashimoto, Michael Hertl, Pascal Joly, and Marcel Jonkman. The headquarters are now located in Sacramento, California. Staff includes Molly Stuart, CEO, and Will Zrnchik, Director of Communications.

PATIENTS

Currently the IPPF lists more than 4500 members, including 2300 in the United States and 2000 abroad, from more than 90 countries, including all 6 continents of the world.

The Web site, www.pemphigus.org, received an average of 16,000 hits; 1800 pages viewed; and 430 visits per day in 2011 (as of June 13, 2011). In 2010, the IPPF received more than 6.4 million

[a] Department of Dermatology, St George Hospital, University of New South Wales, Gray Street, Kogarah, Sydney, NSW 2217, Australia
[b] Department of Dermatology, Perelman Center for Advanced Medicine, Suite 1-330A, 3400 Civic Center Boulevard, Philadelphia, PA 19104, USA
[c] Division of Dermatology, Philadelphia V.A. Medical Center, Philadelphia, PA, USA
[d] International Pemphigus Pemphigoid Foundation, 2701 Cottage Way # 16, Sacramento, CA 85825, USA
[e] Department of Dentistry, New York University, 413 East 53rd Street, New York, NY 10022, USA
* Corresponding author. International Pemphigus Pemphigoid Foundation, 2701 Cottage Way # 16, Sacramento, CA 85825.
E-mail address: david.sirois@nyu.edu

Dermatol Clin 29 (2011) 655–657
doi:10.1016/j.det.2011.06.019
0733-8635/11/$ – see front matter © 2011 Elsevier Inc. All rights reserved.

hits with 1.1 million total pages viewed from 130,000 visitors.

The IPPF provides peer health coaches to aid patients in the navigation of the health care system and recommends dermatologists and other specialists in their area who are experts in autoimmune bullous disease. The IPPF now hosts the largest worldwide registry of pemphigus/pemphigoid patients with biospecimen collection are in the works. Twice a year the IPPF hosts formal meetings with invited speakers. Drs Ahmed, Pandya, Sinha, and Werth have been particularly active with Annual Meetings.

Web forum/town hall meetings are held regularly. Members who have autoimmune bullous disease have their questions answered by one of the IPPF MAB members by conference call or they give a short talk.

Some of the links for IPPF projects:

Home page: www.pemphigus.org/wordpress
Town hall: http://www.pemphigus.org/word press/get-support/townhall

Registry: http://www.pemphigus.org/wordpress/ registry
Support: http://www.pemphigus.org/wordpress/ get-support (includes links to forums, e-mail addresses, and so forth)

There are several national support groups linked to the IPPF:

Australia—Australasian Blistering Diseases Foundation: http://www.blisters.org.au/
Canada—Canadian Pemphigus and Pemphigoid Foundation: www.pemphigus.ca
France—Association Pemphigus & Pemphigoide France: http://pemphigus.asso.fr/
Italy—Associazione Nazionale Pemfigo Pemfigoide Italy: http://www.pemfigo.it
United Kingdom—PEM Friends (UK): http:// www.pemfriends.co.uk/ and the Pemphigus Vulgaris Network: http://www.pemphigus. org.uk/
Japan—Association of Pemphigus Pemphigoid Friends (no Web site listed)

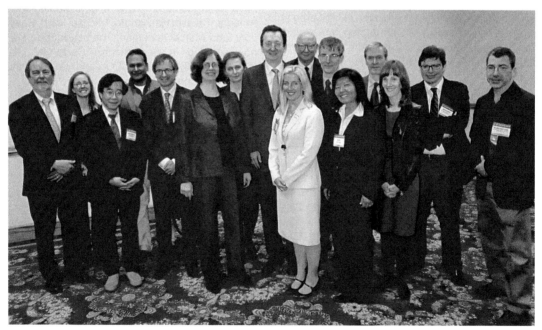

Fig. 1. Members of the MAB of the IPPF (*) who were part of the international outcome measures group at the completion of the definitions and extent measures for bullous pemphigoid[3] at the American Academy of Dermatology meeting in New Orleans, 2011. (*Left to right*) David Woodley (Los Angeles, California), Donna Culton (Chapel Hill, North Carolina), *Takashi Hashimoto (Kurume, Japan), *Animesh Sinha (Buffalo, New York), *Pascal Joly (Rouen, France), *Victoria Werth (Philadelphia, Pennsylvania), Branka Marinovich (Zagreb, Croatia), Luca Borradori (Bern, Switzerland), *Dédée Murrell (Sydney, Australia), *Sergei Grando (Irvine, California), Frederic Caux (Paris, France), Valeria Aoki (Sao Paulo, Brazil), Philippe Bernard (Reims, France), Janet Fairley (Iowa City, Iowa), Jose Mascaro Jr (Barcelona, Spain), and David Rubenstein (Chapel Hill, North Carolina).

OTHER SUPPORT SITES

Pemphigus in remission: http://www.pemphinremission.com/

Pemphigus Group in Spanish: http://www.vivirconpenfigo.blogspot.com/

Social media:

Official IPPF Facebook page: www.pemphigus.org/facebook

Official IPPF Twitter feed: www.pemphigus.org/twitter

DOCUMENTED ACHIEVEMENTS

The MAB members, Victoria Werth, Chair of the MAB, and Dédée Murrell, have coordinated international consensus definitions groups (**Fig. 1**) to work on developing definitions of disease stages and outcome measures for pemphigus and pemphigoid.[1–3]

RECOGNITION

The IPPF has received the American Academy of Dermatology Golden Triangle Award in 2008 and 2009 for its pioneering Web site.

REFERENCES

1. Murrell DF, Amagai M, Barnadas M, et al. Consensus statement on definitions of disease endpoints and therapeutic response for pemphigus. J Am Acad Dermatol 2008;58:1043–6.
2. Rosenbach M, Murrell DF, Bystryn JC, et al. Reliability and convergent validity of two outcome instruments for pemphigus. J Invest Dermatol 2009;129:2404–10.
3. Murrell DF, Daniel BS, Joly P, et al. Definitions and outcome measures for bullous pemphigoid: recommendations by an International Panel of Experts. J Am Acad Dermatol 2011, in press. DOI:10.1016/j.jaad.2011.06.032.

Management of Autoimmune Bullous Diseases in France: A Nationwide Network of 30 Centers

Nicolas Meyer, MD[a,b,*], Carle Paul, MD, PhD[b,c],
Pascal Joly, MD, PhD[d]

KEYWORDS

- Autoimmune bullous diseases • Care • Guidelines
- Reference center

ORGANIZATION OF DERMATOLOGIC HEALTH CARE IN FRANCE

The management of autoimmune bullous disease (AIBD) in France has always been under the guidance of dermatologists. The health care system in France is characterized by a combination of complementary public and private structures. Most dermatologists in France, representing 90% of the 3400 dermatologists practicing in the country, are office-based physicians.[1] It was estimated that in the year 2000, 14 million outpatient consultations were performed by office-based dermatologists. Severe skin diseases as well as skin cancer, including melanoma and skin lymphoma, are mostly taken care of by hospital dermatologists. It has been estimated that inpatients represented more than 100,000 hospital stays during the same period.[2] Since 1958, the academic dermatology departments of the 31 university hospitals have been staffed by full-time hospital physicians. In the year 2000, there were 102 dermatology departments in France (including 51 in university hospitals and 61 in general hospitals), totaling a capacity of 1403 beds.[3] Most of the inpatient capacities are located in academic dermatology departments (in the year 2000, 77% of the 1403 beds of dermatology departments were located in university hospitals), although some nonacademic dermatology departments are very active. AIBDs represent an important group of diseases that are mostly managed by academic and nonacademic dermatology departments. Since 1985, a research group called the French Autoimmune Bullous Disease Group has been created within the French Dermatology Society (Société Française de Dermatologie [SFD]). The French Autoimmune Bullous Disease Group has promoted optimal care for AIBDs and organized clinical trials. Among the landmark studies promoted by the French Autoimmune Bullous Disease Group are the demonstration of the efficacy and safety of topical corticosteroids in bullous pemphigoid (BP),[4] the use of rituximab

Funding sources: none.
Conflict of interest: none.
[a] UMR 1037-CRCT, 20 24 r Pont Saint Pierre, 31052 Toulouse Cedex 3, France
[b] Dermatology Department, Larrey Hospital, chemin de Pouvourville, TSA30030, 31059 Toulouse Cedex 9, France
[c] Paul Sabatier-Toulouse III University, 118 route de Narbonne 31062 Toulouse Cedex 9, France
[d] Dermatology Department, INSERM U905, Rouen University Hospital, 1 Rue de Germont, 76031 Rouen, France
* Corresponding author. Service de Dermatologie, Hôpital Larrey, 24 chemin de Pouvourville TSA30030, 31059 Toulouse Cedex 9, France.
E-mail address: meyer.n@chu-toulouse.fr

Dermatol Clin 29 (2011) 659–662
doi:10.1016/j.det.2011.06.017
0733-8635/11/$ – see front matter © 2011 Elsevier Inc. All rights reserved.

in pemphigus vulgaris,[5] and the identification of risk factors for BP.[6]

AIBD: DEFINITION OF THE DISEASES

AIBDs are a group of rare, acquired disorders characterized by:

- The onset of vesiculobullous lesions on the skin or mucous membranes
- The alteration of cutaneous or mucous membrane components
- The presence of pathogenic autoantibodies targeting structural proteins of the desmosomes and the dermal-epidermal junction (binding of autoantibodies on these desmosomal and hemidesmosomal components disrupts these intercellular or dermal epidermal junctions).

AIBDs are BP, cicatricial pemphigoid, autoimmune pemphigus (AIP), epidermolysis bullosa acquisita, herpetiformis dermatitis, pemphigoid gestationis, and linear IgA dermatosis. AIBDs are separated in 2 groups:

- Intraepidermal AIBD: AIP
- Subepidermal AIBD: all other AIBDs.

Some AIBDs may be severe, especially recalcitrant or relapsing types, leading to treatment side effects and potential lethality.

EPIDEMIOLOGY OF AIBDS IN FRANCE

Most cases of AIBD occur sporadically, without evidence of geographic or familial clustering. Little is known on the epidemiology of AIBD in France. In 1995, a multicentric prospective epidemiologic study was conducted in 3 university hospitals in France.[7] One hundred cases were evaluated over a period of 35 months. The investigators evaluated the overall standardized incidence of subepidermal AIBD to be 10.4 cases per year and per million inhabitants. The most frequent subepidermal AIBD was BP (standardized incidence: 7 cases per million inhabitants per year), which represented 70% of the cases of AIBD. The incidence of other subepidermal AIBD comprised between 0.17 and 0.26 case per year and per million inhabitants. A similar study performed 15 years later in the same regions in France found an incidence rate for BP of 21.7 cases per million persons per year, corresponding to a doubling of the incidence over a 15-year period. Aging of the population may at least in part account for this dramatic increase in disease incidence. The incidence rate of subepidermal AIBD was shown to increase dramatically with age, with up to 224,

329, and 507 cases per million persons per year in the populations aged 75, 80, and 85 years or older, respectively. These results are close to those recently reported by Langan and colleagues[8] in the United Kingdom.

Among AIBDs, the epidemiology of AIP has been extensively studied (reviewed in Ref.[9]). There are 2 basic types of pemphigus: pemphigus vulgaris and pemphigus foliaceus. Although paraneoplastic and drug-induced pemphigus has also been described, its incidence is low. Only sporadic types of pemphigus foliaceus and pemphigus vulgaris have been described in France in contrast to other Mediterranean countries. The incidence of the various types of pemphigus varies from 1 country to another. Sporadic pemphigus vulgaris is the most common in Europe and in the United States, whereas endemic pemphigus foliaceus is more prevalent in Northern Africa, Turkey, and Southern America. Two epidemiologic studies on AIP were conducted in France.[10,11] The first study was conducted in 1995 in the Paris region, the most populated area of northwestern France, and evaluated the incidence of AIP to be 1.7 cases per year and per million inhabitants.[10] The second study was conducted over the 2002 to 2006 period in the region Midi-Pyrénées in the southwestern part of the country. The study included only dermatologist-validated cases of the disease and estimated the incidence of AIP at 1.55 cases per year and per million inhabitants.[11]

In western Europe, 4 studies were conducted on the epidemiology of AIBD between 2000 and 2010.[8,11–13] In a prospective study conducted in 2001 to 2002, Marazza and colleagues[12] evaluated the incidence of BP and AIP in Switzerland. A total of 168 patients were identified. The BP and AIP standardized incidence was estimated at 12.1 and 0.6 cases per year and per million inhabitants, respectively. Similar results were reported by Bertram and colleagues[13] in Germany (Lower Franconia): The most frequent AIBD was BP (standardized incidence = 13.4 cases per year and per million inhabitants). The third study[11] was aimed at evaluating the incidence of AIP in southwestern France, and provided no data on the incidence of other AIBD, and the fourth was registry-based and conducted in the UK by Langan and colleagues.[8] In the study by Langan and colleagues the incidences of BP and pemphigus vulgaris were estimated to be 4.3 cases per year and per 100,000 inhabitants and 0.7 case per year and per 100,000 inhabitants, respectively.

Despite the limited number of studies available, all recent data on the epidemiology of AIBD support that AIBD are rare diseases and that the most frequent of them is BP.

ORGANIZATION OF THE FRENCH NATIONAL NETWORK ON AIBD
Reference and Competence Centers

In 2004 the French Ministry of Health decided to establish and fund reference centers for rare diseases (tertiary care centers), with the aim of improving quality of care and research for orphan diseases. Rare diseases were defined as diseases with a prevalence of less than 50 cases for 10^5 inhabitants. Reference centers were distinguished because of:

- Their ability to establish the correct diagnosis of the orphan diseases

- Their ability to manage the patients properly
- Their research programs and publications on the concerned topic.

The goals of the French references centers are: (1) to develop a national network of competence centers, (2) to establish guidelines for the management of patients, (3) to improve the information of patients, nurses, and physicians on these rare disorders, and (4) to conduct multicenter clinical trials. Two reference centers for the management of AIBDs have been created: the first is in Paris, the other in Rouen (Normandy); this latter tertiary care center is associated with 2 other centers in

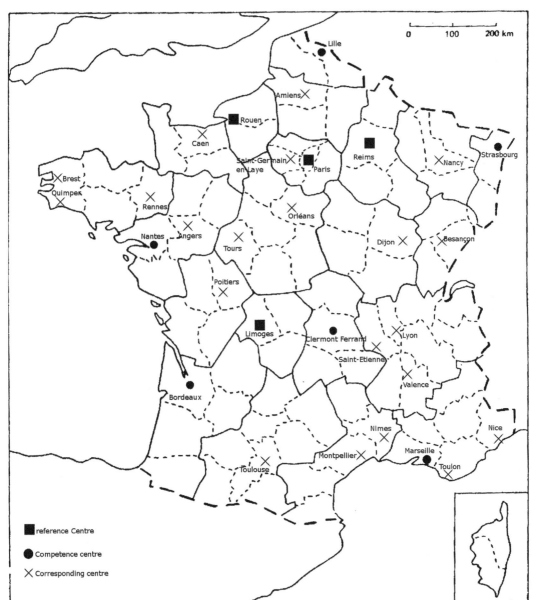

Fig. 1. Geographic location of the AIBD network.

Limoges (Limousin) and Reims (Champagne). A network of 7 competence centers (coordinating 30 corresponding centers) was also established (**Fig. 1**). The missions of the competence centers are: (1) to diagnose and manage patients with autoimmune bullous skin disorders, as close as possible to their home, and (2) to participate in the missions of the national reference center.

French guidelines for the management of BP, pemphigoid gestationis, cicatricial pemphigoid, dermatitis herpetiformis, pemphigus, IgA linear dermatosis, and epidermolysis bullosa acquisita have been created (available on http://www.chu-rouen.fr/crnmba/prive/crnmba_pnds.html; restricted access). Information documents have been printed and are systematically given to patients and nurses, to help them in the understanding of the disease, to explain the usefulness of topical and systemic treatments, and to improve patients' compliance. An evaluation made by reference and competence centers 1 year before the publication of the guidelines showed that the diagnosis and the first-line treatment proposed to patients were in accordance with the guidelines in 97% and 61% of cases, respectively. This evaluation will be done again 2 years after the publication of the guidelines.

Serum analysis and advice for the management of patients is another major task of reference centers. More than 3000 sera are analyzed every year in the laboratories of the reference centers, mainly using immunoblotting and enzyme-linked immunosorbent assays. An average of 300 expert opinions are referred to the reference centers every year. Seventy percent of them originate from France and 30% from Europe and the United States.

Members from the reference centers most often attend the meetings organized by the International Pemphigus and Pemphigoid Patients Association (http://www.pemphigus.org/). Another goal of the French reference centers is to conduct epidemiologic studies. An epidemiologic registry for the 7 AIBDs has been compiled and will be progressively proposed to all French dermatology departments. A Web site (http://www.chu-rouen.fr/crnmba_informations.html) has been created to make available main information documents, guidelines, ongoing clinical studies, publications of the reference centers, and information about reference and competence centers. Two major randomized controlled clinical trials are being performed by French reference and competence centers: (1) evaluation of methotrexate versus topical corticosteroids in the maintenance treatment of BP and (2) the assessment of rituximab as the first line of treatment in patients with pemphigus.

Overall, the national network on AIBD is believed to improve both the diagnosis and management of autoimmune blistering diseases, to provide up-to-date and easily understandable information to patients, nurses and physicians, and to support high-quality clinical trials.

REFERENCES

1. No author listed. Dermatologue. Mode d'emploi. Available at: http://www.syndicatdermatos.org/dermatologue-le-specialiste-des-maladies-de-la-peau-6.html. Accessed October 19, 2010.
2. Roujeau JC. Dermatology in France in 2000. What is the present and future? Ann Dermatol Venereol 2002;129:1261–5.
3. Modeste A-B, Josset V, Hautemanière A, et al. Survey on the activity of hospital departments of dermatology in France. Ann Dermatol Venereol 2002;129:1266–70.
4. Joly P, Roujeau JC, Benichou J, et al. Bullous Diseases French Study Group. A comparison of oral and topical corticosteroids in patients with bullous pemphigoid. N Engl J Med 2002;346:321–7.
5. Joly P, Mouquet H, Roujeau JC, et al. A single cycle of rituximab for the treatment of severe pemphigus. N Engl J Med 2007;357:545–52.
6. Bastuji-Garin S, Joly P, Lemordant P, et al. Risk factors for bullous pemphigoid in the elderly: a prospective case-control study. J Invest Dermatol 2011;131(3):637–43.
7. Bernard P, Vaillant L, Labeille B, et al. Incidence and distribution of subepidermal auto-immune bullous skin diseases in three French regions. Bullous Diseases French Study Group. Arch Dermatol 1995;131:48–52.
8. Langan SM, Smeeth L, Hubbard R, et al. Bullous pemphigoid and pemphigus vulgaris–incidence and mortality in the UK: population based cohort study. BMJ 2008;337:a180.
9. Meyer N, Misery L. Geoepidemiologic considerations of auto-immune pemphigus. Autoimmun Rev 2010;9:A379–82.
10. Bastuji-Garin S, Souissi R, Blum L, et al. Comparative epidemiology of pemphigus between Tunisia and France: unusual incidence of pemphigus foliaceus in young Tunisian women. J Invest Dermatol 1995;104:302–5.
11. Thomas M, Paul C, Berard E, et al. Incidence of auto-immune pemphigus in the Midi-Pyrénées region in 2002-2006. Dermatology 2010;220:97–102.
12. Marazza G, Pham HC, Schärer L, et al. Autoimmune bullous disease Swiss study group. Br J Dermatol 2009;161:861–8.
13. Bertram F, Bröcker EB, Zillikens D, et al. Prospective analysis of the incidence of autoimmune bullous diseases in Lower Franconia, Germany. J Dtsch Dermatol Ges 2009;7:434–40.

Diagnosis and Treatment of Patients with Autoimmune Bullous Disorders in Germany

Enno Schmidt, MD, PhD[a,b,*], Detlef Zillikens, MD[a]

KEYWORDS

- Autoantibody • Bullous • Pemphigus • Pemphigoid
- Therapy

In Germany, 5250 fully trained dermatologists were registered at the end of 2009, including 900 working in hospitals and 4000 in outpatient clinics and private practices (statistics of the German Medical Association; www.bundesaerztekammer.de). Almost all patients with autoimmune bullous disease are initially referred to dermatology departments at university or nonuniversity hospitals for diagnosis and treatment decisions. Most patients are initially treated as inpatients and then allocated to specialized outpatient departments of the hospital or private practices according to the patients' preferences.

At the University of Lübeck and the University of Kiel, specialized interdisciplinary outpatient departments for the treatment of patients with immunobullous diseases have been established in Comprehensive Centers for Inflammation Medicine. In these centers, patients with inflammatory diseases are managed in interdisciplinary teams, including interdisciplinary outpatient clinics and weekly case conferences. This approach facilitates clinical studies, data collection, and biobanking.

Health insurance is compulsory in Germany. It covers all costs for treatment regimens that have been licensed for a particular disease. In addition, for life-threatening diseases, off-label treatments that have been shown to be beneficial are covered.

EPIDEMIOLOGY

The incidence of pemphigus was calculated to be 2.3 new cases per million per year in Germany.[1] With a population of 82.14 million, including 15.57 million inhabitants with a migration background at the end of 2008 (Federal Institute of Statistics, www.destatis.de), about 200 newly diagnosed patients with pemphigus per year are expected in Germany. The age-adjusted incidence of pemphigus vulgaris was 9-fold higher in patients with a migration background compared with native Germans.[1] The incidence of bullous pemphigoid (BP), by far the most frequent autoimmune blistering disease, has been determined to be 13.4 per million per year in a recent prospective study in 2001 and 2002 in Lower Franconia, a well-defined region in

Honoraria for lectures were received from Roche and Fresenius Medical Care (both authors) and from Miltenyi (to E.S.). D.Z. obtained funding for research and development projects from Fresenius Medical Care, Miltenyi, Biotest, and Euroimmun.

Funding: This work was supported in part by the Schleswig-Holstein Cluster of Excellence in Inflammation Research (DFG EXC 306/1).

[a] Department of Dermatology, University of Lübeck, Ratzeburger Allee 160, 23538 Lübeck, Germany
[b] Comprehensive Center for Inflammation Medicine, University of Lübeck, Ratzeburger Allee 160, 23538 Lübeck, Germany
* Corresponding author. Department of Dermatology, University of Lübeck, Ratzeburger Allee 160, 23538 Lübeck, Germany.
E-mail address: enno.schmidt@uk-sh.de

Dermatol Clin 29 (2011) 663–671
doi:10.1016/j.det.2011.06.007

southern Germany, followed by pemphigoid gestationis (2.0 per million per year) and mucous membrane pemphigoid (2.0 per million per year).[2] Based on these data, in 2002, a total of 1830 new patients with immunobullous disorders were estimated. The incidence of BP in Germany has doubled within the last 10 years,[2,3] an observation that may be related to the increasing age of the general population and advances in the diagnostic tools. Because the incidence of BP dramatically increases with age resulting in an incidence of 150 to 190 per million per year for patients who are 80 years and older,[2,4] in 2010, at least 3450 new patients with autoimmune blistering diseases can be expected to be diagnosed in Germany.

SURVEY AMONG SECONDARY AND TERTIARY REFERRAL CENTERS FOR AUTOIMMUNE BULLOUS DISEASES

A standardized questionnaire was sent to all 34 university departments and 38 nonuniversity hospitals with inpatient dermatology departments. The questionnaire consisted of 4 questions about the diagnostic procedures for immunobullous disorders performed in the departments: (1) direct immunofluorescence (IF) microscopy; (2) indirect IF microscopy on monkey esophagus, guinea pig esophagus, human salt-split skin, monkey bladder, rat bladder, and complement binding test on human salt-split skin; (3) commercially available enzyme-linked immunosorbent assay (ELISA) systems, including BP180 NC16A, BP230, desmoglein 1, desmoglein 3, and envoplakin; and (4) in-house ELISA systems and immunoblotting analyses for the detection of autoantibodies against BP180, BP230, laminin 332, type VII collagen, p200 protein, α6 integrin, β4 integrin, desmoplakin I/II, periplakin, and envoplakin. For each test system, the answer yes or no could be marked.

In the treatment section of the questionnaire, first-line therapies for pemphigus vulgaris/foliaceus and BP were requested. In addition to the most frequent therapeutic regimens that could be marked with a cross, other options could be added as free text.

All 34 university departments and 30 of 38 (79%) nonuniversity hospitals with inpatient care for patients with dermatologic problems completed the questionnaire, resulting in a total response rate of 89%.

DIAGNOSIS

All university and 93% nonuniversity departments performed direct IF microscopy. Indirect IF microscopy on monkey/guinea pig esophagus and human salt-split skin was done in 76% and 68% of

university departments and 50% and 23% nonuniversity departments, respectively. Commercial ELISA systems for antidesmoglein and anti-BP180 antibodies were applied in 65% and 76% of university departments and 30% and 37% of nonuniversity departments, respectively. Noncommercial assays for the detection of autoantibodies in immunobullous diseases were used in 19% of dermatology departments, including 21% of university departments and 17% of nonuniversity departments. In addition, in 27% of departments, sera were sent for evaluation to external laboratories, including both university departments of dermatology and private laboratories.

This is the first survey on the diagnostic methods for immunobullous diseases in Germany. This survey reveals that direct IF microscopy is within the standard diagnostic repertoire in almost all dermatologic departments. Detection of serum antibodies by indirect IF microscopy and commercial ELISA systems is also widespread, whereas more sophisticated noncommercial systems are only used in a few specialized departments. A more detailed analysis of the diagnostic standard for immunobullous disorders in Germany is in preparation.

The diagnostic pathway for immunobullous dermatoses at the Department of Dermatology in Lübeck is summarized in **Fig. 1** along with recent reviews.[5,6] Diagnostic criteria used in the authors' department are detailed in **Table 1**.[2]

All diagnostic procedures on both outpatients and inpatients, including the serial determination of circulating autoantibodies during the follow-up period, are covered by the health insurances.

TREATMENT

High-quality controlled prospective clinical trials for the treatment of autoimmune blistering diseases are rare, therefore treatment decisions are mainly guided by published reviews in this field[7–11] or personal experiences. In contrast to the United Kingdom,[12,13] in Germany, no recommendations of the National Society of Dermatology for the treatment of immunobullous disease are available. For mucous membrane pemphigoid, guidelines for both diagnosis and treatment have been published following an international consensus conference.[14] Corticosteroids, dapsone, and cyclophosphamide (for severe cases) are the only drugs licensed for treatment of autoimmune bullous diseases in Germany.

Bullous Pemphigoid

In the present survey, topical clobetasol propionate 0.05% ointment was used as first-line treatment of BP in 68% of university hospitals and 67%

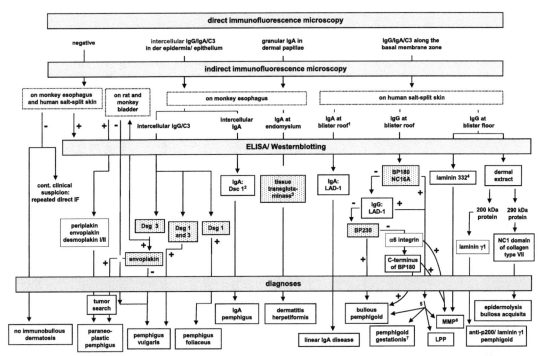

Fig. 1. Diagnostic pathway for immunobullous diseases as applied in the routine autoimmune laboratory of the Department of Dermatology, University of Lübeck. Dsc, desmocollin; Dsg, desmoglein; LAD-1, linear IgA disease antigen 1 (soluble ectodomain of BP180); LPP, lichen planus pemphigoides; MMP, mucous membrane pemphigoid. Dashed boxes indicate commercial ELISA systems. [1]IgA deposits at the blister floor are rare and have been described in variants of anti-laminin 332 mucous membrane pemphigoid and epidermolysis bullosa acquisita. [2]By indirect IF microscopy of Dsc-expressing COS cells. [3]Typical for celiac disease and only in conjunction with positive direct IF microscopy diagnostic for dermatitis herpetiformis. In addition, ELISA systems with epidermal transglutaminase and deamidated gliadin analogous peptides are used. [4]In 25% of patients associated with malignancy, tumor search is strongly recommended. [5]IgG reactivity against BP180 NC16A is associated with various entities. For final diagnosis, additional clinical information is required: pemphigoid gestationis, pregnancy, or postpartum period. [6]Predominance of mucosal lesions required. [7]Complement binding test on human salt-split skin is the most sensitive screening test.

of nonuniversity departments. Lesional application and whole-body application of the topical corticosteroid was used in equal numbers of departments. Systemic corticosteroids of initially 0.5 mg/kg/d to 1.0 mg/kg/d prednisolone equivalent and subsequent tapering were used in 36% and 47% of departments, respectively. Dapsone and azathioprine were the most frequently used corticosteroid-sparing agents, followed by doxycycline/tetracycline, mycophenol, and methotrexate.

In 2007, 32 German departments of dermatology were surveyed on the treatment of BP and pemphigus.[15] For BP, monotherapy with potent topical corticosteroids was used in about a quarter of departments; 75% of the units used systemic corticosteroids, half of them in a dose of less than 1 mg/kg/d prednisolone equivalent and the other half in a dose of 1 to 2 mg/kg/d. Azathioprine was given in 70% of departments as adjuvant immunosuppressant for patients with BP, followed by dapsone in about 20% of clinics.[15]

Compared with the survey by Hofmann and colleagues in 2007,[15] in the present survey, the number of dermatologic departments that used potent topical corticosteroids in the treatment of BP has significantly increased. Systemic corticosteroids are still frequently applied, although doses higher than 1 mg/kg/d are now rarely given. This may be because of the increasing knowledge about the data by Joly and colleagues[16,17] and Rzany and colleagues,[18] showing that BP can be sufficiently controlled by class IV topical corticosteroids in most patients and that the mortality rate increases with the dose of systemic corticosteroids. Most departments, including the authors', applied adjuvant immunosuppressants/immunomodulants for the treatment of BP. This practice may be explained by the 1-year high mortality rate of up to 40% that has been observed with the use of topical corticosteroids alone.[17] This assumption is supported by the authors' retrospective study on the combined use of clobetasol

Table 1
Diagnostic criteria used at the Department of Dermatology, University of Lübeck

Diagnosis	Clinic	Criteria		
		Direct IF Microscopy[a]	Indirect IF Microscopy	ELISA/Immunoblotting
Bullous pemphigoid	Blisters/erosions not predominantly on mucous membranes	IgG>IgA and/or C3 along the BMZ	IgG>IgA at the blister roof[b]	IgG reactivity with BP180
Pemphigoid gestationis	Pregnancy, pruritic skin lesions	IgG and/or C3 along the BMZ	C3 at the blister roof[c]	IgG reactivity with BP180
Mucous membrane pemphigoid[d]	Blisters/erosions not predominantly on mucous membranes	IgG and/or IgA and/or C3 along the BMZ	IgG and/or IgA and/or C3 at the blister roof[b]	IgG and/or IgA reactivity with BP180, laminin 332, or $\alpha_6\beta_4$ integrin
Linear IgA disease	Blisters/erosions not predominantly on mucous membranes	IgA>IgG along the BMZ	IgA>IgG at the blister roof[b]	IgA reactivity with BP180
Dermatitis herpetiformis	Urticarial plaques or vesicles	Granular IgA in dermal papillae	IgA at the endomysium[e]	IgA reactivity with epidermal and/or tissue transglutaminase and/or deamidated gliadin
Epidermolysis bullosa acquisita	Blisters/erosions not predominantly on mucous membranes	IgG and/or IgA and/or C3 along the BMZ	IgG and/or IgA on the blister floor[b]	IgG and/or IgA reactivity with type VII collagen
Anti-p200/laminin γ_1 pemphigoid	Blisters/erosions not predominantly on mucous membranes	IgG and/or C3 along the BMZ	IgG at the blister floor[b]	IgG reactivity with a 200 kDa protein in dermal extract and/or laminin γ_1

Lichen planus pemphigoides	Blisters/erosions and lichenoid papules	IgG and/or C3 along the BMZ	IgG at the blister roof[b]	IgG reactivity with BP180 NC16A
Pemphigus vulgaris	Blisters/erosions on mucous membranes	Intercellular IgG and/or C3 deposits in the epidermis/epithelium	Intercellular IgG deposits in the epithelium[e]	IgG reactivity with desmoglein 3
Pemphigus foliaceus	Blisters/erosions on the skin	Intercellular IgG and/or C3 deposits in the epidermis	Intercellular IgG deposits in the epithelium[e]	IgG reactivity with desmoglein 1
IgA pemphigus	Blisters/erosions/ pustules on the skin	Intercellular IgA deposits in the epidermis	Intercellular IgA deposits in the epithelium[e]	IgA reactivity with desmocollins or desmoglein 3
Paraneoplastic pemphigus[f]	Blisters/erosions on mucous membranes and the presence of a neoplasm	Intercellular IgG and/or C3 deposits in the epidermis/epithelium	Intercellular IgG deposits in the epithelium[e] and IgG in urothelium[g]	IgG reactivity against plakins and/or desmoglein 3 or 1[f]

For diagnostic criteria, "Clinic," "Direct IF Microscopy," and "Indirect IF Microscopy" must be met. In case of negative direct IF, the finding of circulating autoantibodies against the listed antigens is required.

Abbreviation: BMZ, basal membrane zone.

a Of a perilesional biopsy.
b By indirect IF microscopy on 1 M NaCl-split human skin.
c By complement binding test on 1 M NaCl-split human skin.
d According to the criteria of an international consensus conference.[14]
e By indirect IF microscopy on monkey esophagus.
f Detailed in Ref.[35]
g By indirect IF microscopy on monkey or rat bladder.

propionate 0.05% ointment, methylprednisolone (0.5 mg/kg/d), and dapsone (1.0–1.5 mg/kg/d) that resulted in a 1-year high mortality rate as low as 6%.[19] Compared with the survey in 2007, the present use of dapsone has tripled, whereas the administration of azathioprine decreased by half, making dapsone the most frequently used adjuvant medication in BP in Germany at the present time.

The first-line treatments of subepidermal blistering autoimmune diseases in the Department of Dermatology in Lübeck are summarized in **Table 2**.

Pemphigus Vulgaris/Foliaceus

In the present survey on first-line treatments of pemphigus, starting doses of prednisolone equivalents of 1.0 mg/kg/d, 1.5 mg/kg/d, and 2.0 mg/kg/d were applied in 33%, 34%, and 23% of the dermatologic departments, respectively. Systemic corticosteroids were given as IV pulses in 17% of departments. The most frequently used concomitant immunosuppressant was azathioprine (in 84% of departments) followed by mycophenol, IV cyclophosphamide pulses, methotrexate, cyclosporine, and daily oral cyclophosphamide.

Table 2
Standard therapies of immunobullous disorders at the Department of Dermatology, University of Lübeck

Disease	Treatment
Pemphigus	

Pemphigus vulgaris/pemphigus foliaceus	First-line
	   IV dexamethasone pulses (100 mg on 3 consecutive d/mo in prolonging intervals) + azathioprine or mycophenolate
	Second line
	   First-line therapy + immunoadsorption (on 3 consecutive d for 3–4 wk until lesions healed by >90%) + rituximab (2 × 1 g)
	Third line
	   Any of the above (except immunoadsorption) + IVIG (2 g/kg/mo for 3–6 mo)

IgA pemphigus	Dapsone and/or acitretin, additional prednisolone (0.5–1.0 mg/kg/d tapering) if required
Subepidermal Bullous Autoimmune Dermatoses	

Bullous pemphigoid	Mild disease
	   Clobetasol propionate 0.05% ointment (10–30 g/d)
	Moderate disease
	   + Dapsone (1.0–1.5 mg/kg/d)
	Severe disease
	   + Prednisolone (0.5 mg/kg/d tapering) ± immunoadsorption

Pemphigoid gestationis	Class II–III topical corticosteroids ± prednisolone (0.25 mg/kg tapering)
Linear IgA disease	Clobetasol propionate 0.05 ointment ± prednisolone (0.25–0.5 mg/kg tapering) + dapsone (1.0–1.5 mg/kg/d)

Mucous membrane pemphigoid	Without ocular involvement
	   IV dexamethasone pulses (100 mg on 3 consecutive d/mo in prolonging intervals) + dapsone or mycophenolate
	With ocular involvement
	   IV dexamethasone pulses (100 mg on 3 consecutive d/mo in prolonging intervals) + IV cyclophosphamide (500–750 mg/mo) ± cyclophosphamide (50 mg/d by mouth; after clinical remission changed to mycophenolate) ± rituximab (2 × 1 g) ± immunoadsorption

Lichen planus pemphigoides	Prednisolone (0.5 mg/kg/d tapering) + acitretin + bath psoralen plus UV-A
Anti-laminin γ1/p200 pemphigoid	As in BP
Epidermolysis bullosa acquisita	As in pemphigus ± colchicine
Dermatitis herpetiformis	Gluten-free diet + dapsone (1.0–1.5 mg/kg/d)

In 2007, Hofmann and colleagues[15] identified a prednisolone equivalent of less than 1 mg/kg/d as the most frequently administered initial therapy (in 53% of departments) for pemphigus, whereas nearly 40% and 10% of departments used prednisolone equivalents of 1 to 2 mg/kg/d and less than 2 mg/kg/d as starting doses, respectively. Hence, a tendency for higher starting doses of

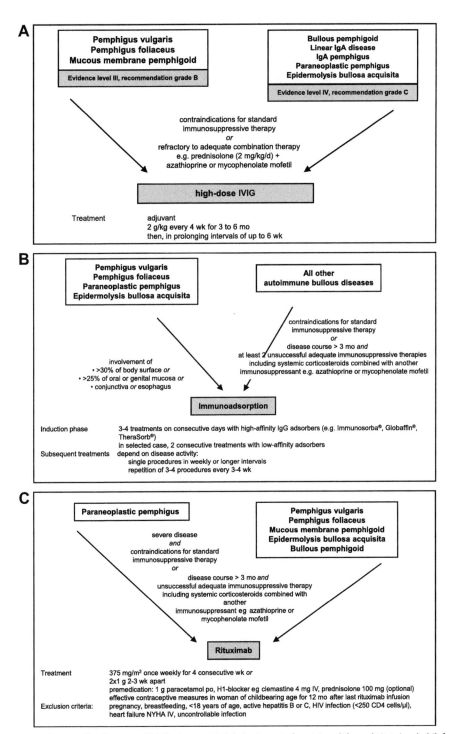

Fig. 2. Recommendations for the use of high-dose IVIG (*A*), immunoadsorption (*B*), and rituximab (*C*) for patients with autoimmune blistering diseases according to consensus conferences of German, Austrian, and Swiss experts. HIV, human immunodeficiency virus; NYHA IV, New York Heart Association IV. (*Data from Refs.*[32–34])

prednisolone is seen in the present survey. In contrast, azathioprine remains by far the most frequent corticosteroid-sparing agent, with 84% in the present study compared with 81% in the 2007 survey.[15]

High-dose IVIG, rituximab, and immunoadsorption were increasingly used for patients with refractory pemphigus. Although the clinical effect of IVIG in the treatment of pemphigus has been demonstrated in a recent placebo-controlled double-blind prospective trial in Japan,[20] increasing evidence for the efficacy of rituximab[21–25] and immunoadsorption[26–31] for these patients is gathered from case series. To investigate efficacy and safety of rituximab and immunoadsorption in pemphigus, multicenter controlled prospective trials have been initiated in Rouen (France) and Lübeck and Marburg (Germany).

With some regional variations, all treatment regimens including IVIG, immunoadsorption, and rituximab will be covered by health insurances when treatment is performed according to the recommendations of German, Austrian, and Swiss experts in this field published in *Journal der Deutschen Dermatologischen Gesellschaft* (*Journal of the German Dermatologic Society*).[32–34] The criteria are summarized in **Fig. 2**. **Table 2** shows the standard regimens for immunobullous diseases at the Department of Dermatology in Lübeck.

In 2010, the first patient support group for patients with autoimmune bullous disease in Germany, the Pemphigus und Pemphigoid Selbsthilfe e.V., was established (www.pemphigus-pemphigoid-selbsthilfe.de).

SUMMARY

Care for patients with autoimmune bullous diseases is generally well established and available in Germany. A relatively large number of dermatologic departments regularly apply the standard diagnostic tools and provide differentiated treatments for these patients. The topical use of potent corticosteroids in BP and the increasing administration of immunoadsorption, rituximab, and IVIG for severe and/or refractory pemphigus reflect the present level of knowledge. This development is fostered because the costs for all adequate diagnostic and therapeutic measures are usually covered by health insurances.

ACKNOWLEDGMENTS

We are grateful to Diana Knuth-Rehr for her valuable assistance with data management. We thank the directors of all 34 university departments of dermatology in Germany and the heads of the following nonuniversity dermatologic clinics (in alphabetical order) for their contribution to this study: Alzenau, Aue, Augsburg, Bayreuth, Berlin Friedrichshain, Bielefeld, Bremen, Darmstadt, Dessau, Dortmund, Dresden, Erfurt, Heilbronn, Hersbruck, Hildesheim, Karlsruhe, Kassel, Krefeld, Lüdenscheid, Ludwigshafen, Minden, München Schwabing, Nürnberg, Oldenburg, Quedlinburg, Recklinghausen, Schwerin, Stuttgart, Wiesbaden, and Zwickau.

REFERENCES

1. Hahn-Ristic K, Rzany B, Amagai M, et al. Increased incidence of pemphigus vulgaris in southern Europeans living in Germany compared with native Germans. J Eur Acad Dermatol Venereol 2002;16:68–71.
2. Bertram F, Brocker EB, Zillikens D, et al. Prospective analysis of the incidence of autoimmune bullous disorders in Lower Franconia, Germany. J Dtsch Dermatol Ges 2009;7:434–40.
3. Zillikens D, Wever S, Roth A, et al. Incidence of autoimmune subepidermal blistering dermatoses in a region of central Germany. Arch Dermatol 1995;131:957–8.
4. Jung M, Kippes W, Messer G, et al. Increased risk of bullous pemphigoid in male and very old patients: a population-based study on incidence. J Am Acad Dermatol 1999;41:266–8.
5. Schmidt E, Zillikens D. Diagnostic and therapy of autoimmune blistering diseases. Dtsch Arztbl Int 2011;108:399–405.
6. Schmidt E, Zillikens D. Modern diagnosis of autoimmune blistering skin diseases. Autoimmun Rev 2010;10:84–9.
7. Goebeler M, Sitaru C, Zillikens D. Blistering autoimmune dermatoses (II): therapy. J Dtsch Dermatol Ges 2004;2:774–91.
8. Mutasim DF. Management of autoimmune bullous diseases: pharmacology and therapeutics. J Am Acad Dermatol 2004;51:859–77.
9. Khumalo N, Kirtschig G, Middleton P, et al. Interventions for bullous pemphigoid. Cochrane Database Syst Rev 2005;3:CD002292.
10. Martin LK, Werth V, Villanueva E, et al. Interventions for pemphigus vulgaris and pemphigus foliaceus. Cochrane Database Syst Rev 2009;1:CD006263.
11. Kasperkiewicz M, Schmidt E. Current treatment of autoimmune blistering diseases. Curr Drug Discov Technol 2009;6:270–80.
12. Harman KE, Albert S, Black MM. Guidelines for the management of pemphigus vulgaris. Br J Dermatol 2003;149:926–37.
13. Wojnarowska F, Kirtschig G, Highet AS, et al. Guidelines for the management of bullous pemphigoid. Br J Dermatol 2002;147:214–21.

14. Chan LS, Ahmed AR, Anhalt GJ, et al. The first international consensus on mucous membrane pemphigoid: definition, diagnostic criteria, pathogenic factors, medical treatment, and prognostic indicators. Arch Dermatol 2002;138:370–9.

15. Hofmann SC, Kautz O, Hertl M, et al. Results of a survey of German dermatologists on the therapeutic approaches to pemphigus and bullous pemphigoid. J Dtsch Dermatol Ges 2009;7:227–33.

16. Joly P, Roujeau JC, Benichou J, et al. A comparison of two regimens of topical corticosteroids in the treatment of patients with bullous pemphigoid: a multicenter randomized study. J Invest Dermatol 2009;129:1681–7.

17. Joly P, Roujeau JC, Benichou J, et al. A comparison of oral and topical corticosteroids in patients with bullous pemphigoid. N Engl J Med 2002;346:321–7.

18. Rzany B, Partscht K, Jung M, et al. Risk factors for lethal outcome in patients with bullous pemphigoid: low serum albumin level, high dosage of glucocorticosteroids, and old age. Arch Dermatol 2002;138:903–8.

19. Schmidt E, Kraensel R, Goebeler M, et al. Treatment of bullous pemphigoid with dapsone, methylprednisolone, and topical clobetasol propionate: a retrospective study of 62 cases. Cutis 2005;76:205–9.

20. Amagai M, Ikeda S, Shimizu H, et al. A randomized double-blind trial of intravenous immunoglobulin for pemphigus. J Am Acad Dermatol 2009;60:595–603.

21. Nagel A, Hertl M, Eming R. B-cell-directed therapy for inflammatory skin diseases. J Invest Dermatol 2009;129:289–301.

22. Joly P, Mouquet H, Roujeau JC, et al. A single cycle of rituximab for the treatment of severe pemphigus. N Engl J Med 2007;357:545–52.

23. Ahmed AR, Spigelman Z, Cavacini LA, et al. Treatment of pemphigus vulgaris with rituximab and intravenous immune globulin. N Engl J Med 2006;355:1772–9.

24. Schmidt E, Goebeler M, Zillikens D. Rituximab in severe pemphigus. Ann N Y Acad Sci 2009;1173:683–91.

25. Schmidt E, Goebeler M. CD20-directed therapy in autoimmune diseases involving the skin: role of rituximab. Expert Rev Dermatol 2008;3:259–78.

26. Schmidt E, Klinker E, Opitz A, et al. Protein A immunoadsorption: a novel and effective adjuvant treatment of severe pemphigus. Br J Dermatol 2003;148:1222–9.

27. Eming R, Rech J, Barth S, et al. Prolonged clinical remission of patients with severe pemphigus upon rapid removal of desmoglein-reactive autoantibodies by immunoadsorption. Dermatology 2006;212:177–87.

28. Shimanovich I, Bohmke AK, Westermann L, et al. Successful treatment of severe pemphigus with the combination of immunoadsorption and rituximab. J Invest Dermatol 2009;129:S97.

29. Shimanovich I, Nitschke M, Rose C, et al. Treatment of severe pemphigus with protein A immunoadsorption, rituximab and intravenous immunoglobulins. Br J Dermatol 2008;158:382–8.

30. Shimanovich I, Herzog S, Schmidt E, et al. Improved protocol for treatment of pemphigus vulgaris with protein A immunoadsorption. Clin Exp Dermatol 2006;31:768–74.

31. Schmidt E, Zillikens D. Immunoadsorption in dermatology. Arch Dermatol Res 2010;302:241–53.

32. Zillikens D, Derfler K, Eming R, et al. Recommendations for the use of immunoapheresis in the treatment of autoimmune bullous diseases. J Dtsch Dermatol Ges 2007;5:881–7.

33. Hertl M, Zillikens D, Borradori L, et al. Recommendations for the use of rituximab (anti-CD20 antibody) in the treatment of autoimmune bullous skin diseases. J Dtsch Dermatol Ges 2008;6:366–73.

34. Enk A, Fierlbeck G, French L, et al. Use of high-dose immunoglobulins in dermatology. J Dtsch Dermatol Ges 2009;7:806–12.

35. Zimmermann J, Bahmer F, Rose C, et al. Clinical and immunopathological spectrum of paraneoplastic pemphigus. J Dtsch Dermatol Ges 2010;8:598–605.

Management of Autoimmune Blistering Diseases in Spain

Ricardo Suárez, MD[a], Agustín España, MD[b],
Josep E. Herrero-González, MD[c], Pilar Iranzo, MD[d],
José M. Mascaró Jr, MD[d],*

KEYWORDS

- Pemphigus • Pemphigoid • Health care • Spain

HEALTH CARE IN SPAIN

The Spanish National Health Care System is a public system that is reasonably efficient and has been considered one of the best in the world. It was ranked seventh according to the World Health Organization in the year 2000,[1] whereas countries like Canada and the United States were ranked 30 and 37, respectively. To become insured people need a social security ("seguridad social") number, which is obtained by either working for an employer (usually a private or public company, who pays, along with the worker, a monthly amount that will provide cover for health care, unemployment, and retirement) or becoming self-employed (in which case, the person pays a monthly amount to be part of the system). Dependents (children and nonworking spouses) are included in the social security card of the worker. The system will continue to cover the health care of the worker when he or she retires (usually at 65 years of age), as well as his or her dependents (ie, nonworking spouses), but not his or her children when they are able to work. Spaniards who are unemployed or are very poor (even if they have never worked) are also usually covered by the system. In this way the system is nearly universal, covering 98.7% of the population.[2]

The Spanish National Health Care System provides primary health care, including general health and pediatric care, outpatient and inpatient surgery, emergency and acute care, and long-term disease management. Prescription drugs require a 40% copayment by the patients, with the exception of retired people (who get medications for free) or hospital medications (such as immunosuppressants or rituximab, which are fully paid by the system). There are some exceptions to this; some medications, creams, moisturizing creams, shampoos, or dressings may not be covered by the system and the patients have to pay the total cost of these products.

The system is a highly decentralized one that gives primary responsibility to the country's 17 autonomous regional governments. The central government provides the money to each autonomous region, and each region decides how to use it, hence health care spending varies from region to region. The regional variation is important because Spaniards usually face many bureaucratic

[a] Department of Dermatology, Hospital General Universitario Gregorio Marañón, Calle del Doctor Esquerdo, 46, 28007 Madrid, Spain
[b] Department of Dermatology, University Clinic of Navarra School of Medicine, University of Navarra, Avenida Pío XII, 36, 31008 Pamplona, Spain
[c] Department of Dermatology, Hospital del Mar, Parc de Salut Mar, Institut Municipal d'Investigació Mèdica, Passeig Marítim, 25-29, 08003 Barcelona, Spain
[d] Department of Dermatology, Hospital Clínic and Barcelona University Medical School, Calle Villarroel 170, 08036 Barcelona, Spain
* Corresponding author.
E-mail address: jmmascaro_galy@ub.edu

Dermatol Clin 29 (2011) 673–676
doi:10.1016/j.det.2011.06.006
0733-8635/11/$ – see front matter © 2011 Elsevier Inc. All rights reserved.

barriers if they try to get nonemergency health care in another part of the country (eg, a consultation in a hospital in Barcelona rather than Madrid).[2]

Spanish patients cannot choose their physicians in the public system, either primary care physicians or specialists. Patients are assigned a general family physician in their area, and if their general physician decides they need a specialist, they will be referred to a specialist who is generally working in a community clinic. Patients do not have direct access to specialists unless they have private health insurance. If patients need a higher specialist standard, they are sent by the community specialist to a community hospital or a large teaching hospital. In general, there are long waiting lists for specialist consultation and nonurgent surgeries.

Private health insurance has expanded in the last few decades in Spain, due to the waiting lists and qualitative problems of the public system. Different companies exist that provide coverage for most routine visits to general physicians, specialists, and procedures. About 12% of Spaniards have mixed coverage (public and private) because the public system is compulsory for everyone. In big cities such as Madrid and Barcelona, the number of privately insured is around 25% of the population.[2] Many go private to avoid waiting lists, and to get simple procedures done in an easy and comfortable way. However, for important diseases (eg, a myocardial infarction or an autoimmune blistering disease [AIBD]) or complicated procedures (eg, organ transplantation), people prefer to make use of the public system, whereby they can usually find the best hospitals and doctors. Most of the large teaching university hospitals in Spain (where the highly specialized clinicians can be found) are public and are part of the system, with some exceptions (eg, the University Clinic of Navarra in Pamplona, which is private although it has agreements with the public system).

EPIDEMIOLOGY AND DIAGNOSIS OF AUTOIMMUNE BLISTERING DISEASES IN SPAIN

There are no official data on the incidence and prevalence of AIBDs in Spain. The figures are probably similar to the ones from other European countries[3,4]: around 40 cases per million persons per year for bullous pemphigoid, and 7 cases per million persons per year for pemphigus vulgaris.[4] In a review of patients diagnosed with pemphigus between 1985 and 2002 (an 18-year period) at the Department of Dermatology of the Hospital Clinic and University Medical School of Barcelona, the

authors found a total of 88 patients (most of them with pemphigus vulgaris).[5] In another review from the same department of patients diagnosed with subepidermal blistering diseases between 2000 and 2005 (a 6-year period) a total of 116 patients were found with the following diagnoses and distribution: 71 with bullous pemphigoid (61%), 23 with dermatitis herpetiformis (20%), 10 with mucous membrane pemphigoid (8%), 6 with epidermolysis bullosa acquisita (5%), 3 with linear IgA bullous dermatosis (3%), 2 with pemphigoid gestationis (2%), and 1 with bullous systemic lupus erythematosus (1%). These data cannot be extrapolated to the rest of Spain, as this institution is a referral center for blistering diseases, and many patients from the region (Catalonia, with 7 million people) are sent here. Similarly, in a revision of AIBD patients treated at Hospital General Universitario Gregorio Marañón in Madrid between 2000 and 2009 (a 10-year period), the authors found a total of 95 patients with the following diagnoses and distribution: 33 with pemphigus vulgaris (35%), 40 with bullous pemphigoid (42%), 13 with dermatitis herpetiformis (14%), 6 with linear IgA bullous dermatosis (6%), and 3 with mucous membrane pemphigoid (3%). In another review of AIBD patients treated at the University Clinic of Navarra in Pamplona from 2000 to now (an 11-year period), the authors found a total of 61 patients with the following diagnoses and distribution: 36 with pemphigus vulgaris (59%), 4 with pemphigus foliaceus (7%), 10 with bullous pemphigoid (16%), 6 with mucous membrane pemphigoid (10%), and 5 with dermatitis herpetiformis (8%). These data are also biased, because mostly patients with severe conditions (like pemphigus) are sent to these hospitals, whereas patients with bullous pemphigoid receive care in their community hospitals.

Recently the authors conducted a mail and e-mail epidemiologic survey on pemphigus vulgaris, involving all hospital dermatologists taking care of patients with AIBD in Spain.[6] Twenty-six dermatology departments answered the survey, covering a population of approximately 10,200,000 people. An estimated incidence of 2.4 cases per million people per year, and a prevalence of 23 cases per million people per year were obtained from this survey.

Most patients with AIBD in Spain are diagnosed based only on clinical and histologic criteria. Immunofluorescence techniques (both direct and indirect) are largely unavailable in most small and middle-sized hospitals. In addition, on many occasions when these techniques are available, they are done in low-volume laboratories by technicians and pathologists with little experience.

Therefore the results are often not very reliable, with false-negative results being common. In addition, histologic diagnosis in many centers is done by general pathologists who have not been trained in dermatopathology and inflammatory dermatoses (and AIBD in particular).

Regarding more sophisticated diagnostic procedures, the enzyme-linked immunosorbent assay (ELISA) is not available to most patients for their diagnosis and follow-up. Except in large university hospitals (such as the authors' institutions in Madrid, Pamplona, and Barcelona), most dermatology departments cannot offer ELISA for Dsg1, Dsg3, and NC16A to their AIBD patients, these techniques being available only at a handful of institutions. Immunoblotting techniques are rarely performed on a routine clinical basis in Spain, even in reference centers, and are only done for research purposes.

MANAGEMENT AND FOLLOW-UP OF AUTOIMMUNE BLISTERING DISEASES IN SPAIN

Patients with AIBD in Spain are usually diagnosed, managed, and followed by dermatologists. However, in recent years some internists are becoming more specialized in "autoimmune diseases" and attempt to take care of patients with cutaneous diseases, including pemphigus, pemphigoid, psoriasis, or other immune-mediated dermatologic diseases. Although this is happening in some large hospital centers, it is fortunately very infrequent. General physicians are not at all involved with patients with AIBD, and always refer them to dermatologists.

Dermatologists outside hospitals (private practice, community public clinics) usually avoid treating AIBD, referring them to hospital-based dermatologists in community hospitals or larger university centers. The problem in many cases is that as AIBDs are relatively rare diseases, there are very few dermatologists who have sufficient experience in managing this type of patient. It is not uncommon to see patients with pemphigus vulgaris who come for a second opinion, who have been managed with systemic steroids but have not received any type of adjunctive immunosuppressant or treatment to prevent osteoporosis (such as calcium, vitamin D, and bisphosphonates).

At present there are no "official" national guidelines for dermatologists to follow regarding the management of AIBD patients. Most dermatologists treat these patients in an ad hoc manner, although they are usually unfamiliar with the administration of systemic steroids or immunosuppressants. It is more common that these patients are referred to tertiary hospitals where there is always somebody familiar with these treatments, although many times they are not experts in AIBD. In the survey that included 26 Spanish dermatology departments managing patients with pemphigus, the authors found that systemic steroids were the standard treatment and that in some instances they were used in very high doses. Immunosuppressant medications were frequently added, azathioprine being the most frequently used, followed by mycophenolate.[6] There was an increasing use of rituximab, whereas plasmapheresis, intravenous cyclophosphamide, and gold salts were used rarely. The preferred regimens in order of frequency were: prednisone 1 mg/kg/d in association with either azathioprine or mycophenolate, followed by rituximab in the case of nonresponsiveness in 20 (77%) of the centers; prednisone 2 to 3 mg/kg/d in association with azathioprine or other immunosuppressants in 2 (8%) of the centers; prednisone up to 1 to 1.5 mg/kg/d in association with cyclophosphamide, methotrexate, gold salts, or rituximab in 1 (4%) of the centers; and other regimens in 3 (12%) of the centers.[6]

In 2008 the authors published a review article in *Actas Dermosifiliográficas*, the official journal of the Spanish Academy of Dermatology, with recommendations for the use of different immunosuppressants and some guidelines for the treatment of the most frequent AIBDs (pemphigus vulgaris, bullous pemphigoid, pemphigoid gestationis, mucous membrane pemphigoid, dermatitis herpetiformis, and linear IgA bullous dermatosis).[7] However, this publication cannot be considered as an "official guideline" for AIBD in Spain.

SPECIALIZED CENTERS, NETWORKS, AND SUPPORT GROUPS FOR AUTOIMMUNE BLISTERING DISEASES IN SPAIN

Only a few centers in Spain, such as the aforementioned institutions, run specialized AIBD clinics, offering adequate diagnostic techniques (immunofluorescence, ELISA), experience with systemic therapies, and available treatment services such as day-care clinics or inpatient dermatology units. In recent years, the authors have created a small network of dermatologists specialized in AIBD in an attempt to optimize the diagnosis and management of patients in Spain (**Fig. 1**). The members of this AIBD network in alphabetical order are Agustin España (University Clinic of Navarra, School of Medicine, University of Navarra, Pamplona), Josep Herrero-González (Hospital del Mar, IMAS, Barcelona), Pilar Iranzo and José M. Mascaró (Hospital Clínic and Barcelona University Medical School,

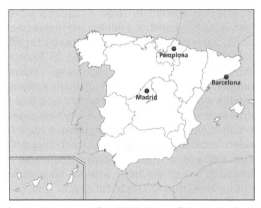

Fig. 1. At present the AIBD Network in Spain has 4 centers in 3 cities (Barcelona, Madrid, and Pamplona) shown as red dots on the map. The map of Spain also shows the country's 17 autonomous regions, all of which have independent health care systems.

Barcelona); and Ricardo Suárez (Hospital General Universitario Gregorio Marañón, Madrid). As a result of this network there have been several presentations and publications in national meetings and journals,[6,7] as well as a 2-day training course for the diagnosis and management of AIBD (organized in the last 2 years in Barcelona by Josep Herrero-González). The network is also currently starting some epidemiologic studies and clinical trials for AIBD in Spain.

Very recently a support group for patients with AIBD was created in Spain, the "Asociacion Española de Penfigo, Penfigoide y Enfermedades Vesiculo-Ampollosas (AEPPEVA)," has created a Web site (http://www.aeppeva.org/), with its headquarters in Burgos. In January 2010, AEPPEVA organized its first meeting in Burgos, to which the authors were invited to give talks for AIBD patients and their families, as well as to participate in patients' colloquia.

SUMMARY

The diagnosis and management of AIBD in Spain is still below desirable standards. Future goals of the authors' AIBD Network would be that all patients can obtain a diagnosis confirmed at least by immunofluorescence techniques, are adequately treated with immunosuppressive regimens avoiding high doses of systemic steroids, and can actively collaborate in clinical and research studies in AIBD in Spain.

REFERENCES

1. The World Health Report. 2000—health systems: improving performance. Geneva (Switzerland): World Health Organization; 2000.
2. Tanner MD. The grass is not always greener: a look at national health care systems around the world. Policy Anal 2008;613:1–48.
3. Zillikens D, Wever S, Roth A, et al. Incidence of autoimmune subepidermal blistering dermatoses in a region of central Germany. Arch Dermatol 1995; 131:957–8.
4. Langan SM, Smeeth L, Hubbard R, et al. Bullous pemphigoid and pemphigus vulgaris—incidence and mortality in the UK: population based cohort study. BMJ 2008;337:160–3.
5. Herrero-González JE, Iranzo P, Benítez D, et al. Correlation of immunological profile with phenotype and disease outcome in pemphigus. Acta Derm Venereol 2010;90:401–5.
6. Suárez-Fernández R, Ciudad C, Alfageme F, et al. Pénfigo vulgar: casuistica española. Poster presentation. 38th Annual Meeting of the Spanish Academy of Dermatology. Málaga (Spain), May 26–29, 2010.
7. Suárez-Fernández R, España-Alonso A, Herrero-González JE, et al. Practical management of the most common autoimmune bullous diseases. Actas Dermosifiliogr 2008;99:441–55.

Autoimmune Blistering Diseases: Incidence and Treatment in Croatia

Branka Marinovic, MD, PhD*, Jasna Lipozencic, MD, PhD,
Ines Lakos Jukic, MD, MSc

KEYWORDS

- Autoimmune blistering diseases • Croatia
- Dermatovenereology • Pemphigus

The Republic of Croatia is a country laying in Central and Southeastern Europe, at the crossroads of the Pannonian Plain, the Balkans, and the Adriatic Sea. Croatia borders Slovenia to the north, Hungary to the northeast, Bosnia and Herzegovina to the southeast, Serbia to the east, and Montenegro to the southeast (**Fig. 1**). The population of Croatia is estimated to be 4.5 million inhabitants, with 1.2 million of them living in Zagreb, the capital of Croatia. Dermatovenereology in Croatia has a long tradition, with the first Department of Dermatovenereology in Croatia having opened in Zagreb in 1894. Because Croatia was a part of the Austro-Hungarian Empire and because of its geographic location in Central Europe, approach to dermatovenereology is based on Central European dermatovenereology traditions, with treatment of many patients still on in-patient wards. There are 4 medical schools in Croatia (in Zagreb, Split, Rijeka, and Osijek) and 5 university departments of dermatovenereology (one of them is part of a school of dental medicine). In other towns in Croatia, some hospitals have dermatology units.

If a diagnosis of autoimmune bullous disease (AIBD) is suspected, the patient is referred to one of the university departments because of their ability to establish the diagnosis. The diagnosis of AIBD is based on clinical, histopathologic, and immunopathologic findings. Most of the patients from Northern and Eastern Croatia are referred to the Department of Dermatology and Venereology

of the University of Zagreb School of Medicine. To the best of the authors' knowledge, it is only at this department in Zagreb that the complete diagnostic algorithm of AIBD is performed (histopathology, immunofluorescence studies, and ELISA).[1–4] The Department of Dermatology and Venereology, University Hospital Centre Zagreb also has a specific unit for children, which has been appointed a national referral center for epidermolysis bullosa by the Ministry of Health and Social Welfare of the Republic of Croatia. Hence, that department is a center of expertise in blistering diseases. The authors have analyzed patient records from the department from 2005 to 2010. In that period of time, the authors diagnosed 41 new pemphigus cases and 44 new pemphigoid cases. As indicated previously, patients from Northern and Eastern Croatia gravitate to Zagreb, so there is an estimated population of 2.2 million inhabitants. According to these data, the annual incidence for the pemphigus group of diseases is 3.7 new cases per million and 4 new cases of the pemphigoid group of diseases per million. In the pemphigus group of patients, 27 (66%) were women and 14 (34%) were men. In the pemphigoid group of patients, there were 23 (52%) women and 21 (48%) men. In the Dalmatian region of Croatia, on the eastern Adriatic coast, which is part of the Mediterranean, in the same period of time, there were 14 new pemphigus cases and 20 new pemphigoid cases. Because the estimated population

Department of Dermatology and Venereology, University Hospital Centre Zagreb, School of Medicine, University of Zagreb, Salata 4, 10000 Zagreb, Croatia
* Corresponding author.
E-mail address: branka.marinovic@kbc-zagreb.hr

Dermatol Clin 29 (2011) 677–679
doi:10.1016/j.det.2011.07.003

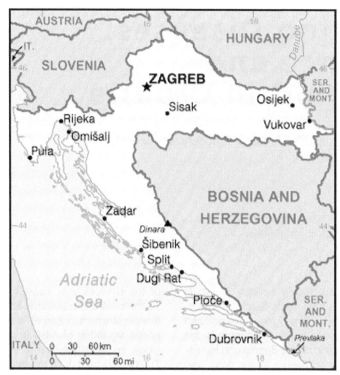

Fig. 1. Map of Croatia.

of Dalmatia is 900,000, the annual incidence of the pemphigus group of diseases in this area is 3.1 per million and 4.4 new cases of pemphigoid group of diseases per million. The incidences of these two diseases are not dissimilar, given that in many countries, pemphigoid is more common than pemphigus. The life expectancy in Croatia for men is 71 years and for women is 78 years. Because pemphigoid predominantly affects the elderly population, the authors do not believe these patients are dying of other causes before the development of pemphigoid, which may occur in poorer countries.

All laboratory procedures, including ELISA for detecting autoantibodies against desmoglein 1, desmoglein 3, BP180, BP230, and tissue and epidermal transglutaminase, are covered by obligatory health insurance possessed by all Croatian citizens. Sera from patients who have been hospitalized in other university departments are referred to the Department of Dermatology and Venereology, University Hospital Centre Zagreb, School of Medicine, University of Zagreb for ELISA testing. After a diagnosis of AIBD is established, the treatment is started. Almost all patients with the pemphigus group of diseases and the majority of patients with the pemphigoid group of diseases are hospitalized, which enables quick and complete assessment of patients' overall medical status to identify risks of developing complications

from steroids and other systemic drugs. Patients with mild forms of pemphigoid are treated in the outpatient clinic. The standard therapy for the pemphigus group of diseases includes prednisone, usually 1 mg/kg (for pemphigus vulgaris). Azathioprine is usually given as adjuvant treatment, although there are some patients in whom mycophenolic acid is introduced. In refractory cases intravenous immunoglobulin is given. Plasmapheresis, an effective treatment, has been used for only a few patients. The authors have no experience with biologic drugs, such as rituximab, because of limited indications for this drug covered by health insurance companies. Patients with the pemphigoid group of diseases (bullous pemphigoid) are treated with corticosteroids, usually starting with prednisone (0.5 mg/kg) with accentuation of topical corticosteroid therapy. Only a few refractory patients have been on adjuvant therapy also. Patients with dermatitis herpetiformis Duhring and linear IgA dermatosis are initially treated with dapsone, but this drug has not been registered in Croatia, so patients have to buy it themselves.

After control of AIBD is achieved, patients are released from the department and then regularly controlled and carefully followed up in the outpatient clinic, usually monthly, with special attention to possible side effects of long-term corticosteroid therapy. All medications and procedures, which are recommended by a dermatologist, are prescribed by a competent general practitioner. Some of the most interesting cases cured and diagnosed in the Department were discussed and published in dermatologic journals.[5–8] Unfortunately, there are no AIBD support groups in Croatia. Since 2007 the authors have been collecting data concerning patients with AIBD (a project supported by Ministry of Science of the Republic of Croatia) and are investigating the possible association of certain HLA class II alleles and haplotypes with pemphigus vulgaris in Croatia. The aim of this study is to analyze HLA associations and to investigate any differences between patients from central Croatia and those from Dalmatia. Future goals are to participate in multicenter studies because this is the only possibility for further investigation for these rare diseases.

REFERENCES

1. Marinovic B, Fabris Z, Lipozencic J, et al. Comparison of diagnostic value of indirect immunofluorescence assay and desmoglein ELISA in the diagnosis of pemphigus. Acta Dermatovenerol Croat 2010;18: 79–83.

2. Lakos Jukic I, Marinovic B. Sensitivity of indirect immunofluorescence test in the diagnosis of pemphigus. Acta Dermatovenerol Croat 2004;12:162–5.

3. Marinovic B, Lakos Jukic I. Autoimmune blistering diseases in childhood. Acta Dermatovenerol Croat 2002;10:33–7.

4. Ljubojevic S, Lipozencic J, Brenner S, et al. Pemphigus vulgaris: a review of treatment over a 19-year period. J Eur Acad Dermatol Venereol 2002;16:599–603.

5. Pastar Z, Rados J, Lipozencic J, et al. Case of concurrent epidermolysis bullosa acquisita and anti-p200 pemphigoid—how to treat it? Int J Dermatol 2007;46:295–8.

6. Marinovic B, Mokos Bukvic Z, Basta-Juzbasic A, et al. Atypical clinical appearance of pemphigus vulgaris on the face: case report. Acta Dermatovenerol Croat 2005;13:81–4.

7. Marinovic B, Basta-Juzbasic A, Bukvic Mokos Z, et al. Coexistence of pemphigus herpetiformis and systemic lupus erythematosus. J Eur Acad Dermatol Venereol 2003;17:316–9.

8. Pasic A, Ljubojevic S, Lipozencic J, et al. Coexistence of psoriasis vulgaris, bullous pemphigoid and vitiligo: a case report. J Eur Acad Dermatol Venereol 2002;16:426–7.

Prevalence and Treatment of Pemphigus in Iran

Cheyda Chams-Davatchi, MD

KEYWORDS

- Autoimmune bullous disease • Pemphigus • Treatment
- Management

Autoimmune bullous diseases (ABD) are a group of diseases caused by autoantibodies against the dermoepidermal junction and desmosome, cleaving the skin and mucous membrane. The clinical forms and the prevalence seem to be different from one continent to another.

Since 1984, patients with bullous disease have been seen in our ABD Research Center. In a study from March 1997 to February 2006, 1402 cases of ABD were seen in our center. At this time, the population of Iran was approximately 72.5 million with 8 million in Tehran. Pemphigus vulgaris (PV) was the most frequent ABD at 81.2% (95% confidence interval [CI] 79%–83.1%); followed by 11.6% bullous pemphigoid (95% CI 10.05%–13.4%) and 4.4% pemphigus foliaceus (95% CI 3.5%–5.6%). Much rarer were pemphigoid gestationis 0.7% (95% CI 0.4%–1.3%), mucous membrane pemphigoid 0.7% (95% CI 0.4%–1.3%), epidermolysis bullosa acquisita 0.5% (95% CI 0.2%–1.1%), linear IgA disease 0.4% (95% CI 0.2%–1%), paraneoplastic pemphigus 0.2% (95% CI 0.04%–0.67%), IgA pemphigus 0.2% (95% CI 0.04%–0.67%), and pemphigus erythematosus 0.1% (95% CI 0%–0.45%). Our center is the major referral center for ABDs in Iran.[1]

Patients with pemphigus were registered using a predefined computer-based data chart and saved into an electronic database. They were followed at the Pemphigus Research Unit regularly, and the database was updated subsequently. The diagnosis was based on clinical manifestations, the histologic pattern, and direct immunofluorescence (DIF). The analysis of the database,

performed in 2007, showed 1782 cases of pemphigus. The male/female ratio was 1:1.44. The mean age was 42 ± 19 years with 95% CI of 41.9 to 43.1. Familial pemphigus were found in 1.5% (95% CI 1%–1.4%) and juvenile pemphigus in 2.7% (95% CI 2%–3.6%) of the cohort.

The major clinical form of the disease was PV observed in 1606 patients (91.1%, CI 1.4). PV has different phenotypes: (1) the mucous membrane alone phenotype was seen in 19%; (2) skin and mucous membrane together phenotypes in 69%; (3) the skin alone phenotype in 12%.

The other clinical forms of the disease were: pemphigus foliaceus, which was seen in 7% (95% CI 5%–9%); pemphigus vegetans 2.6% (95% CI 1.7%–3.5%); and a few cases of drug-induced pemphigus, paraneoplastic pemphigus, and IgA pemphigus.[2]

Our group studied the frequency of HLA class II alleles (DRB, DQA1, and DQB1) and haplotypes in 52 Iranian non-Jewish patients with PV and in 180 normal individuals as the control group. The results of our study showed that 36.5% of the patients with PV carry the HLA-DRB1*04, DQA1* 0301, DQB1*0302 haplotype versus 5.5% in the control group (P<.0001). In the patients, 25% carry the HLA-DRB1*1401, DQA1*0104, DQB1*0502 haplotype versus 4.4% in the control group (P<.0001). Ashkenazi Jewish PV carry the DRB1*040, DQB1*0302 haplotype. Our findings suggest that the susceptibility complex of PV histocompatibility class II alleles in non-Jewish Iranians patients with PV is the same as the Ashkenazi Jewish PV.[3] A previous study reported the same finding and

Department of Dermatology, Autoimmune Bullous Disease Research Center, Razi Hospital, Tehran University for Medical Sciences, Vahdat Eslami Square, Tehran 11996, Iran
E-mail address: cheyda@davatchi.net

Dermatol Clin 29 (2011) 681–683
doi:10.1016/j.det.2011.06.011
0733-8635/11/$ – see front matter © 2011 Elsevier Inc. All rights reserved.

concluded that they probably derive from the same ancestor.[4]

In a study done in 2005, the prevalence of pemphigus in Iran was found to be about 30 per 100,000 inhabitants. The incidence per 100,000 inhabitants per year was 1.6 in Tehran and 1 for Iran.[5] An average of 4 new cases per week are seen in the ABD Research Center in Tehran.

Our treatment strategy is to start prednisolone, an indispensable drug for pemphigus, plus cytotoxic drugs. Prednisolone is started at 2 mg per kg of body weight per day (total dose not going over 120 mg/d). Then, as soon as no new blisters appear and the lesions are dried, the total dose is reduced by one-third. Then every 3 days or every other day, the dose of prednisolone is reduced by 5 mg to reach 30 mg per day. Then prednisolone is gradually tapered by 1.25 mg per week to reach 15 mg per day, and then every 2 weeks to reach 7.5 or 5 mg per day. After 6 months, if DIF[6] and enzyme-linked immunosorbent assay (ELISA) are negative, the dose of prednisolone is reduced to 2.5 mg and then the treatment is stopped.[7]

In addition to steroid, a cytotoxic drug is added to the regimen. Azathioprine was shown to be efficient.[8,9] We start our patients at 2.5 mg per kg per day, or mycophenolate mofetil 2 g per day. Thiopurine S-methyltransferase activity is not measured routinely before using azathioprine (not available in Iran).[10] Mycophenolate mofetil is a more expensive drug than azathioprine, and some patients cannot afford it, but it is a very efficient drug in some patients and is well tolerated[7–9,11,12] If azathioprine has side effects, or is not efficient, it is changed to mycophenolate mofetil, or vice versa . If azathioprine and mycophenolate are not effective, the patients is switched to oral cyclophosphamide 100 mg/d for 3 to 6 months. Oral cyclophosphamide has important side effects in treatment of long duration, especially in young patients. If cyclophosphamide is not efficient, rituximab (anti-CD20 antibody)[13–15] or IVIg[16–18] is used but they are expensive and few patients can afford these drugs.

In cases of complete remission, if the disease is dependent on steroids, more than 15 mg prednisolone daily, other drugs, including dapsone, methotrexate gold are tried. They sometimes seem efficient, although there is no evidence.

Some patients on a minimum dose of 5 to 7.5 mg/d of prednisolone relapse frequently, but localized to the face or head, and always in the same place. These patients receive triamcinolone acetonide intralesionally every week diluted as 20 mg/mL in lidocaine. As pemphigus foliaceus, can also be severe, this is treated in the same way as PV. In pregnant patients, the starting dose of prednisolone is 30 mg per day, plus application 15 g of corticosteroid on normal skin when the disease is severe. In juvenile patients, we prefer prednisolone plus dapsone. If the disease is severe and does not respond, azathioprine or mycophenolate mofetil is used.

In conclusion, early treatment and adequate drugs adapted for each patient are the mainstay of treatment. It is worthwhile reaching the minimum possible level of corticosteroid whenever possible. Patient education and prevention of relapses and complications are essential. The patient must avoid triggers (stress being the most important), infections especially herpes simplex, and drugs and vaccinations that induce pemphigus. Possibly avoidance of some food and toxic substances are also important in the management of these patients.

Pemphigus seems to be more frequent in Iran, with a more severe phenotype and younger patients. Multicenter studies are warranted to find the best and most cost-effective treatment.

REFERENCES

1. Daneshpazhooh M, Chams-Davatchi C, Payandemehr P. Spectrum of autoimmune bullous diseases in Iran: a 10-year review. Presented at 18th EADV Congress, October 7–10, 2009, Berlin/Germany. p. 152.
2. Chams-Davatchi C, Daneshpazhooh M, Esmaili N. Analysis of 1782 pemphigus. Presented at 21st World Congress of Dematology, October 1–5, 2007, Buenos Aires (Argentina);75:1190.
3. Shams S, Amirzargar AA, Yousefi M, et al. HLA class II (DRB, DQA1 and DQB1) allele and haplotype frequencies in the patients with pemphigus vulgaris. J Clin Immunol 2009;29:175–9.
4. Mobini N, Yunis EJ, Alper CA. Identical MHC markers in non-Jewish Iranian and Ashkenazi Jewish patients with pemphigus vulgaris; possible common central Asian ancestral origin. Hum Immunol 1997;57:62–7.
5. Chams- Davatchi C, Valikhani M, Daneshpazhooh M, et al. Pemphigus: analysis of 1209 cases. Int J Dermatol 2005;44:470–6.
6. Balighi K, Taheri A, Mansoori P, et al. Value of direct immunofluorescence in predicting remission in pemphigus vulgaris. Int J Dermatol 2006;45:1308.
7. Abasq C, Mouquet H, Gilbert D. ELISA testing of anti-desmoglein 1 and 3 antibodies in the management of pemphigus. Arch Dermatol 2009;145:529–35.
8. Chams-Davatchi C, Esmaili N, Daneshpazhooh M, et al. Randomized controlled open-label trial of 4 treatment regimens for pemphigus vulgaris. J Am Acad Dermatol 2007;57:622–8.
9. Martin LK, Werth V, Villanueva E. Interventions for pemphigus vulgaris and pemphigus foliaceus. Cochrane Database Syst Rev 2009;1:CD006263.

10. Firooz A, Ghandi N, Hallaji Z, et al. Role of thiopurine methyltransferase activity in the safety and efficacy of azathioprine in the treatment of pemphigus vulgaris. Arch Dermatol 2008;144:1143–7.

11. Beissert S, Minouni D, Kanvar AJ, et al. Treating pemphigus vulgaris with prednisone and mycophenolate mofetil: a multicenter, randomized, placebo-controlled trial. J Invest Dermatol 2010;130:2041–8.

12. Chams-Davatchi C, Nonahal Azar R, Daneshpazooh M, et al. Open trial of mycophenolate mofetil in the treatment of resistant pemphigus vulgaris. Ann Dermatol Venereol 2002;129:23–5.

13. Joly P, Mouquet H, Roujeau JC, et al. A single cycle for the treatment of severe pemphigus. N Engl J Med 2007;357:545–52.

14. Schmidt E, Goebeler M, Zillikens D. Rituximab in severe pemphigus. Ann N Y Acad Sci 2009;1173:683–91.

15. Hertl M, Zilikens D, Borradori L, et al. Recommendations for the use of rituximab (anti-CD20 antibody) in the treatment of autoimmune bullous skin diseases. J Dtsch Dermatol Ges 2008;6:366–73.

16. Lolis M, Toosi S, Czernick A, et al. Effect of intravenous immunoglobulin with or without cytotoxic drugs on pemphigus intercellular antibodies. J Am Acad Dermatol 2011;64(3):484–9.

17. Green MG, Bystryn JC. Effect of intravenous immunoglobulin therapy on serum levels of IgG1 and IgG4 antidesmoglein 1 and antidesmoglein 3 antibodies in pemphigus vulgaris. Arch Dermatol 2008;144:1621–4.

18. Amagai M, Ikeda S, Shimizu H, et al. A randomized double-blind trial of intravenous immunoglobulin for pemphigus. J Am Acad Dermatol 2009;60: 595–603.

Pemphigus Treatment in Japan

Akiko Tanikawa, MD, PhD,*, Masayuki Amagai, MD, PhD

KEYWORDS

- Pemphigus • Japan • Epidemiology • PDAI • ELISA

Pemphigus is a group of autoimmune blistering diseases characterized by blisters and erosive lesions on the skin and mucous membranes due to loss of cell and cell adhesion of keratinocytes. In 2010, new Japanese guidelines for the management of pemphigus were published for dermatologists. Systemic corticosteroid are the gold standard and the first choice of treatment of pemphigus. Desmoglein 1 (Dsg1) and desmoglein 3 (Dsg3) are the target antigens in pemphigus.[1]

According to a report from a research project of the Ministry of Health, Labour and Welfare of Japan, the incidence of pemphigus in Japan was 4085 in 2007. The male-to-female ratio was 1:1.5. The average age of onset of the disease was approximately 60 years with a peak in the 50s. Among different subtypes in pemphigus; pemphigus vulgaris was 65%, pemphigus foliaceus 23%, pemphigus erythematosus 6%, pemphigus vegetans 2%, and the unclassified subtype 4%. Among the total Japanese cases, 5.0% were in the severe group, 20.4% in the moderate group, and 74.0% in the mild group, as evaluated by the Japanese disease severity score.[2] In contrast, when focusing on new cases per year, 20.6% were in the severe group, 45.2% in the moderate group, and 34.2% in the mild group.

In 2010, new Japanese guidelines for the management of pemphigus were published for dermatologists[3] and their English version will be published soon. In Japan, the gold standard and the first choice of treatment of pemphigus, as accepted worldwide, are systemic corticosteroids.

The treatment protocol has two major phases: consolidation and maintenance. The consolidation phase indicates the initial phase of the treatment to control the disease activity (to minimize new blister formation and start to withdraw prednisolone [PSL] dosages, usually 2 to 4 weeks after the initial treatment); the maintenance phase is defined as the period when the disease is under control and the PSL is being reduced (early phase, PSL 60 to 20 mg/day; and late phase, PSL <20 mg/day). The definition and treatment goals follow the statement of the International Pemphigus Committee in 2008,[4] namely to reduce the disease activity rapidly by using different therapeutic options and to control disease activity with minimal corticosteroid dosing (PSL $\leq$0.2 mg/kg/day or PSL $\leq$10 mg/day). The choice of adjuvant therapy in Japan is strongly influenced by the insurance system. High-dose intravenous immunoglobulin (IVIG) is an effective therapeutic option for refractory pemphigus. In Japan, a randomized double-blind controlled trial for high-dose IVIG for pemphigus was performed and demonstrated that a single cycle with high-dose IVIG successfully suppresses the disease activity of steroid-resistant pemphigus.[5] Based on this study, IVIG has been covered by national insurance in Japan since 2009. Corticosteroid pulse therapy and plasmapheresis are other options used during the consolidation phase. As adjuvant therapies, immunosuppressants, such as azathioprine, cyclosporine, cyclophosphamide, and methotrexate, are considered steroid-sparing agents.

Department of Dermatology, Keio University School of Medicine, 35 Shinanomachi Shinjuku-ku, Tokyo 160-8582, Japan
* Corresponding author.
E-mail address: tanikawa@sc.itc.keio.ac.jp

Dermatol Clin 29 (2011) 685–686
doi:10.1016/j.det.2011.07.004
0733-8635/11/$ – see front matter © 2011 Elsevier Inc. All rights reserved.

The guidelines also recommend the pemphigus disease area index (PDAI) as a new measure to evaluate pemphigus disease activity.[3] In Japan, ELISA has been widely used not only for making serologic diagnosis but also for monitoring disease activity. The cost for ELISA is covered by national insurance. In the consolidation phase, when active lesions still exist, the disease activity is evaluated by PDAI, whereas in the maintenance phase, when no active lesions are seen, ELISA provides a useful indicator for guidance in reducing corticosteroids.[6] By using a combination of the PDAI and ELISA, pemphigus can be managed in a more objective and efficient way.

Although rituximab and mycophenolate mofetil are widely recognized as efficient drugs for refractory cases of pemphigus,[7] they are not yet approved in Japan. Government approval requires independent clinical trials to be conducted in Japan. On the other hand, Japan has a unique system to cover essentially all the medical costs, including inpatient care, for patients with 56 intractable diseases. Pemphigus is approved as one of the intractable diseases.

ACKNOWLEDGMENTS

This work was partly supported by Health and Labour Sciences Research Grants for Research on Measures for Intractable Diseases from the Ministry of Health, Labour and Welfare of Japan.

REFERENCES

1. Amagai M. Pemphigus. In: Bolognia JL, Jorizzo JL, Rapini RP, et al, editors. Dermatology. 2nd edition. Spain: Mosby; 2008. p. 417–29.
2. Immamura S. A form for the diagnosis of pemphigus. Annual Report of the Intractable Skin Disease Study Group. Japan: Ministry of Welfare and Health of Japan; 1991. p. 12 [in Japanese].
3. Committee for Guidelines for the Management of Pemphigus Disease, Amagai M, Tanikawa A, et al. Guidelines for the management of Pemphigus. Jpn J Dermatol 2010;120(7):1443–60.
4. Murrell DF, Dick S, Ahmed AR, et al. Consensus statement on definitions of disease, end points, and therapeutic response for pemphigus. J Am Acad Dermatol 2008;58:1043–6.
5. Amagai M, Ikeda S, Shimizu H, et al. A randomized double-blind trial of intravenous immunoglobulin for pemphigus. J Am Acad Dermatol 2009;60:595–603.
6. Tanikawa A. Managing pemphigus with PDAI (Pemphigus Disease Area Index), a new measure for disease activity in pemphigus. Clin Dermatol 2011; 65:110–3.
7. Faurschou A, Gniadecki R. Two courses of rituximab (anti-CD20 monoclonal antibody) for recalcitrant pemphigus vulgaris. Int J Dermatol 2008;47:292–4.

The Autoimmune Blistering Diseases in Australia: Status and Services

Benjamin S. Daniel, BA, BCom, MBBS, MMed (Clin Epi)[a,b],
Andrew Dermawan[a,b],
Dédée F. Murrell, MA, BMBCh, FAAD, MD, FACD[c,*]

KEYWORDS
- Autoimmune blistering diseases • Pemphigus
- Bullous pemphigoid

The term autoimmune bullous disease (AIBD) refers to a heterogeneous group of blistering conditions with varying rates of mortality and morbidity. A strong genetic component is proposed, supported by differing prevalence rates between countries. Australia, the smallest continent and the sixth largest country, has a population of just more than 22 million people,[1] with the majority living in the eight major state and territory capitals of Canberra, Sydney, Melbourne, Brisbane, Perth, Adelaide, Hobart, and Darwin (**Fig. 1**).

In 2008, there were more than 78,900 registered medical practitioners in Australia, with more working in major cities than rural and remote areas.[2] A shortage of rural doctors has resulted in reduced facilities and services to the rural and remote areas. To counter this, the various federal governments have developed programs and incentives to recruit, relocate, and maintain health practitioners in rural and remote locations. These issues now influence medical student selection, specialty training, and salaries.[3,4] Most, if not all, medical practitioners in Australia have had some exposure to rural locations as part of their career. Technological advances have recently been used to deliver health care to rural areas. Teledermatology in Australia was first reported in 1999[5] and its use has increased owing to an expansion of technology and commonwealth funding.[6] Despite the paucity of published reports regarding the diagnosis of blistering diseases with teledermatology,[7] its use in Australia is promising for the provision of dermatologic services to patients in rural locations without access to a dermatologist.

There are more than 130 Aboriginal and Torres Strait islander doctors in Australia[8] treating indigenous and nonindigenous patients. There is marked inequality between indigenous and nonindigenous health in both rural and urban areas, sparking a recent commitment from the commonwealth government to increase funding and introduce measures to close the life-expectancy gap between the two groups.[9] The true incidence of AIBD amongst Aboriginal Australians is unknown, probably owing to isolation, itinerant lifestyles, lack of facilities, and cultural differences. Only one reported case of bullous pemphigoid has been reported in an Aboriginal Australian, though it is likely there are many others with an AIBD who have not been diagnosed.[10]

[a] Department of Dermatology, St George Hospital, Gray Street, Kogarah, Sydney, NSW 2217, Australia
[b] Faculty of Medicine, University of New South Wales, Sydney, NSW 2052, Australia
[c] Department of Dermatology, St George Hospital, University of New South Wales, Gray Street, Kogarah, Sydney, NSW 2217, Australia
* Corresponding author.
E-mail address: d.murrell@unsw.edu.au

Dermatol Clin 29 (2011) 687–690
doi:10.1016/j.det.2011.07.002

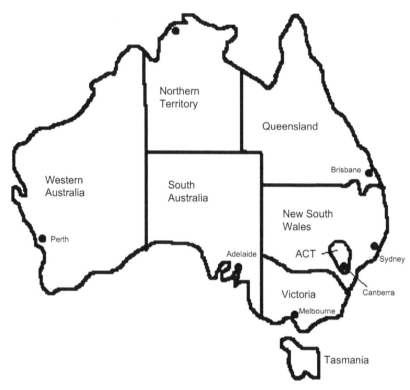

Fig. 1. Australia, the smallest continent and the sixth largest country.

AIBD REGISTRY

Because of limited data about AIBD in Australia, a registry has been set up to determine the frequency, mortality, and associated conditions. It is expected the registry will aid research in Australia by providing epidemiologic data, as well as by maintaining an up-to-date database with patient contact details.

The main purpose of a medical registry is to collect and categorize extensive amounts of data and information about a disease. The data can then be analyzed to facilitate research into the cause, pathogenesis, and prognosis of a disease. Registries play a significant role in the advancement of research in rare diseases such as AIBD by creating a greater awareness of the disease as well as providing an acceptable means to approach government and other institutions for financial and social aid.[11] In general, registries are either hospital-based or population-based.[12] Hospital-based registries gather information about patients who have attended a hospital. The AIBD registry in Australia is based on the Australian Epidermolysis Bullosa Registry, which was developed in 2006.[13] Ethical approval for the development and maintenance of a registry for AIBD was obtained in 2008. Patients with an AIBD are invited to participate in this registry. Participation involves providing their names, contact details, and medical history, as well as giving permission to access their medical records from hospitals or other clinicians. This permission is vital in confirming the diagnosis, assessing the incidence of disease, and investigating the cause and potential triggers. The registry allocates each patient a registry number so that he or she becomes de-identified for research purposes. Audits of the registry are regularly performed to identify inappropriate collection methods and ensure reliable data.[14]

Most patients in the Australian AIBD registry are recruited from the practices of dermatologists in Australia. The practice of Professor Dédée F. Murrell, situated in Sydney since 1996, has provided the most patients to date. This practice has a specialist bullous clinic treating patients from all of Australia. Other dermatologists who have interests in AIBD and have contributed to the registry include Drs Belinda Welsh, Christopher McCormack, and George Varigos, all from Melbourne, Victoria, about 850 km from Sydney. It is the authors' intention to publish more extensively when there are a sufficient number of patients included because, currently, the AIBD registry includes only 37 patients.

The Australasian College of Dermatologists (ACD), (www.dermcoll.asn.au/) is the professional body that oversees the training and education of dermatologists in Australia. In 1997, there were 258 practicing dermatologists, 92% of whom worked in capital cities and major urban centers. In 2005, there were 385 members of the ACD.[15] To determine the number of patients with AIBD seen in a given year, a survey was distributed among the members of the ACD who use an online web server to discuss professional issues; it was then posted. In 2011, an online survey was completed by eight dermatologists. The response rate was too low to make definitive claims; however, it is clear that there are some dermatologists see fewer than 10 cases of AIBD per year and refer them to specialist clinics, and several who stated that they had not seen any AIBD patients in the past 12 months.

DIAGNOSIS AND MANAGEMENT

Skin biopsies are routinely performed by Australian dermatologists and sent to local or specialty laboratories for dermatopathologic evaluation. Direct immunofluorescence on perilesional skin and indirect immunofluorescence testing are typically available at laboratory centers in the major capital centers, in particular the Skin and Cancer Foundation Australia located in Sydney, Melbourne, and Brisbane. Antidesmoglein antibody testing, however, is not routinely available apart from a research laboratory at Westmead Hospital in Sydney, where it is part of a collaborative research project with the authors' group.

Immunosuppressive agents to treat AIBD,[16] such as systemic corticosteroids and azathioprine, are commonly prescribed and accessible via Medicare in Australia, though special approval is required for the use of intravenous immunoglobulin.[17] Other medications, in particular mycophenolate and rituximab, are not currently covered on Medicare. Australian private medical insurance typically does not provide adequate coverage for expensive medications. Some teaching hospital dermatology departments are able to cover the costs of these drugs, subject to approval by each hospital's drug committee, but this tends to be restricted to patients residing within the local area. These medications are not subsidized by the Australian government for the indication of AIBD. The cost is borne by patients or hospitals, unlike the cost of the same drugs when used for patients receiving transplants and patients with cancer. These patients have been known to remain on high doses of corticosteroids for many months while trying to find another hospital specialist, such as an immunologist, in their local area who could provide these drugs.

PATIENT SUPPORT GROUP

A patient support group called the Australasian Blistering Diseases Foundation (ABDF), www.blisters.org.au, was founded in 2007 by Professor Murrell and Dr Linda Martin, to provide education, support, research, and advocacy for all patients with any blistering condition and their caretakers. Most members are patients with AIBD or genetic blistering diseases (eg, epidermolysis bullosa), and their relatives and caretakers, although health professionals and members of the community also join. The ABDF is instrumental in supporting research in bullous disorders and providing patients with the opportunity to participate in research and view the latest results. Annual charity fun-runs are organized to promote a greater awareness of the ABDF, simultaneously raising funds to support research. The ABDF recently received a grant to fund an epidermolysis bullosa nurse at St George Hospital.

SUMMARY

Though the exact epidemiology of autoimmune bullous disorders in Australia is unknown, a registry and patient support group has been developed to investigate the incidence, geographic distribution, and possible trigger factors of disease, while catering to the needs of patients and/or caregivers. The current focus is the expansion of the registry by generating an increased awareness among dermatologists. There is ongoing research into precipitating factors, diagnostic methods, and therapeutic agents for AIBD.

REFERENCES

1. Available at: http://www.abs.gov.au/ausstats/abs@.nsf/94713ad445ff1425ca25682000192af2/1647509ef7e25faaca2568a900154b63!OpenDocument. Accessed August 5, 2011.
2. AIHW. Medical labour force 2008. Cat. no. AUS 131. Canberra (Australia): AIHW; 2010.
3. Somers GT, Jolly B, Strasser RP. The SOMERS index: a simple instrument designed to predict the likelihood of rural career choice. Aust J Rural Health 2011;19(2):75–80.
4. Henry JA, Edwards BJ, Crotty B. Why do medical graduates choose rural careers? Rural Remote Health 2009;9(1):1083.
5. Tait CP, Clay CD. Pilot study of store and forward teledermatology services in Perth, Western Australia. Australas J Dermatol 1999;40(4):190–3.
6. Muir J, Lucas L. Tele-dermatology in Australia. Stud Health Technol Inform 2008;131:245–53.

7. Feldman SR, Vallejos QM, Whalley LE, et al. Blistering eruption in a Latino migrant farmworker. J Agromedicine 2007;12(4):81–5.

8. O'Mara P. Close the gap: Australian indigenous doctors' association. Med J Aust 2009;190(10):607.

9. Eades SJ, Taylor B, Bailey S, et al. SEARCH Investigators. The health of urban Aboriginal people: insufficient data to close the gap. Med J Aust 2010;193(9):521–4.

10. Lo S, Mollison LC, Kumar A. Bullous pemphigoid in an Aborigine. Australas J Dermatol 1993;34(2):41–4.

11. Roos LL, Nicol JP. A research registry: uses, development, and accuracy. J Clin Epidemiol 1999;52(1):39–47.

12. Naldi L, Chatenoud L. Registry research in dermatology. Dermatol Clin 2009;27(2):185–91, vii.

13. Kho YC, Rhodes LM, Robertson SJ, et al. Epidemiology of epidermolysis bullosa in the antipodes: the Australasian Epidermolysis Bullosa Registry with a focus on Herlitz junctional epidermolysis bullosa. Arch Dermatol 2010;146(6):635–40.

14. Willis CD, Jolley DJ, McNeil JJ, et al. Identifying and improving unreliable items in registries through data auditing. Int J Qual Health Care 2011;23(3):317–23.

15. ACD annual report. 2006. Available at: http://www.dermcoll.asn.au/downloads/ACD_annualreport06.pdf. Accessed July 5, 2011.

16. Daniel BS, Murrell DF. The actual management of pemphigus. G Ital Dermatol Venereol 2010;145(5):689–702.

17. Smith SD, Dennington PM, Cooper A. The use of intravenous immunoglobulin for treatment of dermatological conditions in Australia: a review. Australas J Dermatol 2010;51(4):227–37.

Autoimmune Bullous Diseases in Austria

Martin Laimer, MD*, Gabriela Pohla-Gubo, PhD,
Lukas Kraus, MD, Elke Nischler, MD, J.W. Bauer, MD,
V. Ahlgrimm-Siess, MD, Helmut Hintner, MD

KEYWORDS

- Autoimmune bullous diseases • Austria • Epidemiology
- Registry • Diagnosis • Therapy

AUTOIMMUNE BULLOUS DISEASES

Autoimmune bullous diseases (AIBD) refer to a group of rare (ie, orphan disease) tissue-specific autoimmune disorders targeting the structural and functional integrity of skin and mucous membranes. Driven by genetic susceptibility, both the humoral and cellular immune systems are synergistically involved in the pathogenesis of these potentially life-threatening entities. As a unifying feature, circulating autoantibodies induce intraepidermal, junctional (in lamina lucida of the basement membrane zone [BMZ]), or dermolytic (below lamina densa of the BMZ) cleavage, leading to characteristic cutaneous blisters and erosions. This process is supposed to occur by mechanisms of steric hindrance or induction of inflammatory signal transduction cascades as well as apoptotic pathways.[1]

Many AIBD have a chronic, relapsing, and often progressive course, and extensive disease may be complicated by scarring, superinfections, multisystemic involvement, and catabolism. This process causes significant morbidity (as for example by blindness, **Fig. 1**) and even mortality (also by side effects of therapy), as well as considerably high costs because treatment and regular follow-ups may be expensive (eg, €2200 for 500 mg rituximab), intensive, and lifelong. Current treatment modalities, including corticosteroids and corticosteroid-sparing adjuvant immunosuppressive or immunomodulatory agents, are effective, but a remarkable side-effect profile may limit their applicability. Moreover, most of the drugs have never been evaluated in large controlled studies, due to the rareness of AIBD.

Therefore, collecting data of affected individuals in national and international registries on AIBD, covering clinical, diagnostic, and therapeutic data as well as biobanking, should provide a comprehensive database to facilitate clinical and investigative studies as a further step toward better patient care.

EPIDEMIOLOGY OF AIBD IN AUSTRIA

Currently lacking an integrative administrative approach in Austria, exact data on the national epidemiology of AIBD are largely missing. Between 1990 and 2007, the authors' own departmental registry in Salzburg, serving a catchment area of about 650,000 inhabitants from Salzburg, neighboring districts of Upper Austria, and Bavaria, enrolled a total of 270 AIBD patients (**Fig. 2**). About 50% of these patients were (newly) diagnosed for bullous pemphigoid (BP) and another 10% for each pemphigus disease (including pemphigus vulgaris [PV], and pemphigus foliaceus [PF]), cicatricial (mucous membrane) pemphigoid (CP) and epidermolysis bullosa acquisita (EBA). The remainder were classified as suffering from dermatitis herpetiformis Duhring (DHD, 7%), linear IgA dermatosis (LAD, 4%), lichen ruber pemphigoides (LRP, 3%) and, even more rarely, gestational

Disclosures: The authors declare no conflict of interest. This work was supported by the "Verein zur Förderung der Universitätsklinik für Dermatologie Salzburg (St-Johanns-Spital)".

Department of Dermatology, Paracelsus Medical University Salzburg, Muellner Hauptstrasse 48, A-5020 Salzburg, Austria
* Corresponding author.
E-mail address: m.laimer@salk.at

Dermatol Clin 29 (2011) 691–698
doi:10.1016/j.det.2011.06.001

derm.theclinics.com

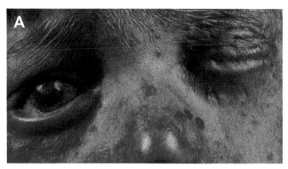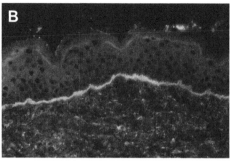

Fig. 1. (A) Blindness in a boy with IgA epidermolysis bullosa acquisita. (B) Linear band of IgA in the basement membrane of a biopsy of clinically normal-appearing skin (direct immunofluorescence with anti-IgA antibody, original magnification ×400).

pemphigoid (GP, 2%), IgA pemphigus (IgA-P, 1%), and paraneoplastic pemphigus (PNP, <1%).

These epidemiologic data correspond overall to published incidence rates, while the calculated higher frequency of EBA (0.22/100.000 vs 0.017–0.026 in the literature) and a lower incidence of DHD (0.2 vs 0.98–10) most probably reflect statistical limitations attributable to the small study population.

Comparability of epidemiologic studies, even when referring to matchable study populations,[2] is limited because of rareness of disease, small cohort sizes, and inconsistent study sampling, as well as differences in observation periods, diagnostic algorithms, immunogenetic background, and procedures of referral management (eg, general practitioner vs dermatologist).

With regard to the authors' registry, the calculated total incidence rate for AIBD in the land of Salzburg is 2.13/100,000. It is significantly lower in rural (1.64) compared with urban areas (3.08). This statistic is supposed to reflect varying numbers of unreported cases, as yet undefined environmental causes, differences in lifestyle, health-seeking behavior, and sociodemographic conditions. As about 17% of the registered patients are non-native Austrians of mostly Mediterranean descent who mainly live within urban areas, racial predilection due to a more sensitive genetic background (human leukocyte antigen class II allele profile) may be another important modifying factor of the regional AIBD incidence.

During the observation period of 17 years, the total number of cases admitted per year had gradually increased along with generally anticipated higher incidence rates. The latter possibly reflect the increased life expectancy of the general population that predisposes for diseases of the elderly, an increase in genetically susceptible non-native Austrians, advances in diagnostic tools (increase in diagnostic sensitivity and specificity, eg, in prodromal or atypical stages), and increased consciousness of these diseases (eg, consistent inclusion of GP in the differential diagnosis in all pregnant patients with long-standing pruritic skin lesions[2]).

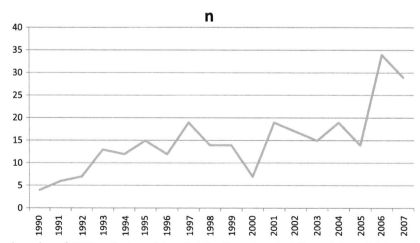

Fig. 2. Annual number of AIBD patients registered at the Department of Dermatology, Salzburg, between 1990 and 2007 (total 270).

In 2008, the authors performed a survey among all university and nonuniversity hospitals with inpatient dermatology departments to assess the frequency of AIBD in Austria for 2006. Methodologically, screening for AIBD patients was based on direct and indirect immunofluorescence study results indicative of AIBD, which were obtained from departmental and associated diagnostic laboratories in this year. Immunofluorescence data were then correlated with the most recent medical report. Anonymously registered and categorized for a specific AIBD, every patient's definitive diagnosis had to be confirmed according to the requirements of the authors' own departmental registry, that is, by correlation of clinical presentation, histology, and specific immunopathological findings in direct and indirect immunofluorescence, autoantibody serology, or immunoblotting.

In this study, 370 patients were enrolled nationwide who had been diagnosed for PV (73), pemphigus vegetans (Pveg, 2), PF (20), pemphigus erythematosus (PE, 1), PNP (2), BP (205), CP (4), GP (5), LAD (4), LRP (8), EBA (6), and DHD (49) (**Fig. 3**).

Of note, in this population, although only individually counted (exclusion of double reports), no differentiation was made between newly diagnosed individuals or patients with known, mostly long-lasting AIBD and disease relapse or those under control. However, this survey provided a quantitative estimate on the distribution of AIBD entities in Austria that in terms of incidence again roughly corresponded to published epidemiologic data (reviewed in Ref.[2]).

Intended to foster the establishment of an Austrian registry covering relevant data of all patients diagnosed or treated for AIBD in national dermatologic centers, this study, however, also clearly demonstrated the obstacles and limitations of such an initiative. Thus, one major finding was the lack of national standardization of data acquisition, registration, archivation, and administration on AIBD as a prerequisite for the implementation of a registry. Likewise, user-friendly (electronic) access to databases, continuous usage of a universal nomenclature and classification system (eg, coding according to the International Statistical Classification of Diseases and Related Health Problems, ICD-10), adherence to defined diagnostic criteria, and standardized discriminative diagnostic algorithms were inconsistently and sometimes insufficiently implemented among the participating institutions. Considering the vision to establish international archives to cover also very rare subentities, these problems are likely to become even more evident and thus should be primarily addressed by future strategies.

This approach, however, is one major prerequisite to the comprehensive characterization of disease causes and pathogenic pathways as well as a multidisciplinary support devoted to the principles of medical best practices and state-of-the-art care.

The value of AIBD registries is manifold. Studies such as the one presented here

- provide data on the prevalence of distinct (entity-specific) clinical symptoms and comorbidities to assess activity, course, drug-specific therapeutic efficacy, and side-effect profile as well as importance of preventive multidisciplinary care (eg, topical steroids in BP; osteoporosis and prescription of bisphosphonates);
- facilitate the identification and development of clinical parameters to quantitatively and qualitatively measure disease activity, clinical response, or relapses as well as subjective impairment (eg, entity-specific mean time of hospitalization; autoimmune bullous skin disorder intensity score);
- determine age of onset and gender and race predilection of AIBD;
- assess the specificity and sensitivity of distinct diagnostic tools to improve diagnostic algorithms[3] and identification of patients at risk;
- facilitate the design of novel immunomodulatory therapeutic approaches[4];

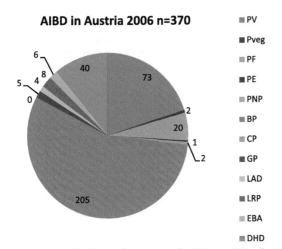

AIBD in Austria 2006 n=370

■ PV
■ Pveg
■ PF
■ PE
■ PNP
■ BP
■ CP
■ GP
■ LAD
■ LRP
■ EBA
■ DHD

Fig. 3. Distribution of registered AIBD entities in Austria in 2006. CP, cicatricial (mucous membrane) pemphigoid; DHD, dermatitis herpetiformis Duhring; EBA, epidermolysis bullosa acquisita; GP, gestational pemphigoid; IgA-P, IgA pemphigus; LAD, linear IgA dermatosis; LRP, lichen ruber pemphigoides; PE, pemphigus erythematosus; PF, pemphigus foliaceus; PNP, paraneoplastic pemphigus; PV, pemphigus vulgaris; Pveg, pemphigus vegetans.

- allow to monitor laboratory values such as total protein level, blood sedimentation rate, or mean steroid dosage to assess therapy efficacy, therapy side effects, or compliance;
- elucidate predisposing and prognostic factors that lead to break of autotolerance and critically affect clinical features and final disease outcome, including race-specific genetic polymorphisms affecting inflammatory and tissue repair response, drugs, infections, or environmental factors; and
- provide epidemiologic data for the distribution of resources within the public health care system.

AIBD DIAGNOSIS IN AUSTRIA

The population of Austria, currently counting about 8.36 million inhabitants (Statistics Austria, www.statistik.at), is served by approximately 700 registered dermatologists working in hospitals, outpatient clinics, and private practices.

For multidisciplinary diagnostic and therapeutic measures (and adequate financial reimbursement), the majority of patients with complex AIBD, after seeing the family doctor or family dermatologist, is initially referred to one of currently 19 dermatology departments at university (8) or nonuniversity (11) hospitals, and are mostly treated as inpatients. The average time of hospitalization of AIBD patients in Salzburg is currently 10 to 13 days and this has gradually decreased in the last decade, which is primarily attributable to the efficacy of newly available therapeutics even in very severe AIBD subvariants.

Follow-up is done either in specialized outpatient clinics at the departments ("Spezialambulanz," "Spezialsprechstunde") or private practices with expertise. Thereby, a generally well-established care system for AIBD patients is available nationwide.

In correlation with the clinical presentation, routine (standard) diagnostic procedures for AIBD are available at almost all university and nonuniversity departments of dermatology as well as several associated laboratories. The techniques adhere to international practice guidelines and include the investigation of specimens from recent, intact blisters including surrounding perilesional tissue, clinically normal-appearing, non–sun-exposed skin (inner aspect of upper arm) or serum, with subsequent assessment by:

- Histology
- Immunofluorescence studies,[5] ie,
  - Direct immunofluorescence microscopy (perilesional and often also clinically uninvolved, sun-protected skin)
  - Indirect immunofluorescence microscopy (intercellular space pattern, BMZ pattern, endomysial antibody pattern)
  - Direct and indirect salt-split skin test
- Immunoserology using extracts from epidermis and cultured keratinocytes or recombinant epidermal and dermal adhesion and structural proteins as substrate (in Salzburg also in collaboration with Professor Hashimoto, Department of Dermatology, University School of Medicine, Kurume, Japan[6]).

Considering AIBD with a heterogeneous immune profile, screening is still broadly based on immunofluorescence studies because of their high sensitivity, although the latter may be compromised by varying (to low) amounts of circulating autoantibodies, especially in GP, CP, and EBA.

Commercially available enzyme-linked immunoassay (ELISA) systems are widely used to detect antibodies targeting BP180 NC16A, BP230, desmoglein 1 and 3, and tissue transglutaminase, as well as recombinant envoplakin and periplakin, with high specificity and sensitivity.[7]

In specialized laboratories, ELISA systems and immunoblotting analyses are available for detection of additional autoantibodies as, for example, against laminin 332, type VII collagen, p200 protein (laminin γ1 chain[8]), α6 integrin, β4 integrin, desmoplakin I/II, and the soluble ectodomain of type XVII collagen (LAD-1). In an academic setting, ELISA sensitivity is further increased up to 100% when various recombinant proteins encompassing various portions of the index antigen(s) (eg, NC16A domain, COOH-terminal portion, entire ectodomain, extracellular portions of BP230 in BP) are used in combination.[9]

ELISA systems require only 10 to 20 µL of serum and have several other advantages, including multiple sample testing that is rapid and easy to perform; better standardization compared with immunofluorescence assays; quantitative measurement and direct comparison of sera (standard amounts to coat wells; spectrophotometer); autoantibody isotyping for correlation with clinical activity and prognosis (PV, BP); and recognition (detection) of the tertiary and quaternary structure of antigens (conformational epitopes), as the assay is performed under native conditions and without denaturation (as with sodium dodecyl sulfate in Western blotting).[10]

Thus, this method is increasingly replacing immunoblot and immunoprecipitation techniques (eg, recombinant forms of BP180/230 expressed in prokaryotic or eukaryotic systems), which are technically much more demanding and solely available in specialized laboratories. Only in tricky cases, such as in elderly patients with itchy skin eruptions and nonspecific histologic findings, circulating antibodies to the basement membrane, reactivity with BP180 and BP230, but without evidence for deposits of immunoreactants in skin as assessed by immunofluorescence,[11] are more sensitive techniques such as immunoelectron microscopy used in a few specialized academic institutions.

Concomitantly, relevant differential diagnoses, including infectious and other immunologic causes of blistering (bullous impetigo, staphylococcal scalded skin syndrome, erythema exsudativum multiforme, erosive lichen ruber of mucous membranes, bullous drug eruption, and so forth) as well as hereditary bullous diseases must of course be ruled out according to a diagnostic algorithm.[3]

Exact diagnosis of AIBD is accompanied by specific staging procedures to assess causative, permissive, or associated diseases (**Table 1**).

AIBD THERAPY IN AUSTRIA

High-quality controlled, prospective clinical trials for the treatment of AIBD, addressing issues such as optimal dosage of corticosteroid and adjuvants or long-term side effects, are largely absent, due to the rarity of the disease.[12] Thus, the spectrum of therapeutics licensed for the treatment is highly limited and off-label use is routine. Treatment decisions are mainly guided by published reviews, the few accessible guidelines of national or international societies of dermatology, and personal experience, rather than evidence (**Table 2**).[13,14] This situation again underscores the importance to foster efforts for the implementation of AIBD registries.

Systemic corticosteroids remain the main standard therapy for most AIBDs, and are most frequently used. However, susceptibility to (induction of latent) infections, arterial hypertension, diabetes, gastrointestinal ulcers, osteoporosis, aseptic bone necrosis, and thromboembolism, as well as dosage correlating with lethality, must be

Table 1
Checklist for specific staging of selected AIBD

Disease	Check Specific Staging For
PNP	• Paraneoplastic autoimmune multiorgan syndrome (respiratory and gastrointestinal tract) • Internal malignancies, malignant lymphoproliferative and hematologic disorders • Epitope spreading: Dsg3, Dsg1, desmoplakin I and II, evoplakin, periplakin, plectin, BP230, 170-kDa protein, desmocollins 1–3, etc
IgA pemphigus	• Benign and malignant monoclonal IgA gammopathies and gastrointestinal disorders
BP	• Malignancies (discussed, age- rather than disease-related)[11]: digestive tract, urinary bladder, lung, lymphoproliferative disorders • Autoimmune diseases (rheumatoid arthritis, Hashimoto thyroiditis, dermatomyositis, lupus erythematosus, autoimmune thrombocytopenia) • Psoriasis, lichen planus, neurologic disorders[25–28] • Epitope spreading within BP180 and BP230 • High IgG ELISA-BP180 NC16A titers as putative indicator for increased relapse risk[29]
Antiepiligrin mucous membrane pemphigoid	• Solid cancer[30]
GP	• Choriocarcinoma, hydatiform mole
DHD	• Autoimmune disorders (autoimmune thyroiditis, type I diabetes, lupus erythematosus, Sjögren disease, vitiligo) • Gut lymphomas associated with long-standing CD (and possibly DHD)
EBA	• Bullous systemic lupus erythematosus • Systemic diseases (inflammatory bowel disease)[31,32]
LAD	• Inflammatory bowel disease, sclerosing cholangitis

Table 2
Standard therapeutic modalities for selected AIBD at the Department of Dermatology, Salzburg

Disease	Therapy Standards
Pemphigus diseases	1. Topical and systemic corticosteroids, doxycycline for desquamative gingivitis 2. Corticosteroid-sparing adjuvant immunosuppressive or immunomodulatory agents such as azathioprine (AZA), mycophenolate mofetil (MMF), dapsone (for PF) 3. Intermittent steroid pulse therapy, rituximab (primary option in PNP), optionally in combination with immunoadsorption techniques,[a] or high-dose intravenous immunoglobulins (IVIG) 4. Cyclophosphamide-dexamethasone pulse therapy
BP	1. Topical steroids (clobetasol propionate 0.05%) for mild and localized BP variants 2. Systemic corticosteroids 3. Corticosteroid-sparing adjuvant immunosuppressive or immunomodulatory agents such as AZA, MMF, dapsone 4. Pulse corticosteroid therapy, plasmapheresis,[a] photopheresis,[a] rituximab combined with immunoapheresis or IVIG, pulse cyclophosphamide
DHD	1. Dapsone, sulfonamides (sulfapyridine, sulfamethoxypyridazine) 2. Gluten-free diet
EBA	Oral corticosteroids, immunosuppressive agents such as AZA, methotrexate, or cyclophosphamide (inflammatory variants); dapsone and prednisone (childhood EBA) Colchicine; adjuvant rituximab and IVIG, in combination with immunosuppressives, immune adsorption/plasmapheresis,[a] and extracorporeal photochemotherapy[33–39,a]

[a] Unavailable therapy in Salzburg; patients with indication are referred to the Department of Dermatology, Medical University, Vienna.

considered and sufficiently addressed by regular controls and preventive measures under long-term treatment.[15,16] Reluctance to lesional (sometimes whole body) application of class IV topical corticosteroids in BP,[17] despite favorable data on efficacy and tolerability obtained with the highest level of evidence,[18–20] may reflect a selected cohort of usually more severely affected inpatients at dermatologic departments, but also common reservations about the study concept and protocol as well as its implementation in daily routine.

Corticosteroid-sparing adjuvant immunosuppressive or immunomodulatory agents such as azathioprine (thiopurine methyltransferase![21]) and mycophenolate mofetil are concomitantly used to reduce the cumulative steroid dose and associated mortality rate while maintaining efficacy, although they themselves may cause severe side effects and comorbidity necessitating rigid pre-, inter-, and post-therapy monitoring.

Access to advanced therapeutic modalities such as immunoadsorption techniques is rather limited and only available in few university departments.

In Austria, federal health insurance usually covers all costs of diagnostic procedures and treatment regimes that have been approved for the particular disease or are performed according to published expert recommendations.[22–24] In life-threatening diseases or in the absence of alternatives, off-label treatments will also be reimbursed when there is a consensus on effectiveness, that is, published data implying a therapeutic benefit.

SUMMARY

Dermatologic departments and/or associated laboratories in Austria apply standard diagnostic and therapeutic modalities to provide state-of-the-art diagnosis and treatment of AIBD. Most of the affected individuals are initially treated as inpatients, while follow-up is done either in specialized outpatient clinics at dermatologic departments of the hospital or in private practices with expertise. Thereby, a generally well-established care system for AIBD patients is available nationwide. Concomitant expenditures are usually covered by federal health insurance.

Considering the significant morbidity and mortality, but also rareness of AIBD, national and international standardization of AIBD administration in registries is a major requirement for further improvement in patient care.

ACKNOWLEDGMENTS

The authors thank the chairmen (in alphabetical order) of all Austrian university and nonuniversity dermatologic departments that participated in the epidemiologic survey of 2006: Werner Aberer (Graz), Josef Auböck (Linz), Peter Fritsch (Innsbruck), Herbert Hönigsmann (Vienna), Wolfgang Jurecka (Vienna), Helmut Kerl (Graz), Georg Klein (Linz), Paul Mischer (Wels), Robert Müllegger (Wiener Neustadt), Wolf Pachinger (Klagenfurt), Hubert Pehamberger (Vienna), Klemens Rappersberger (Vienna), Andreas Steiner (Vienna), Georg Stingl (Vienna), Robert Strohal (Feldkirch), Franz Trautinger (St Pölten), Beatrix Volc-Platzer (Vienna).

REFERENCES

1. Marchenko S, Chernyavsky AI, Arredondo J, et al. Antimitochondrial autoantibodies in pemphigus vulgaris: a missing link in disease pathophysiology. J Biol Chem 2010;285(6):3695–704.
2. Bertram F, Bröcker EB, Zillikens D, et al. Prospective analysis of the incidence of autoimmune bullous disorders in Lower Franconia, Germany. J Dtsch Dermatol Ges 2009;7(5):434–40.
3. Nischler E, Klausegger A, Hüttner C, et al. Diagnostic pitfalls in newborns and babies with blisters and erosions. Dermatol Res Pract 2009;2009:320403.
4. Di Bisceglie MB, Lucchese A, Crincoli V. Pemphigus: the promises of peptide immunotherapy. Immunopharmacol Immunotoxicol 2009; 31(4):509–15.
5. Pohla-Gubo G, Kraus L, Hintner H. Role of immunofluorescence microscopy in dermatology. G Ital Dermatol Venereol 2011;146(2):127–42.
6. Lanschuetzer CM, Pohla-Gubo G, Schafleitner B, et al. Telepathology using immunofluorescence/immunoperoxidase microscopy. J Telemed Telecare 2004;10(1):39–43.
7. Probst C, Schlumberger W, Stöcker W, et al. Development of ELISA for the specific determination of autoantibodies against envoplakin and periplakin in paraneoplastic pemphigus. Clin Chim Acta 2009;410(1–2):13–8.
8. Dainichi T, Kurono S, Ohyama B, et al. Anti-laminin gamma-1 pemphigoid. Proc Natl Acad Sci U S A 2009;106(8):2800–5.
9. Desai N, Allen J, Ali I, et al. Autoantibodies to basement membrane proteins BP180 and BP230 are commonly detected in normal subjects by immunoblotting. Australas J Dermatol 2008;49(3):137–41.
10. Kim G, Chen M, Hallel-Halevy D, et al. Epidermolysis bullosa acquisita. In: Hertl M, editor. Autoimmune diseases of the skin. Pathogenesis, diagnosis, management. 3rd edition. Vienna (NY): Springer; 2011. p. 113–36.
11. Di Zenzo G, Laffitte E, Zambruno G, et al. Bullous pemphigoid: clinical features, diagnostic markers, and immunopathogenic mechanisms. In: Hertl M, editor. Autoimmune diseases of the skin. Pathogenesis, diagnosis, management. 3rd edition. Vienna (NY): Springer; 2011. p. 65–96.
12. Martin LK, Werth V, Villanueva E, et al. Interventions for pemphigus vulgaris and pemphigus foliaceus. Cochrane Database Syst Rev 2009;1:CD006263.
13. Chan LS, Ahmed AR, Anhalt GJ, et al. The first international consensus on mucous membrane pemphigoid: definition, diagnostic criteria, pathogenic factors, medical treatment, and prognostic indicators. Arch Dermatol 2002;138(3):370–9.
14. Nischler C, Sadler E, Lazarova Z, et al. Ocular involvement in anti-epiligrin cicatricial pemphigoid. Eur J Ophthalmol 2006;16(6):867–9.
15. Liu Z, Sui W, Zhao M, et al. Subepidermal blistering induced by human autoantibodies to BP180 requires innate immune players in a humanized bullous pemphigoid mouse model. J Autoimmun 2008;31(4):331–8.
16. Patsatsi A, Vyzantiadis TA, Chrysomallis F, et al. Medication history of a series of patients with bullous pemphigoid from northern Greece—observations and discussion. Int J Dermatol 2009;48(2):132–5.
17. Hofmann SC, Kautz O, Hertl M, et al. Results of a survey of German dermatologists on the therapeutic approaches to pemphigus and bullous pemphigoid. J Dtsch Dermatol Ges 2009;7(3):227–33.
18. Joly P, Roujeau JC, Benichou J, et al. A comparison of two regimens of topical corticosteroids in the treatment of patients with bullous pemphigoid: a multicenter randomized study. J Invest Dermatol 2009;129(7):1681–7.
19. Joly P, Roujeau JC, Benichou J, et al, Bullous Diseases French Study Group. A comparison of oral and topical corticosteroids in patients with bullous pemphigoid. N Engl J Med 2002;346(5):321–7.
20. Rzany B, Partscht K, Jung M, et al. Risk factors for lethal outcome in patients with bullous pemphigoid: low serum albumin level, high dosage of glucocorticosteroids, and old age. Arch Dermatol 2002; 138(7):903–8.
21. Oender K, Lanschuetzer CM, Laimer M, et al. Introducing a fast and simple PCR-RFLP analysis for the detection of mutant thiopurine S-methyltransferase alleles TPMT*3A and TPMT*3C. J Eur Acad Dermatol Venereol 2006;20(4):396–400.
22. Zillikens D, Derfler K, Eming R, et al. Recommendations for the use of immunoapheresis in the treatment of autoimmune bullous diseases. J Dtsch Dermatol Ges 2007;5(10):881–7.
23. Hertl M, Zillikens D, Borradori L, et al. Recommendations for the use of rituximab (anti-CD20 antibody) in the treatment of autoimmune bullous skin diseases. J Dtsch Dermatol Ges 2008;6(5):366–73.

24. Enk A, Fierlbeck G, French L, et al. Use of high-dose immunoglobulins in dermatology. J Dtsch Dermatol Ges 2009;7(9):806–12.

25. Chan LS, Vanderlugt CJ, Hashimoto T, et al. Epitope spreading: lessons from autoimmune skin diseases. J Invest Dermatol 1998;110(2):103–9.

26. Leung CL, Zheng M, Prater SM, et al. The BPAG1 locus: alternative splicing produces multiple isoforms with distinct cytoskeletal linker domains, including predominant isoforms in neurons and muscles. J Cell Biol 2001;154(4):691–7.

27. Steiner-Champliaud MF, Schneider Y, Favre B, et al. BPAG1 isoform-b: complex distribution pattern in striated and heart muscle and association with plectin and alpha-actinin. Exp Cell Res 2010;316(3): 297–313.

28. Laffitte E, Burkhard PR, Fontao L, et al. Bullous pemphigoid antigen 1 isoforms: potential new target autoantigens in multiple sclerosis? Br J Dermatol 2005;152(3):537–40.

29. Bernard P, Reguiai Z, Tancrède-Bohin E, et al. Risk factors for relapse in patients with bullous pemphigoid in clinical remission: a multicenter, prospective, cohort study. Arch Dermatol 2009;145(5):537–42.

30. Egan CA, Lazarova Z, Darling TN, et al. Anti-epiligrin cicatricial pemphigoid: clinical findings, immunopathogenesis, and significant associations. Medicine (Baltimore) 2003;82(3):177–86.

31. Chan LS, Woodley DT. Pemphigoid: bullous and cicatricial. In: Lichtenstein LM, editor. Current therapy in allergy, immunology and rheumatology. 5th edition. St Louis (MO): AS Fauci Mosby; 1996. p. 93.

32. Lohi J, Leivo I, Tani T, et al. Laminins, tenascin and type VII collagen in colorectal mucosa. Histochem J 1996;28(6):431–40.

33. Gordon KB, Chan LS, Woodley DT. Treatment of refractory epidermolysis bullosa acquisita with extracorporeal photochemotherapy. Br J Dermatol 1997; 136(3):415–20.

34. Saha M, Cutler T, Bhogal B, et al. Refractory epidermolysis bullosa acquisita: successful treatment with rituximab. Clin Exp Dermatol 2009;34(8):e979–80.

35. Schmidt E, Benoit S, Bröcker EB, et al. Successful adjuvant treatment of recalcitrant epidermolysis bullosa acquisita with anti-CD20 antibody rituximab. Arch Dermatol 2006;142(2):147–50.

36. Crichlow SM, Mortimer NJ, Harman KE. A successful therapeutic trial of rituximab in the treatment of a patient with recalcitrant, high-titre epidermolysis bullosa acquisita. Br J Dermatol 2007;156(1):194–6.

37. Niedermeier A, Eming R, Pfütze M, et al. Clinical response of severe mechanobullous epidermolysis bullosa acquisita to combined treatment with immunoadsorption and rituximab (anti-CD20 monoclonal antibodies). Arch Dermatol 2007;143(2):192–8.

38. Gammon WR, Briggaman RA. Epidermolysis bullosa acquisita and bullous systemic lupus erythematosus. Diseases of autoimmunity to type VII collagen. Dermatol Clin 1993;11(3):535–47.

39. Chen M, Marinkovich MP, Veis A, et al. Interactions of the amino-terminal noncollagenous (NC1) domain of type VII collagen with extracellular matrix components. A potential role in epidermal-dermal adherence in human skin. J Biol Chem 1997;272(23): 14516–22.

Treatment of Chronic Bullous Disease of Childhood

Emily M. Mintz, MD, Kimberly D. Morel, MD*

KEYWORDS

- Chronic bullous disease of childhood • Bullous
- Linear IgA • IgA • Treatment

Chronic bullous disease of childhood (CBDC) is generally a self-limited disease of prepubescent children that resolves within months to years. However, as discussed in the previous issue of *Dermatologic Clinics,* the disease is associated with significant morbidity and usually requires systemic therapy. Treatment is aimed at controlling blistering while avoiding adverse reactions. There are several anecdotal reports of treatment options, but controlled or comparative studies are lacking.

Dapsone is considered the drug of choice and is begun at a low dose (<0.5 mg/kg) and slowly increased until blistering and symptoms are controlled (usually 2 mg/kg/day). Dose-related adverse effects include hemolysis (especially in the setting of glucose-6-phosphate dehydrogenase [G6PD] deficiency) and methemoglobinemia, which manifests as cyanosis, dyspnea, lethargy, and headache. A benign hemolysis is expected, and a compensatory reticulocytosis occurs.[1,2] Idiosyncratic adverse reactions include agranulocytosis, peripheral neuropathy, hepatitis, gastrointestinal upset, cutaneous hypersensitivity reactions, and dapsone hypersensitivity syndrome. Initial laboratory evaluation should include a complete blood count (CBC) with differential; liver function tests; renal function tests, including urinalysis; and a G6PD level. A CBC should be monitored frequently during the first 3 months of treatment, and additional blood work must be done periodically thereafter.[3]

Sulfapyridine (150 mg/kg although pediatric dosage is not well-established) is another first-line agent[2] and is associated with adverse reactions similar to those of dapsone but generally less severe.[3] This drug is no longer readily available in the United States but may be provided on a compassionate basis through Jacobus Pharmaceutical Company (telephone: 609-921-7447). Other sulfonamides may also be of benefit. Dapsone and sulfonamides may be combined for improved efficacy without additive side effects.[1] The addition of systemic corticosteroids may be needed for symptomatic control at the onset of the disease and periodically during flares but long-term use is discouraged given the plethora of adverse effects. Topical corticosteroids may be used in combination with the systemic therapies described herein.

Children with G6PD deficiency in whom dapsone and sulfapyridine are contraindicated should be treated with an alternative agent. Colchicine, which exerts its antiinflammatory effects by inhibiting neutrophil motility, adhesiveness, and chemotaxis, has been shown to be an effective option. Systemic corticosteroids may be used in combination with colchicine initially but should be tapered over a few weeks such that patients are maintained on colchicine monotherapy, usually at a dosage of 0.5 mg twice daily. Side effects at this dosage are usually absent, but dosage-dependent gastrointestinal disturbances may occur at higher dosages. Colchicine should not be used in patients with blood

The authors have no funding support to disclose.
Department of Dermatology, Columbia University, 161 Fort Washington Avenue, 12th Floor, New York, NY 10032, USA
* Corresponding author.
E-mail address: km208@columbia.edu

Dermatol Clin 29 (2011) 699–700
doi:10.1016/j.det.2011.08.013

dyscrasias or serious gastrointestinal, renal, hepatic, or cardiac disorders. Blood work should be monitored periodically during treatment.[4–6]

Antibiotics may also be of benefit in patients who are not candidates for standard therapy. Successful treatment with erythromycin, presumably through its antiinflammatory actions, has been described.[7] Erythromycin as a solo therapy is unlikely to provide sustained improvement in CBDC, but its administration on initial patient evaluation may lead to early improvement while awaiting further work-up.[8] Gastrointestinal upset is a common side effect of erythromycin therapy, but serious adverse reactions are uncommon. Successful treatment with dicloxacillin and oxacillin, both at dosages of 50 mg/kg daily, has been described. Potential side effects include gastrointestinal intolerance, urticaria and other allergic reactions, and occasionally transient hepatic dysfunction.[2] Improvement with trimethoprim-sulfamethoxazole[9] has been reported in a single patient. Treatment with antibiotics does not require blood monitoring, which is particularly advantageous in the treatment of children.

CBDC has historically been treated with liquid arsenicals with variable response.[10,11] Historical treatments also included a gluten-free diet because CBDC was initially thought to be a variant of dermatitis herpetiformis. Not unexpectedly, most patients found no improvement with this dietary restriction.[11,12] Resection of the diseased rectal stump led to improvement in a child with CBDC associated with ulcerative colitis who failed prednisolone, cyclosporine, and thalidomide.[13] Nicotinamide in combination with dapsone was effective in a child with CBDC.[14] Nicotinamide and tetracycline have been effective in adults with linear immunoglobulin A (IgA) disease,[15] but tetracycline antibiotics are contraindicated in young children. Intravenous immunoglobulin[16,17] and immunoadsorption[18] have led to favorable outcomes in adults with refractory linear IgA disease but have not been used in the treatment of CBDC.

REFERENCES

1. Guide SV, Marinkovich MP. Linear IgA bullous dermatosis. Clin Dermatol 2001;19(6):719–27.
2. Siegfried EC, Sirawan S. Chronic bullous disease of childhood: successful treatment with dicloxacillin. J Am Acad Dermatol 1998;39(5): 797–800.
3. Hall RP III, Mickle CP. Dapsone. In: Wolverton SE, editor. Comprehensive dermatologic drug therapy. 2nd edition. Philadelphia: Elsevier Inc; 2007. p. 239–57.
4. Banodkar DD, Al-Suwaid AR. Colchicine as a novel therapeutic agent in chronic bullous dermatosis of childhood. Int J Dermatol 1997;36(3):213–6.
5. Knable AL Jr, Davis LS. Miscellaneous systemic drugs. In: Wolverton SE, editor. Comprehensive dermatologic drug therapy. 2nd edition. Philadelphia: Elsevier Inc; 2007. p. 477–9.
6. Zeharia A, Hodak E, Mukamel M, et al. Successful treatment of chronic bullous dermatosis of childhood with colchicine. J Am Acad Dermatol 1994;30(4): 660–1.
7. Cooper SM, Powell J, Wojnarowska F. Linear IgA disease: successful treatment with erythromycin. Clin Exp Dermatol 2002;27(8):677–9.
8. Farrant P, Darley C, Carmichael A. Is erythromycin an effective treatment for chronic bullous disease of childhood? A national survey of members of the British Society for Paediatric Dermatology. Pediatr Dermatol 2008;25(4):479–82.
9. Edwards S, Wojnarowska F. Chronic bullous disease of childhood in three patients of Polynesian extraction. Clin Exp Dermatol 1990;15(5):367–9.
10. Grant PW. Juvenile dermatitis herpetiformis. Trans St Johns Hosp Dermatol Soc 1968;54(2):128–36.
11. Wojnarowska F. Chronic bullous disease of childhood. Semin Dermatol 1988;7(1):58–65.
12. Wojnarowska F, Marsden RA, Bhogal B, et al. Chronic bullous disease of childhood, childhood cicatricial pemphigoid, and linear IgA disease of adults. A comparative study demonstrating clinical and immunopathologic overlap. J Am Acad Dermatol 1988;19(5 Pt 1):792–805.
13. Handley J, Shields M, Dodge J, et al. Chronic bullous disease of childhood and ulcerative colitis. Pediatr Dermatol 1993;10(3):256–8.
14. Khanna N, Pandhi RK, Gupta S, et al. Response of chronic bullous dermatosis of childhood to a combination of dapsone and nicotinamide. J Eur Acad Dermatol Venereol 2001;15(4):368.
15. Chaffins ML, Collison D, Fivenson DP. Treatment of pemphigus and linear IgA dermatosis with nicotinamide and tetracycline: a review of 13 cases. J Am Acad Dermatol 1993;28(6):998–1000.
16. Khan IU, Bhol KC, Ahmed AR. Linear IgA bullous dermatosis in a patient with chronic renal failure: response to intravenous immunoglobulin therapy. J Am Acad Dermatol 1999;40(3):485–8.
17. Letko E, Bhol K, Foster CS, et al. Linear IgA bullous disease limited to the eye: a diagnostic dilemma: response to intravenous immunoglobulin therapy. Ophthalmology 2000;107(8):1524–8.
18. Kasperkiewicz M, Meier M, Zillikens D, et al. Linear IgA disease: successful application of immunoadsorption and review of the literature. Dermatology 2010;220(3):259–63.

Index

Note: Page numbers of article titles are in **boldface** type.

Dermatol Clin 29 (2011) 701–707
doi:10.1016/S0733-8635(11)00154-9
0733-8635/11/$ – see front matter © 2011 Elsevier Inc. All rights reserved.

derm.theclinics.com

United States Postal Service
Statement of Ownership, Management, and Circulation
(All Periodicals Publications Except Requestor Publications)

1. Publication Title
Dermatologic Clinics of North America

2. Publication Number
0 0 0 - 7 0 5

3. Filing Date
9/16/11

4. Issue Frequency
Jan, Apr, Jul, Oct

5. Number of Issues Published Annually
4

6. Annual Subscription Price
$317.00

7. Complete Mailing Address of Known Office of Publication *(Not printer) (Street, city, county, state, and ZIP+4®)*
Elsevier Inc.
360 Park Avenue South
New York, NY 10010-1710

Contact Person
Amy S. Beacham
Telephone *(Include area code)*
215-239-3687

8. Complete Mailing Address of Headquarters or General Business Office of Publisher *(Not printer)*
Elsevier Inc., 360 Park Avenue South, New York, NY 10010-1710

9. Full Names and Complete Mailing Addresses of Publisher, Editor, and Managing Editor *(Do not leave blank)*

Publisher *(Name and complete mailing address)*
Kim Murphy, Elsevier, Inc., 1600 John F. Kennedy Blvd. Suite 1800, Philadelphia, PA 19103-2899

Editor *(Name and complete mailing address)*
Stephanie Donley, Elsevier, Inc., 1600 John F. Kennedy Blvd. Suite 1800, Philadelphia, PA 19103-2899

Managing Editor *(Name and complete mailing address)*
Barton Dudlick, Elsevier, Inc., 1600 John F. Kennedy Blvd. Suite 1800, Philadelphia, PA 19103-2899

10. Owner *(Do not leave blank. If the publication is owned by a corporation, give the name and address of the corporation immediately followed by the names and addresses of all stockholders owning or holding 1 percent or more of the total amount of stock. If not owned by a corporation, give the names and addresses of the individual owners. If owned by a partnership or other unincorporated firm, give its name and address as well as those of each individual owner. If the publication is published by a nonprofit organization, give its name and address.)*

Full Name	Complete Mailing Address
Wholly owned subsidiary of	4520 East-West Highway
Reed/Elsevier, US holdings	Bethesda, MD 20814

11. Known Bondholders, Mortgagees, and Other Security Holders Owning or Holding 1 Percent or More of Total Amount of Bonds, Mortgages, or Other Securities. If none, check box. ☑ None

Full Name	Complete Mailing Address
N/A	

12. Tax Status *(For completion by nonprofit organizations authorized to mail at nonprofit rates) (Check one)*
The purpose, function, and nonprofit status of this organization and the exempt status for federal income tax purposes:
☐ Has Not Changed During Preceding 12 Months
☐ Has Changed During Preceding 12 Months *(Publisher must submit explanation of change with this statement)*

PS Form 3526, September 2007 (Page 1 of 3 (Instructions Page 3)) PSN 7530-01-000-9931 PRIVACY NOTICE: See our Privacy policy in www.usps.com

---

13. Publication Title
Dermatologic Clinics of North America

14. Issue Date for Circulation Data Below
July 2011

15. Extent and Nature of Circulation

			Average No. Copies Each Issue During Preceding 12 Months	No. Copies of Single Issue Published Nearest to Filing Date
a. Total Number of Copies *(Net press run)*			1050	1200
b. Paid Circulation (By Mail and Outside the Mail)	(1)	Mailed Outside-County Paid Subscriptions Stated on PS Form 3541. *(Include paid distribution above nominal rate, advertiser's proof copies, and exchange copies)*	286	260
	(2)	Mailed In-County Paid Subscriptions Stated on PS Form 3541 *(Include paid distribution above nominal rate, advertiser's proof copies, and exchange copies)*		
	(3)	Paid Distribution Outside the Mails Including Sales Through Dealers and Carriers, Street Vendors, Counter Sales, and Other Paid Distribution Outside USPS®	144	155
	(4)	Paid Distribution by Other Classes Mailed Through the USPS (e.g. First-Class Mail®)		
c. Total Paid Distribution *(Sum of 15b (1), (2), (3), and (4))*			430	415
d. Free or Nominal Rate Distribution (By Mail and Outside the Mail)	(1)	Free or Nominal Rate Outside-County Copies Included on PS Form 3541	87	103
	(2)	Free or Nominal Rate In-County Copies Included on PS Form 3541		
	(3)	Free or Nominal Rate Copies Mailed at Other Classes Through the USPS (e.g. First-Class Mail)		
	(4)	Free or Nominal Rate Distribution Outside the Mail (Carriers or other means)		
e. Total Free or Nominal Rate Distribution *(Sum of 15d (1), (2), (3) and (4))*			87	103
f. Total Distribution *(Sum of 15c and 15e)*			517	518
g. Copies not Distributed *(See instructions to publishers #4 (page #3))*			533	682
h. Total *(Sum of 15f and g)*			1050	1200
i. Percent Paid *(15c divided by 15f times 100)*			83.17%	80.12%

16. Publication of Statement of Ownership
☐ If the publication is a general publication, publication of this statement is required. Will be printed in the October 2011 issue of this publication. ☐ Publication not required

17. Signature and Title of Editor, Publisher, Business Manager, or Owner
(signature) Amy S. Beacham — Senior Inventory Distribution Coordinator
Date September 16, 2011

I certify that all information furnished on this form is true and complete. I understand that anyone who furnishes false or misleading information on this form or who omits material or information requested on the form may be subject to criminal sanctions (including fines and imprisonment) and/or civil sanctions (including civil penalties).

PS Form 3526, September 2007 (Page 2 of 3)

Moving?

Make sure your subscription moves with you!

To notify us of your new address, find your **Clinics Account Number** (located on your mailing label above your name), and contact customer service at:

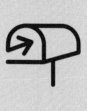

Email: journalscustomerservice-usa@elsevier.com

800-654-2452 (subscribers in the U.S. & Canada)
314-447-8871 (subscribers outside of the U.S. & Canada)

Fax number: 314-447-8029

Elsevier Health Sciences Division
Subscription Customer Service
3251 Riverport Lane
Maryland Heights, MO 63043

Printed and bound by CPI Group (UK) Ltd, Croydon, CR0 4YY

03/10/2024

01040356-0009